Essentials of
Disease in Wild Animals

T0321473

Essentials of
Disease in Wild Animals

Gary A. Wobeser

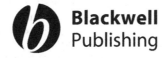

Blackwell
Publishing

Gary A. Wobeser, DVM, PhD, is a professor in the Department of Veterinary Pathology at Western College of Veterinary Medicine, University of Saskatchewan. He enjoys an excellent reputation among his peers and is one of the leading thinkers and researchers in wildlife medicine.

Blackwell Publishing Professional
2121 State Avenue, Ames, Iowa 50014, USA

Orders: 1-800-862-6657
Office: 1-515-292-0140
Fax: 1-515-292-3348
Web site: www.blackwellprofessional.com

Blackwell Publishing Ltd
9600 Garsington Road, Oxford OX4 2DQ, UK
Tel.: +44 (0)1865 776868

Blackwell Publishing Asia
550 Swanston Street, Carlton, Victoria 3053, Australia
Tel.: +61 (0)3 8359 1011

Upper left-hand photo courtesy of National Scenic Byways Online and the US-Fish and Wildlife Service.

Upper right hand photo courtesy of Erwin C. Nielsen/Painet Inc and the Illinois Department of Natural Resources.

First edition, 2006

Library of Congress Cataloging-in-Publication Data

Wobeser, Gary A.
   Essentials of disease in wild animals / Gary A. Wobeser.— 1st ed.
      p. cm.
   Includes bibliographical references.
   ISBN-10: 0-8138-0589-9
   ISBN-13: 978-0-8138-0589-4
   1. Wildlife diseases. I. Title.

SF996.4W62 2006
639.9′64—dc22

                                        2005008945

The last digit is the print number: 9 8

This book is dedicated to three mentors: A. Bruce Stephenson, wildlife biologist, who introduced me to field research and showed me that farm boy skills were applicable to working with wild animals; Lars H. Karstad, wildlife disease specialist, who welcomed me to the then new field of wildlife diseases and gave me the freedom to explore and make mistakes; N. Ole Nielsen, veterinary pathologist and "Green Dean," who has been a tireless advocate for incorporation of environmental thinking into veterinary medicine.

Contents

Preface

I began this book because I perceived that many of those who are being called upon to work with disease in wild animals lack experience or training in the general features of disease as they relate to wild animals. Unfortunately, disease has not been part of most training programs in biology and ecology so that individuals from that background have little knowledge of the range of factors that cause disease, the effects of disease agents on individual animals, or how disease agents move through populations and persist in the environment. Physicians, veterinarians, and public health specialists are familiar with the medical aspects of disease but often have little understanding of the ecology or natural history of wild animals, or experience in thinking about disease as a natural component of ecosystems. Theoretical ecologists, mathematicians, and population biologists can model how disease should behave quantitatively within populations, but they may have little experience with the medical aspects (physiology, anatomy, immunology, pathology) of disease, or with the practicalities of wildlife management.

There is no introductory level book about disease in wild animals that deals with basic subjects such as the nature of disease, what causes disease, how disease is described and measured, how diseases spread and persist, and the effects of disease on individual animals and populations. It is presumptuous of any individual to attempt to deal with all aspects of disease, and my intent is not to try to discuss any particular disease in detail.

This book developed from a graduate class in wildlife diseases that I have taught periodically over the past 30 years. The class began as a survey of the important diseases of western Canadian wildlife in which I dealt with viral, bacterial, fungal, parasitic, and toxic diseases of specific species. My approach was a rather standard veterinary one, concentrating on individual causative agents and their effect on the individual animal, in terms of the clinical disease and pathology that they produced. I initially placed relatively little emphasis on why disease occurred, or on the complex interactions that occur among disease agents, the environment, and host populations.

Embedded in my early approach was the notion that disease was somehow unique and different from other ecological factors and, as such, had more to do with medicine than with ecology. I also must admit that disease often was treated as a harmful phenomenon that should be "fought" or "managed" at every opportunity. (This was a residue of evangelical zeal from my veterinary training!) As time advanced, my interest and the class content became concerned more with general aspects of health in wild animals, such as how and why various diseases occur in wild animals, why animals and parasites appear to get along better in some situations than in others, and the effects of disease on populations rather than on individuals. There was a growing realization on my part that disease is one ecological factor among many and that disease can never be considered satisfactorily in isolation.

I have been fortunate to have been influenced during my career by many wildlife managers and ecologists. Some took a very pragmatic approach to disease while others tried to put disease into a larger ecological and evolutionary framework. From the first group, I have learned about natural history, observation, and the practicalities of working with wild animals. From the second group, I have learned that the features we observe in animals—such as their behavior, reproductive strategies, habitat selection, and susceptibility to various mortality factors—should be considered in terms of lifetime fitness, selective advantage, differential survival, and evolution.

Acknowledgments

I am indebted to the many colleagues and students who have contributed information and inspiration for this book. I am very grateful to my departmental home for allowing me to pursue an interest in wildlife diseases for many years and to the Department of Pathobiology, Ontario Veterinary College, University of Guelph for its hospitality while I was preparing the manuscript. I particularly thank my wife, Amy, for her continuous encouragement and enthusiasm.

Essentials of
Disease in Wild Animals

1
Introduction

The study of disease in wild animals is a relatively new scientific discipline when compared to the study of disease in humans or domestic animals. During the first half of the twentieth century a small number of scientists began pioneering studies of diseases such as tularemia and plague in wild rodents (McCoy 1911; McCoy and Chapin 1912), avian botulism in waterfowl (Kalmbach and Gunderson 1934), and rinderpest in African antelope (Carmichael 1938) and Elton (1931) reviewed epidemic diseases of wild animals. Formation of an international scientific body, the Wildlife Disease Association, in 1951 marked the beginning of more organized study of disease in wild animals, but most of the people involved in the early years of that organization would have identified themselves as members of some other discipline, such as virology, toxicology, parasitology, ecology, and pathology, who worked with wild animals rather than as wildlife disease specialists. During the past two decades, there has been a huge increase in interest in the subject. Scientists from a wide spectrum of disciplines including conservation biology, wildlife management, veterinary medicine, agriculture, public health, theoretical ecology, toxicology, animal behavior, and human medicine have become interested, on an unprecedented scale, in the particulars of disease in wild animals.

There are several reasons for this sudden increase in interest and involvement. A major factor has been a burgeoning awareness of the involvement of wild animals in infectious diseases of humans. Despite earlier optimism that infectious diseases in humans could be eliminated or controlled, it is now clear that infections have not been vanquished. "Emerging infectious diseases" have become a medical growth industry. New human diseases continue to be discovered and many old foes have returned with a vengeance because of environmental and demographic changes, declines in public health activities, and evolution of resistant organisms. Public health officials and physicians have been forced to deal with wild animals by the discovery that most of the emerging infectious diseases of humans are diseases that are shared with animals (zoonoses), and that wild animals have a central role in many of these conditions (table 1.1). Many other important human diseases in addition to those shown in table 1.1, including severe acute respiratory syndrome (SARS), Ebola disease, and Marburg virus infection, are believed to originate in wildlife, although the specific wild animal has not been identified to date. Many well-established human diseases that continue to cause problems including plague, tularemia, Lassa fever, rabies, and influenza are linked directly to wild animals.

Veterinarians and agriculturists also have developed a great interest in wild animals, because of the involvement of free-ranging animals in many diseases of domestic animals (table 1.2). Some of the associations between wild animals and diseases of domestic animals have been known for many years, but, in other instances, the role of wild animals in the disease did not become apparent until there was effective control of the disease in domestic animals. As an example, rabies in much of North America was thought of as a disease for which the domestic dog was the principal animal host; however, when rabies in dogs was controlled by vaccination and leash laws, it became obvious that the disease was not going to disappear, because it was still cycling in wild carnivores and bats. As the disease was studied further, it was discovered that there was not one rabies virus, as had been thought, but many strains, each circulating in one principal wild species. Thus, in North America, different strains of rabies virus occur in skunks, foxes, and raccoons as well as several strains in bats.

Table 1.1 Emerging Diseases of Humans in Which Wild Animals Are Important

Disease in humans	Causative agent	Wild species involved
Viruses		
Hantavirus pulmonary syndrome	Sin Nombre virus and many other New World hantaviruses	Rodents
Hemorrhagic fever with renal syndrome	Puumala virus and other Old World hantaviruses	Rodents
West Nile fever	West Nile virus	Birds
Hemorrhagic fevers (Argentinean, Bolivian, Brazilian, Venezuelan)	Arenaviruses	Rodents
Australian bat lyssavirus infection	Lyssavirus similar to rabies virus	Bats
Bacteria		
Human granulocytic ehrlichiosis	*Ehrlichia phagocytophila*	Rodents, cottontail rabbits
Monocytic ehrlichiosis	*Ehrlichia chaffeensis*	White-tailed deer
Lyme disease	*Borrelia burgdorferi*	Rodents, birds, deer
Cardiopathy, endocarditis	*Bartonella* spp.	Rodents
Cestodes (tapeworms)		
Alveolar echinococcosis	*Echinococcus multilocularis*	Fox, rodents
Nematodes (roundworms)		
Visceral larva migrans	*Baylisascaris procyonis*	Raccoons

Note: An emerging disease is one whose incidence in humans has increased recently or that threatens to increase in the near future. Included are previously unrecognized infections, new infections as a result of a change in a previously recognized causative agent, infections spreading to new areas or populations, and old infections that are reemerging because of deterioration in control or public health measures.

Some diseases that have been eliminated from domestic animals continue to occur in wildlife. For instance, cattle in most of North America are free of brucellosis caused by *Brucella abortus* but remnant pockets of infection in bison and elk in a few locations are considered to be a risk to national eradication programs.

Similarly, the occurrence of Newcastle disease in double-crested cormorants is considered a risk to North American poultry from which the disease has been eliminated (Kuiken 1999). The persistence of disease in wild animals has stymied efforts to eradicate some diseases of domestic livestock. The best documented of these is bovine tuberculosis caused by *Mycobacterium bovis*. Efforts to eradicate this disease in domestic cattle have stalled in England and Ireland because of tuberculosis in badgers, in New Zealand because of the disease in brushtail possums, and in parts of the United States and Canada because of infection in wild deer and elk. New disease problems involving wild animals continue to be discovered, for example, paratuberculosis, a disease of domestic ruminants caused by *Mycobacterium paratuberculosis*, is now known to occur in a wide variety of nonruminant wild animals that may

pose a risk to domestic livestock (Beard et al. 2001; Daniels et al. 2003).

Conservation biologists have become increasingly concerned about disease because of recognition that disease may play an important role in the survival of threatened or endangered species (Daszak et al. 2000; Cleaveland et al. 2001). Disease may limit captive breeding and release programs, and have devastating effects on small populations. Examples include the impact of avian malaria and poxvirus on indigenous Hawaiian birds (Atkinson et al. 1995), the near eradication of the black-footed ferret by canine distemper (Williams et al. 1988), the possible role of chytrid fungi and iridoviruses in declining amphibian populations worldwide, avian vacuolar myelinopathy in bald eagles and other species (Fischer et al. 2003), and rabies and canine distemper in Ethiopian wolves (Laurenson et al. 1998).

Wildlife managers have been forced to become more involved with disease for several reasons. There has been considerable pressure to manage wild species as part of control programs for diseases that may spread to humans and livestock, such as rabies, *Echinococcus multilocularis* infection, bovine

Table 1.2 Diseases of Domestic Animals in Which Wild Animals Are a Source of Infection

Disease	Domestic animal(s)	Wild animal(s)
Viral		
Hendra virus infection[1]	Horse	Fruit bats
Nipah virus infection	Pig	Fruit bats
Louping ill	Sheep	Red grouse, mountain hare
Malignant catarrhal fever	Cattle	Wildebeest
Foot-and-mouth disease	Cattle, sheep, pigs	African buffalo
Classical swine fever	Pigs	Wild boar
Newcastle disease	Poultry	Cormorants, other birds
Avian influenza	Poultry	Wild waterbirds
Bacterial		
Bovine tuberculosis	Cattle, deer	Badger, brushtail possum, white-tailed deer, elk, bison
Brucellosis	Cattle	Bison, elk
Anaplasmosis	Cattle, sheep and goats	Wild ruminants
Leptospirosis	Cattle, pigs, dogs	Different forms of *Leptospira* occur in a number of wild hosts
Protozoa and helminths		
Theileriosis	Cattle	African buffalo, eland
Cytauxzoonosis	Domestic cat	Bobcat
Hydatid disease (*Echinococcus granulosus*)[1]	Horse, sheep	Fox, dingo, macropods
Liver fluke (*Fascioloides magna*)	Cattle, sheep	White-tailed deer, elk
Meningeal worm (*Parelaphostrongylus tenuis*)	Llama, sheep, goat	White-tailed deer

[1]May also affect humans.

tuberculosis, and West Nile virus infection. Currently, there is considerable public concern and pressure for action in North America to deal with the expanding known geographic distribution of chronic wasting disease in deer and elk. Managers also have become concerned about the effects of disease on wild species per se. Recent examples of disease-related phenomena that appear to have had a serious effect on wild animals include a precipitous population crash of vultures in Pakistan caused by poisoning with an antiinflammatory medication used widely in cattle (Oaks et al. 2004); population declines of house finches as a result of eye infections caused by the bacterium *Mycoplasma gallisepticum* (Dhondt et al. 1998); massive die-offs of seals caused by morbillivirus infection (Kennedy 2001); loss of lions in the Serengeti to canine distemper (Roelke-Parker et al. 1996); extirpation of the Allegheny wood rat in part of its range by a raccoon parasite (Logiudice 2003); and the spread of bovine tuberculosis in African buffalo, other ungulates, and carnivores in Kruger National Park (Caron et al.

2003). Wildlife managers also have become more aware that their actions can contribute to disease problems ranging from simple things such as muscle injury (capture myopathy) as a result of capture and handling animals to the introduction of new diseases as a result of translocating diseased animals.

Toxicologists have been interested in wild animals for many years and effective control measures have been developed for some diseases such as those caused by organochlorine insecticides, mercurial seed dressings, and lead shot. Some of the emphasis in wildlife toxicology has shifted from the more overt poisons to compounds, such as endocrine-disrupting chemicals (Ottinger et al. 2002), that may have sublethal effects on immune function, behavior, and reproduction. Contaminants of various types often appear to interact with other potential disease-causing agents, closing the gap between infectious and noninfectious diseases. For instance, during an outbreak of phocine distemper (caused by a morbillivirus), seals from the heavily polluted Baltic Sea appeared to be most severely affected (Kennedy

1990) and seals fed contaminant-laden fish from the Baltic had reduced immune function compared to seals fed fish from the less-contaminated Atlantic (Swart et al. 1994). Contaminants also may interact synergistically with other mortality factors such as predation (Relyea 2003).

Interest in disease in wild animals also has increased for an entirely different reason. There has been an explosion of academic attention to various aspects of disease in wild animals by ecologists, behaviorists, population biologists, and modelers. Many of these scientists are interested in aspects of the coevolution of disease agents and animals, and the theoretical rather than the pragmatic features of disease. Their work is providing a theoretical framework for understanding host-parasite evolution, virulence, and the population effects of disease.

IS DISEASE IN WILD ANIMALS TRULY BECOMING MORE IMPORTANT?

All of the attention outlined above suggests that disease in wild animals is becoming more important or significant. One should ask if this is because there really is more disease or if disease has just become more apparent because more people are looking for it. Some of the apparent increase in disease is a result of greater surveillance. The hantaviruses provide a good example of this phenomenon. The discovery that one hantavirus, Sin Nombre virus from deer mice, caused fatal hantavirus pulmonary syndrome (HPS) in humans in a small focus in the United States (Nichol et al. 1993) led to a huge search for similar viruses. In less than a decade, more than 25 different hantaviruses, each with its own specific rodent host, have been identified in North, Central, and South America (Mills and Childs 2001). Many of these viruses have been linked to human disease. There is no evidence that these are truly new entities. The viruses have been present but unrecognized in rodents, and the human disease, which also has been present, has now been given a name (HPS) and its cause has been identified.

Some diseases do appear to have become more common or prevalent. For instance, it is unlikely that massive die-offs of waterfowl similar to those that have occurred during the past three decades as a result of avian cholera would have gone unrecognized earlier in the century, but the disease was not known to occur in wild birds in North America prior to 1943 and widespread large outbreaks have only been recognized since the mid-1970s (Friend and Franson 1999). Eye infections of house finches caused by *Mycoplasma gallisepticum* appear to be a completely new disease that has spread widely in North America since it was first recognized in 1994 (Dhondt et al. 1998). Canine parvovirus 2, which infects several wild canid species, appears to have arisen from a virus of cats and spread rapidly in domestic dogs and wild canids around the world about 1978 (Barker and Parrish 2001). West Nile virus is a new transplant to the New World that has spread rapidly with major consequences for wild birds, horses, and humans.

It is safe to predict that disease in its many manifestations will become even more significant for wild animals in the future and that there will be increasing pressure on wildlife biologists to "manage" disease. New emerging diseases of humans will continue to be linked to wild animals as pressure from the expanding human population brings humans and wild animals into ever closer contact. The rapid movement of humans means that an individual exposed to an infection in a wild animal in a remote part of the world can be in the middle of a city on another continent before the disease becomes apparent. The rapid and extensive movement of exotic animals for the pet, zoo, and game farm industries means that infected individuals can mingle with humans and traditional domestic animals in unexpected ways, as occurred in the introduction of monkeypox to the United States in 2003 (CDC 2003).

New diseases of domestic animals also will emerge that will be linked to wild animals. For instance, within the past decade three new viral diseases (Hendra virus that infects horses and humans, Nipah virus that infects pigs and humans, and Menangle virus that infects domestic pigs) have been discovered in fruit bats. Continued pressure on land for agriculture and urban development will intensify contact and exchange of disease between domestic animals and the wild animals that live in residual areas of natural habitat. The concern about some diseases such as bovine tuberculosis is that wild animals are a source of infection for domestic animals. There is also concern for transmission of disease from domestic to wild animals, as has occurred with transmission of canine distemper virus from dogs to the Ethiopian wolf (Laurenson et al. 1998), African wild dog (Alexander and Appel 1994), lions in the Serengeti (Packer et al. 1999), and seals in Lake Baikal (Mamaev et al. 1995).

The interrelationships among wild animals, domestic animals, and humans may be complex. In some situations, domestic animals may be an intermediary by which diseases from wild animals reach humans. This occurred in Malaysia in 1999. A previously unrecognized virus of wild fruit bats became established in domestic pigs by some unknown route. There was no evidence of transmission from bats to humans, or of human to human spread, but 265 humans developed encephalitis (inflammation of the brain) in the outbreak. Of the affected people, 93% had worked with pigs and 105 died of so-called Nipah disease (WHO 2001). Approximately 900,000 pigs were killed to control the disease. Influenza presents a potentially even more dangerous situation. Wild waterbirds carry an array of all known subtypes of influenza A virus and shed the virus in their droppings. The virus can survive in surface water for an extended period. Influenza viruses recombine readily to form novel viruses and the great waves of human influenza that sweep around the world (pandemics) result from formation of a new strain. Although influenza strains from birds can infect humans directly, as occurred in Hong Kong in 1997 and is occurring in several Asian countries as this is written, the pandemic strains that affected humans around the world in the 20th century resulted from reassortment that occurred in pigs infected with both a strain from humans and a strain from birds (Kida 2003). Thus, pigs served as an intermediary between birds and humans. The combination of wild waterbirds, intensive poultry production, intensive pig production, and dense human populations that occurs in some areas of the world provides the ideal milieu for generation of new influenza viruses.

The discussion above dealt with infectious diseases that are shared by people, domestic animals, and wild animals. Disease also is likely to have a greater direct effect on wild species in the future. New agricultural and industrial practices will result in exposure of wild animals to new contaminants, often with unexpected results. For example, introduction of "second-generation" anticoagulants for control of rats and mice has resulted in secondary poisoning of carnivores. Acidification of soils by acid rain may be leading to calcium deficiency in passerine birds and cadmium poisoning of mammals. Some diseases that are unimportant currently are likely to become significant because of continued human pressure on natural habitats. Diseases are like weeds in that both thrive in disturbed environments. Just as weeds have great difficulty gaining a foothold in an established forest or grassland, diseases have difficulty being perpetuated in stable systems, but both weeds and some forms of disease quickly invade and proliferate following disturbance.

Human history is replete with examples in which pestilence has followed social and environmental disruption. It is useful in this regard to compare human and wild animal populations. Improvements in sanitation, shelter, nutrition, and water supply have been central to the control of important infectious and noninfectious diseases of humans. When these improvements are disrupted by social or natural disasters, disease follows rapidly. Few wild animals live in undisturbed environments or in circumstances in which the level of sanitation, shelter, nutrition, or the quality of water have improved. Diseases such as measles have emerged in epidemic form in human populations as a result of the large, dense populations that occur in cities. Refuges on which wild waterfowl are crowded together for months and artificial feeding areas on which some wild species congregate seem very like cities to me, but they are cities without the benefit of sewage disposal, clean water, and the immunization programs that protect us from many diseases. It should not be surprising that avian cholera has emerged in the past few decades on these refuges, or that tuberculosis has become a self-sustaining infection among artificially fed white-tailed deer (Miller et al. 2003), or that salmonellosis occurs among passerine birds congregated at bird feeders (Daoust et al. 2000; Refsum et al. 2003).

STUDY OF WILDLIFE DISEASES: AN INTERFACE AREA

The study of wildlife diseases is an interface area (fig. 1.1) that can be approached from many different perspectives. The great diversity of interest in diseases of wild animals is healthy because disease usually is complex and beyond the expertise of any one discipline. For example, I am part of a group struggling to develop an appropriate strategy for the management of bovine tuberculosis in elk and deer within and outside a national park, and in cattle in the vicinity of the park. In developing this plan, wildlife managers, conservation ecologists, geographers, agriculturalists, foresters, rural sociologists, veterinarians, modelers, biometricians, historians, and laboratory scientists have made a significant contribution, because their skills are complementary.

It is my perception that many of those who are being called upon to work with disease in wild animals lack experience or training in the general features of disease as they relate to wild animals. Unfortunately, disease has not been part of most training programs in biology and ecology so that individuals from that background have little knowledge of the range of factors that cause disease, the

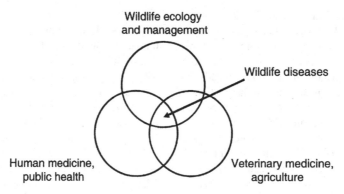

Fig. 1.1. Disease in wild animals occurs at the interface among human medicine, veterinary medicine, and ecology.

effects of disease agents on individual animals, or how disease agents move through populations and persist in the environment. Physicians, veterinarians, and public health specialists are familiar with the medical aspects of disease but often have little understanding of the ecology or natural history of wild animals, or experience in thinking about disease as a natural component of ecosystems. Theoretical ecologists, mathematicians, and population biologists can model how disease should behave quantitatively within populations but may have little experience with the medical aspects (physiology, anatomy, immunology, pathology) of disease, or with the practicalities of wildlife management.

In the chapters ahead, I will discuss the nature of disease, what causes disease, how disease is described and measured, how diseases spread and persist, and the effects of disease on individual animals and populations. It is presumptuous of any individual to attempt to deal with all aspects of disease, and my intent is not to try to discuss any particular disease in detail. I will use examples from wild species to provide basic information about the nature of disease in its many forms and the range of factors that result in disease. I hope to provide some familiarity with the vocabulary of disease (e.g., the difference between infection and disease, and between prevalence and incidence), some understanding of the intricacies of detecting disease (e.g., the specificity and sensitivity of tests), and the difference between humoral and cell-mediated immunity. I will stress that all disease, regardless of cause, begins at the cellular level, and that changes at the cellular level result in functional changes in the individual that have population effects. If nothing else, I hope that the reader will gain an appreciation that disease is one environmental feature among many that affect animals, and that it is impossible to understand dis-

ease without considering the interactions among disease agents and with other factors such as nutrition, predation, climate, and reproduction.

Over the past few decades, technical books have appeared that describe many individual diseases that occur in wild animals. Some deal with a single species, such as *Diseases and Parasites of White-tailed Deer* (Davidson et al. 1981); groups of related species, such as *Diseases of Wild Waterfowl* (Wobeser 1997); or larger taxa, such as *Infectious Diseases of Wild Mammals* (Williams and Barker 2001) and *Parasitic Diseases of Wild Mammals* (Samuel et al. 2001); or diseases that occur in a geographical area, for example, *Parasites and Diseases of Wild Birds in Florida* (Forrester and Spalding 2002). These are excellent references on clinical, epidemiological, and pathologic features of important diseases with a heavy emphasis on game species and on diseases that cause conspicuous mortality. *Ecology of Infectious Diseases in Natural Populations* (Grenfell and Dobson 1995) and *The Ecology of Wildlife Diseases* (Hudson et al. 2001) deal with more general aspects of infectious disease in wild animals with a particular emphasis on mathematical aspects of disease in populations as demonstrated in models.

A feature of most books that deal with wildlife disease is a distinct separation of subject matter based on causation. Noninfectious diseases caused by poisons and contaminants are almost never discussed together with infectious diseases. Noninfectious diseases caused by factors such as nutrition, aging, and genetic defects have received almost no attention. Diseases caused by living organisms usually are separated into those caused by "little" organisms (viruses, bacteria, fungi) and those caused by larger organisms that are visible to the naked eye such as fleas, lice, and various worms. (Protozoa seem to float between the two main groups.)

Diseases caused by the little organisms (*microorganisms*) are usually termed *infectious,* and diseases caused by the larger animals are generally referred to as *parasitic.* However, at the ecological level, all of the infectious agents are parasites and diseases caused by both big and little organisms are infectious.

I have tried to incorporate both infectious and noninfectious conditions in the discussion throughout this book, because the two types of disease occur together in nature, because the basic principles are the same, and because I believe that there is merit in trying to use the same ecological construct for looking at disease of all types. Wild animals seldom are exposed to just one disease-causing agent at a time, or to just infectious or just noninfectious factors. As a simple example, Pawelczyk et al. (2004) examined one tissue (blood) from common voles by one method (light microscopy). They identified at least five different microscopic organisms, including some that generally are classified as parasites and some that are considered infectious agents. At the instant that they were sampled, about 50% of the voles had two agents visible in their blood and 1% was infected concurrently with four different agents. One can assume that these voles also were infected with a range of infectious agents in tissues other than blood, that they had agents that were not visible with the light microscope, and that they carried residues of potentially harmful substances in their tissues, because that is the "usual" situation in wild animals. The voles may or may not have been suffering dysfunction as a result of these agents.

Different types of disease-causing agents often interact and many diseases are caused by combinations of agents rather than by a single factor. Noninfectious factors affect the ability of animals to respond appropriately to infectious agents and infections may compound or confound the effects of abiotic factors. As a diagnostic pathologist, I often have been confronted with dead animals that had elevated residues of several classes of chemicals, greater than usual numbers of worms, evidence of exposure to one or more viruses, infection with potentially damaging bacteria such as *Salmonella* spp., and evidence of malnutrition. In such situations, selecting any one of the chemicals, parasites, bacteria, viruses, or nutrition as the main cause of the problem is naive.

I have tried to insinuate some basic life history theory in various parts of this book. The most important single feature is that natural selection favors evolution of physiological mechanisms to ensure optimal allocation of limited resources to competing activities. "Success" is the result of making the most appropriate trade-offs, and disease is all about resources and trade-offs. Infectious agents and host animals must both make trade-offs. Bacteria, viruses, and larger parasites trade off the amount of nutrients that they can extract from an animal against the probability of being transmitted to another animal. If they are too greedy and cause too much damage to their host, they may compromise their own survival and fitness. Similarly, host animals make many trade-offs related to disease (e.g., should they graze in a lush area where worm larvae are abundant or move to another area where parasites are less numerous but the plants are less nutritious? Should they use resources to resist a disease or put those resources toward growth and reproduction in the hope that the disease won't occur or that they can survive its effects? Should they allocate resources toward reproduction now if doing so compromises their resistance to disease and decreases the chance of surviving to reproduce again later? How many resources should they allocate to resisting the effects of one disease agent compared to those devoted to defense against another agent?).

Most of my experience has been in the cooler parts of North America so that many of the examples I use reflect my familiarity with that environment. I have tried to incorporate references to work dealing with experimental systems for studying basic aspects of disease and mathematical modeling of disease situations, because I believe that theory developed by laboratory studies of creatures such as *Daphnia* and field studies such as those of wild rodent populations infected with cowpox virus are relevant for understanding and management of problems such as West Nile virus infection and bovine tuberculosis.

From time to time, I will make reference to Aldo Leopold, the "father" of wildlife management in North America, because many of his views on the place of disease in wild animal ecology, as expressed in *Game Management* (Leopold 1933), remain relevant. When referring to research on disease he wrote, "It is a pity that the narratives of scientific exploration in this field—as fantastic a romance as any Arabian Nights—should either be masked by such technical verbiage as to mean nothing to the thinking layman, or translated for the popular press in such kindergarten terms as to be no longer true." My sincere hope is that I can avoid either extreme in discussing disease.

SUMMARY

- The study of disease in wild animals is a recent phenomenon.

- There has been a great increase in effort in this discipline because of the recognition of the involvement of wild animals in diseases of humans and domestic animals, the impact of disease on wildlife management and conservation biology, the recognition of new forms of environmental contamination, and the academic interest in disease as an ecological factor.

- Disease in wild animals will become even more important because of environmental, agricultural, and demographic changes as a result of growing human populations that will increase contact between wild animals, humans, and domestic animals and that will further degrade natural habitats.

- The study of disease in wild animals must be multidisciplinary because of its complexity.

- Wild animals are affected by a range of infectious and noninfectious factors that occur together and that interact. To consider only one or the other type of cause is to understand only part of the picture.

- Disease is an ecological entity that should be considered in terms of life history theory and that is intimately intertwined with resources and trade-offs.

2
What Is Disease?

The word "disease" is used so commonly in everyday conversation that each person has his or her own understanding of its meaning. That understanding is highly variable depending upon one's particular perspective. For most people who live in an urban setting, reference to disease usually relates to the human condition, as in "she died of heart disease," "alcoholism is a disease," or "gum disease is a serious problem that needs attention." I find it interesting that the examples that came to mind while writing the above were all noninfectious entities related in some way to lifestyle. This reflects my perspective as a member of a society in which most infectious causes of human disease have been removed from everyday thought. In contrast, if I were writing this book from the perspective of someone dealing with human ailments in some of the poorest parts of the developing world, the examples that would spring to mind would be diseases resulting from communicable infections, parasitism, malnutrition, and perinatal conditions (Murray and Lopez 1997).

If one lives in a rural community, many everyday references to disease relate to livestock or to crops. In veterinary medicine, one also sees a disparity in the type of disease that is important based on the purpose for which the animals are kept and the level and intensity of management of the animals. The diseases of pet animals (dogs and cats) are similar to those of their owners, with the added factor of many genetic disorders related to human selection for traits that have negative survival value. The owner of a large herd of intensively managed dairy cows usually is most concerned about so-called production diseases. These are conditions that result in decreased milk yield or lower conversion of feed into milk, or that extend the time period between calves from each cow. This same type of production disease is important in intensively managed pig and poultry operations. Most of these conditions, as in diseases of humans in affluent societies, are related to the lifestyle of the cows, pigs, and chickens. However, the animals have little choice in the food they eat, the amount that they exercise, or the company that they keep, unlike their human counterparts. In contrast, many of the disease problems of less intensively managed livestock such as beef cattle or sheep living on range relate to various infectious agents, poor nutrition, and intoxications from plants. The ecological concept of *fitness* as it relates to lifetime reproductive success has no meaning in most domestic species, because the animals seldom are allowed to live their full life span or to reproduce at will.

Because the perception of what constitutes disease is highly variable, it is difficult to find a definition for the word that is inclusive enough to encompass both the irritation of receding gums (i.e., "gum disease") and a condition such as botulism that may kill 500,000 waterfowl on a single lake. It also is difficult to find a definition that is specific enough to clearly separate disease from conditions that we usually do not think of as disease. For instance, if a snowshoe hare dies as a result of severe intestinal damage caused by parasitic worms, most people would consider this to be an example of disease. If another hare were killed by a great horned owl, we generally would consider this to be an example of predation rather than of disease. However, in each of these situations, another species extracted nutrients for its own use from the hare and in doing so caused its death. This makes the dividing line between predation and disease seem a bit hazy. The difference seems to be that the owl acted without accomplices and did the job quickly, while many worms were involved, each taking just a bit from the hare, and they did so over a period of time.

We can extend this example a little further and assume that both hares had worms but in the second hare the intestinal injury caused by the worms was not so severe that the hare died because of the worms. (This would represent the more normal "parasitic" situation.) However, the worms are extracting nutrients from the hare by feeding on intestinal cells and on blood from shallow wounds in the intestinal lining, and the hare is responding by producing inflammatory cells and antibodies to defend itself against the worm and by trying to repair the injury. Thus, the worms represent a *cost* to the hare. The second hare may have been able to *compensate* for this cost by eating more to provide both for its own increased needs (for resistance and repair) and for the needs of its uninvited lodgers, but, in doing so, it may have to spend an extra hour each day foraging for food. Hares that are moving are more vulnerable to predators than hares that are sitting motionless and hidden, and hares that are nutritionally stressed may be able to allocate less resources to antipredator behavior than well-fed hares. If the hare was killed by an owl during the extra hour of activity, should we attribute its death to disease (parasitism) or to predation? One could argue that the basic or underlying cause of death was parasite-induced injury (disease) that made the hare more vulnerable to the owl and that predation was only the proximate cause of death. We might extend this example and hypothesize that heavily parasitized individuals within the hare population are more susceptible to predation than unparasitized hares and that parasitism could be an important component in the ecology of hares and of their evolution.

A similar example is the severely emaciated coyote that has stopped hunting and has removed most of its hair coat in a frantic attempt to reduce the intense irritation caused by *Sarcoptes scabei* mange mites (fig. 2.1). When this distracted, starving animal wanders into the path of a passing automobile or ventures into a farmyard and is killed by the dog, should its death be attributed to disease or to simple bad luck?

Because disease comes in many forms with degrees of severity, and has many causes, I think it can be defined most adequately in terms of the effect on normal functions of the individual. The definition that I prefer is that disease includes "any impairment that interferes with or modifies the performance of normal functions, including responses to environmental factors such as nutrition, toxicants, and climate; infectious agents; inherent or congenital defects; or combinations of these factors" (Wobeser 1981).

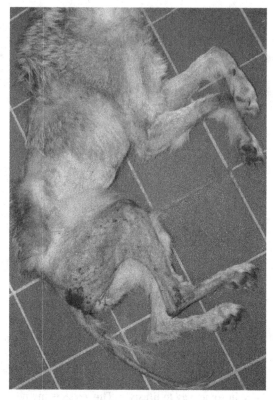

Fig. 2.1. Coyote with severe hair loss as a result of infestation with the mange mite *Sarcoptes scabei*. Severely infected coyotes are usually emaciated and many have secondary bacterial skin infection. Some die of starvation and others die as a result of misadventure (hit by car, killed by dog, shot by farmer) because of abnormal behavior.

Implicit within this definition are four concepts:

1. *Disease is measured in terms of impairment of function rather than by the death of individuals.* This distinction is important because death often has been the endpoint used to evaluate disease in wild animals but not all dysfunctions lead to death. For instance, a condition that results in reduced milk production by female elk so that their calves grow less well is disease, as is infestation with mites that causes a bird to be less attentive to its nest and, hence, results in poor reproductive success. The animals did not die of disease in either of these examples. I find it easiest to think in terms of a continuum between two endpoints: absolute health (a state in which all functions are optimal) and death, which occurs when functions are so severely compromised that life is impossible (fig. 2.2). Between these two points there is a region of

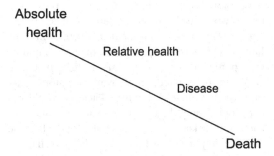

Absolute
health

Relative health

Disease

Death

Fig. 2.2. Disease is any impairment that interferes with normal functions and occupies a region on a continuum between absolute health and death. Defining the precise point where relative health ends and mild disease begins is difficult.

relative health that blends imperceptibly into a region that we can define as disease. The degree of functional impairment and, hence, the seriousness of disease increases as an animal's state moves from left to right along this continuum. Trying to define exactly where health ends and disease begins is similar to trying to define when people become old. Aging is a process that proceeds at different rates in individuals, and people become old at different stages of their life. Similarly, the degree of dysfunction that occurs as a result of any insult is highly variable. Death, the ultimate endpoint of both disease and aging, is easier to define than progress along the process.

If we return to the hare-worm example, the location of a hare on this continuum depends upon many factors including the number of worms present, the type of worms and their ability to cause damage, the hare's ability to resist and repair injury, and environmental factors that determine the quality and availability of food. Hares with only a few worms, of a type that causes only mild injury, will be in a high degree of relative health, particularly in a year when food is abundant. Those hares with many parasites that damage the intestine extensively may have severely compromised function, and some might die as a result, particularly in years when food is hard to find.

2. Factors that cause disease may be either *intrinsic,* such as an inherited defect in an animal's vascular plumbing or degenerative changes associated with aging, or *extrinsic,* such as a virus, bacterium, or contaminant that enters its body and causes injury.

3. *Disease may result from factors acting alone or in combination.* Much of what we currently know about disease in wild animals relates to conditions in which one factor, acting more or less alone, results in obvious impairment and often death. However, such diseases are likely the exception rather than the rule, and, on more thorough examination, most conditions will be found to involve several interrelated and interacting factors. Often the relationship among causative factors is extremely complex.

4. *Many different functions may be impaired.* Some effects of impaired function may be obvious, others may be so subtle that they are difficult to detect or may not be evident within the current generation. However, this does not mean that subtle functional impairments are of negligible importance. Until recently, disease in wild animals received little attention except when a condition in a wild species spread to humans or to domestic animals. There has been relatively little interest in the effect of disease on the wild animals themselves. The attitude among many biologists who study and manage wild animals has been that disease is unimportant except, perhaps, for conditions such as botulism and avian cholera in waterfowl or viral hemorrhagic disease of wild deer that may cause spectacular die-offs. As a friend once said of wild animals, "If their feet are in the air and their eyes are closed they have disease; otherwise they are healthy." Jansen (1964) summarized this attitude to disease in a different way: "Insufficient attention is paid to the infectious and parasitic diseases of wildlife until some outbreak of disease, no matter whether in wildlife or domestic animals, when the importance of disease or infestation of wildlife is overestimated."

Two groups of scientists have been interested in the occurrence of disease in wild animals but they have approached the phenomenon from different directions. One group has been interested in conditions that have "management implications," because the disease causes conspicuous die-offs or because it may also affect humans or domestic animals. They have worked predominantly with larger animals, particularly the birds and mammals that are hunted as game. Emphasis has been on identifying the cause of individual conditions, describing the clinical and pathologic effects of the disease on the individual animal, and identifying the factors that led to the occurrence of obvious disease. Diseases have usually been considered as separate entities and on a short-term basis, in order to answer questions such as, "Why did avian botulism kill 30,000 ducks on this wetland in 1997?" The ultimate goal has been to identify methods to prevent or reduce the impact of the disease in a specific time or place. Because of the activity of these scientists, there are excellent catalogues of "important" conditions that occur in many wild species. This group has paid little attention to subtle forms of disease or to interactions among various diseases, and there has been relatively little attention to developing theory about how disease operates at the population level.

Another group, working from a more theoretical and mathematical perspective, has been probing disease as a variable that influences the overall ecology and evolution of species. Its work often has involved smaller species, and the emphasis has been on developing a strong theoretical framework for considering disease, in its broadest sense, as an ecological and evolutionary force. There has been relatively little cross-pollination between the two groups, which is unfortunate, because the value of combining studies to understand the effect of the disease on the individual with a strong emphasis on the theoretical basis for what is observed has been demonstrated in detailed studies of a parasite of red grouse in the United Kingdom (Hudson et al. 1992b).

INJURY AND REACTION TO INJURY

The causes of disease and the way the body responds to injury will be discussed at length in later chapters. In this initial overview of disease, it is important to introduce a concept proposed by Forbus (1943), who stated that disease "does not exist except as a reaction to injury." Stated in another way, disease results from the body's reaction to injury rather than from the injury itself. When injury occurs to a cell or tissue, powerful forces come into action to resolve the injury, and it is these reactions that result in the clinical manifestations or dysfunctions that we recognize as disease. For instance, when you have a sliver in your finger, there may be temporary loss of function of the digit because of pain. This dysfunction fits the definition of disease (although of a minor sort). The pain and loss of function result from pressure on nerves from the swelling of the tissue because of increased blood flow, leakage of fluid, and influx of white blood cells into the area, and from the release of powerful chemical mediators that occur in response to the

sliver rather than any direct effect of the tiny splinter of wood itself. When bacteria such as *Mannheimia (Pasteurella) haemolytica* penetrate into the lung of a bighorn sheep, they occupy such a minuscule portion of the volume of the lung that they cause no direct interference with respiratory function. (Approximately 1 billion bacteria would occupy only about 1 cubic centimeter of volume if carefully stacked [Schaechter et al. 1993].) It is the massive outpouring of fluid, white blood cells, and protein into the lung, which occurs in an attempt to neutralize and destroy the bacteria, that fills the alveoli and airways so that air cannot enter the lung and impairs respiratory function, sometimes fatally. Similarly, when a coyote or a wombat becomes infested with *Sarcoptes scabei,* the mites are confined to the outer layers of the skin and appear to cause little actual damage; however, the mites and their secretions are recognized by the body as foreign substances and this stimulates powerful inflammatory and immune responses. It is this response that causes the intense pruritus (itchiness) that drives the animal to cease normal activities such as hunting or feeding while it chews and scratches away all the fur that it can reach.

The conundrum in all diseases is that although the responses to injury are protective and designed to destroy or neutralize invaders and to repair tissue injury, the same processes are costly to the animal and inherently dangerous. There is always a delicate balance between the degree of response needed to resolve the injury and an excessive response that is damaging or fatal. The reaction to injury is truly a two-edged blade.

DISEASE NOMENCLATURE

Within the broad definition of disease, animals that have similar dysfunctions can be grouped together and said to be affected by a specific disease. This grouping and categorization is an important first step toward understanding a disease, because it allows one to separate a particular condition from other conditions that also may be affecting the animals. Defining and naming a disease is a gradual and continual process that often proceeds from a broad descriptive term to a very specific name. When a disease is first recognized, a general term such as *respiratory disease* may be used, as in "bighorn sheep in this area of British Columbia have respiratory disease." This name might be based on nothing more than the observation of coughing sheep. Although the descriptive term is general, it clearly indicates the body system that is involved (the respiratory tract), and it may be sufficient to differentiate what is happening in these particular sheep from what might be occurring in sheep elsewhere. As affected sheep are examined more closely, it may become apparent that there is severe inflammation of the lungs and that the term *pneumonia* (inflammation of the lungs) is appropriate. Inflammation may result from many different causes including parasitic worms, bacteria, viruses, or some combination of all of these. There are different types of pneumonia that have characteristics familiar to pathologists. As the morphological features of the affected lungs are determined, the name might be refined to *fibrinous pneumonia,* which would signal to a pathologist that a particular type of inflammatory process is involved, or to *verminous pneumonia,* if parasitic worms are prominent in the lung lesions. This level of definition can be very useful, as it may allow one to differentiate the disease in a particular group of sheep from one that occurred in the same area in the past or to conclude that the disease is the same as one seen previously in the same or some other area. (In the latter case management that was used in the past may be appropriate in the present situation.) Finally, as the cause of the disease becomes apparent, the name of the causative agent may be incorporated into the name, for example, fibrinous pneumonia caused by *Mannheimia haemolytica* or verminous pneumonia of bighorn lambs caused by *Protostrongylus stilesi.*

There is no consistent method for applying names to diseases. Some diseases have been named for the location where they were discovered, such as Newcastle disease, a viral disease of birds, named for Newcastle, England, and tularemia, a bacterial disease that principally affects rodents and rabbits, named for Tulare County, California. Some diseases have been named for the person who discovered them. A disease first described in laboratory mice is called Tyzzer's disease in honor of its discoverer E. E. Tyzzer. Fortunately, naming diseases for an individual or location is less common in animal diseases than in diseases of humans, because neither the location nor the discoverer's name are particularly helpful or easy to remember.

Names that describe some recognizable feature of the disease are much more useful. Bluetongue is the name of a viral disease that often causes swelling and congestion of the tongue of affected sheep. Necrotic enteritis is used for a disease caused by overgrowth of certain bacteria that results in death (necrosis) of intestinal tissue and inflammation of the intestine (enteritis) in a variety of species. Other names describe how the disease occurs within a population, for example, epizootic hemorrhagic disease of deer is a disease that may occur in sudden unexpected outbreaks *(epizootics)* and is characterized by the occurrence of conspicuous hemorrhages. Enzootic ataxia is a disease of sheep and deer in some areas of the world caused by a deficiency of copper; its name is derived from its regular and predictable *(enzootic)* occurrence in the area and because the animals have a staggering gait *(ataxia)* as a result of damage to their nervous system. Many diseases are named after the causative agent, for example, aspergillosis is the name used for a disease caused by infection with fungi of the genus *Aspergillus* and haemonchosis is used for disease in ruminants caused by intestinal nematodes of the genus *Haemonchus.*

Disease nomenclature is replete with eccentricities and historical remnants. For instance, both the name of the disease botulism and that of the causative bacterium *Clostridium botulinum* are derived from Latin *botulus* for sausage, because human poisoning was associated with ingestion of toxin produced by the bacterium in improperly preserved sausages. The name has little relevance to the disease that occurs in wild waterbirds that have never seen a sausage! A disease in wild rodents caused by one bacterium in the genus *Yersinia (Y. pestis)* is called plague while diseases that are very similar to plague but are caused by other members of the same genus are lumped together under the term "yersiniosis." Cholera is a disease of humans characterized by severe diarrhea that is caused by the bacterium *Vibrio cholera.* Avian cholera is a disease of birds, in which diarrhea is not a feature, caused by a bacterium *Pasteurella multocida,* which is not related to the organism causing the human disease.

The name of a disease often changes as new information is gathered. Paul Errington used hemorrhagic disease, based on pathologic changes seen in affected animals, to describe a condition in wild muskrats. Others began to call the condition Errington's disease to indicate that they were seeing the disease that Errington had described. Karstad et al. (1971) discovered that the pathology of the disease in muskrats was identical to that of a disease of laboratory mice named after E. E. Tyzzer, and Tyzzer's disease of muskrats became standard usage. The bacteria causing Tyzzer's disease in different species are not identical, so we can anticipate new names for this condition in the future. Ironically, hemorrhagic disease applied by Errington is most descriptive of the disease.

THE COST OF DISEASE

Most of the attention to disease in wild animals has been directed toward the relatively few conditions that cause conspicuous illness or death. Other less-dramatic conditions often have been considered to be unimportant. This underassessment of the significance of disease results from having insensitive techniques for detecting and measuring the effect of disease.

One major difficulty lies in trying to detect sick or dead individuals among free-living animals. In contrast to humans who can monitor their own health and domestic animal populations that are watched carefully by their owners, wild animals seldom are observed in detail by anyone concerned about their health. Wild animals that have some form of dysfunction often hide so that they become even less visible. When diseased wild animals are detected, they are anonymous (unless captured and marked) so that it usually is impossible to follow an individual over time to determine whether it remains disabled, recovers, or succumbs. Even when animals die as a result of disease, it can be extremely difficult to find their carcasses to assess how many have died or why they died.

Two studies that measured the ease with which dead birds can be detected illustrate this problem. Researchers in Texas measured the proportion of dead ducks that would be detected during searches of a marsh. They were interested in two diseases: avian cholera, a disease that kills birds rapidly, and lead poisoning, which results in prolonged illness. For the study, 100 duck carcasses were distributed in a marsh; 50 were placed in open water to mimic birds that died of avian cholera and 50 were placed in vegetation to mimic birds that had hidden while sick because of lead poisoning. Thirty minutes after the carcasses were put in place, eight searchers (who were unaware of placement of the birds) searched the marsh for dead birds. They found 6 of the 50 birds in open water and none of the 50 birds in cover. The search effort in this study was much more intense than that used in routine surveillance for the effects of disease, leading to the conclusion that "casual searches would result almost invariably in negative findings even though large numbers of birds actually died" (Stutzenbaker et al. 1986).

My wife and I used a different method to study the detection of bird carcasses (Wobeser and Wobe-

ser 1992). We placed 50 one-day-old domestic chick carcasses each day for 5 days in predetermined random locations on a 1 ha area of grass pasture to simulate a severe die-off of small birds. We searched randomly chosen plots equal to 10% of the area each day, and for 5 days following the end of the die-off. Despite having placed 250 carcasses on the 1 ha area, we found only 1 carcass suitable for necropsy. This confirmed the observation by Stutzenbaker et al. (1986) that the carcasses of wild animals are "quickly assimilated into the environment."

It usually is even more difficult to detect animals experiencing sublethal forms of disease, such as impaired reproduction, subtle behavioral changes, or decreased growth rate. As an example of a sublethal effect that would be difficult to detect, cowpox virus caused no overt signs of disease and did not affect the survival of wild voles and mice but reduced their fecundity by about 25% by increasing the mean time to first litter by 20–30 days (Feore et al. 1997). This disease could have a significant effect on the lifetime reproduction of such short-lived species, but its effect would be invisible without intense surveillance. Some causes of disease such as contaminants may act as selective agents that result in loss of genetic diversity (Nacci et al. 2002), an effect that would be extremely difficult to detect. Orlando and Guillette (2001) suggested that measures of central tendency may not always be good indicators of the effect of stressors such as contaminants on populations and that the degree of variance of different features also may be important.

Although many agents that cause disease may not cause conspicuous illness in wild animals, these agents still have a cost to the animal that may be important to the biology of the species (Yuill 1987). It is difficult to identify and quantify the cost of disease or to compare the relative costliness of different conditions. One problem lies in finding a unit of measurement or "currency" that can be used to evaluate different types of cost and to relate the cost to the probable effect on an animal or population. A few ecologists have advocated using *energy* as a currency for evaluating the cost of disease (Munger and Karasov 1989; Delahay et al. 1995). Energy is used here in the sense of the ability or capacity to do work (Odum 1993). Energy is "the single common denominator of life on earth, that is something that is absolutely essential and involved in every action large or small" (Odum 1993) and "any physiological dysfunction is likely to have energetic consequences" (Delahay et al. 1995).

The amount of energy that an animal can acquire

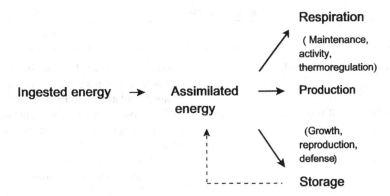

Fig. 2.3. The partitioning of energy in an animal. Two basic features are important: energy use cannot exceed energy intake, and use of energy for one purpose decreases the energy available for all other purposes.

depends upon the amount and quality of food available, the animal's feeding activity, and the efficiency with which nutrients are extracted by its digestive system. The energy that is assimilated is allocated to *respiration* (maintenance of structural and functional elements, activity, and thermoregulation), *production* (growth, reproduction, and defense responses), and *storage* (fig. 2.3).

Any change in the amount of energy that can be acquired alters the amount available for allocation, and any change in how energy is allocated to one function changes the amount that is available for other functions. Decreased intake of energy for example, because of reduced digestive efficiency, must be offset either by consumption of more food or by decreased energy use. Increased use of energy for one purpose necessarily results in less energy being available for other uses unless energy intake can be increased. For example, mounting an immune response requires energy and has been shown to impair growth in several species of birds (Soler et al. 2002). How energy is allocated among various functions is one of the classical trade-offs in ecology (Stearns 1992). It is likely that there is no absolute rule for the priority that is given to various uses of energy. Coop and Kyriazakis (1999) proposed that growth, pregnancy, and lactation had a higher priority than immunity in ruminants, but the relative value of various functions is likely to be highly variable in different situations. Individuals vary in their ability to acquire and utilize resources so that they may make different life-history allocations of resources (Reid et al. 2003).

One of the most common physiologic responses in many diseases is a lack of desire to eat (inappetence). Many people may even experience nausea when confronted with food while they are ill. A second common response in many diseases is increased body temperature. Fever is a part of the defense system against invading organisms but it involves a dramatic increase in energy usage. In humans, energy-consuming enzymes speed up by 13% with every degree rise in body temperature (Keusch 1993). Thus, a sick animal may be using energy at an increased rate because of fever while its intake of energy is decreased by inappetence. This state can only be maintained through some combination of increased usage of stored energy (if any is available) and reduced allocation of energy to other activities such as growth or reproduction. If there is a severe energy deficit, all uses are effected. Examples of how various diseases may affect energetics are shown in table 2.1.

Many disease agents affect energy balance in more than one way. *Sarcoptes scabei* is a tiny mite that causes the disease sarcoptic mange by living and burrowing in the skin of infected animals. We see this condition on a regular basis in coyotes, wolves, and red foxes in western Canada, and it occurs in many other species including wild ibex in Europe and wombats in Australia. Although the mites are confined to the epidermis (the outer layer of the skin), their presence and excretions cause severe irritation so that infested animals continually worry and chew their skin, often removing most of the hair that can be reached and causing many self-inflicted wounds. There is a severe inflammatory response, with protein-rich fluids and cells exuding through the damaged skin and collecting as a crust on the surface (fig. 2.4). Because of the intense itchiness, the animals stop foraging for food. Energy intake is reduced dramatically while at the same time

Table 2.1 How Individual Disease Conditions May Affect Energy Availability and Use

Effect of disease	Examples
Decreased energy intake because of inappetence	Ascarid nematodes in children[1], gastrointestinal nematodes in reindeer[2], cecal nematodes in red grouse[3], malaria in Hawaiian birds[4]
Reduced intake because of impaired mobility	Muscle atrophy resulting from malnutrition during winter in ungulates, degenerative joint disease in many species.
Decreased digestive efficiency	Intestinal tapeworms in white-footed mice[5], enteritis of many types including paravoviral infection in canids, *Mycobacterium paratuberculosis* infection in ruminants, and cecal nematodes in red grouse[6]
Reduced intake because of altered behavior	Sarcoptic mange in coyotes, caribou moving to snow to avoid flies, sheep eating less nutritious pasture to avoid parasites[7]
Increased energy for thermoregulation	Loss of fur in mange, oiling of feathers.
Increased energy demand because of fever	Many infectious diseases[8]
Increased energy use because of altered behavior	Caribou moving to avoid flies, increased grooming and preening
Increased energy for inflammatory, immune, and repair functions	Most diseases
Increased loss of nutrients in excretions	Many kidney diseases, e.g., renal coccidiosis and leptospirosis, many diseases in which diarrhea occurs.

[1]Hadju et al. (1996).
[2]Arneberg et al. (1996).
[3]Shaw and Moss (1990).
[4]Atkinson et al. (1995).
[5]Munger and Karasov (1989).
[6]Shaw and Moss (1990).
[7]Hutchings et al. (1999).
[8]Kluger (1979).

they expend extra energy in scratching and chewing at themselves, in producing inflammatory cells and secretions to battle the mites, and for thermoregulation because of the condition of their coat. Energy that could have been used for growth and reproduction, or stored, is expended. The damaged skin is a poor barrier to other disease agents, so that mange often is complicated by invasion of *Staphylococcus aureus* bacteria. (Immune function and other host resistance factors are also affected adversely by energy shortage but this has not been investigated in coyotes.)

Many mangy animals submitted to our laboratory have expended their energy reserves and only a raddled hulk remains. We diagnose starvation as the proximal cause of death in these animals. Some coyotes that still may have energy reserves die from a variety of traumatic misadventures (hit by cars,

killed by dogs, shot by farmers) presumably because they are less wary than normal as a result of having less than normal energy to expend in avoiding trouble. The survival time of red foxes with mange was about one-fifth that of uninfected foxes (Newman et al. 2002).

Petroleum oil, one of the most common contaminants encountered by waterbirds, serves to demonstrate that noninfectious diseases also have energetic effects. The most obvious effect of exposure to oil is soiling of the plumage or pelage (fig. 2.5) resulting in loss of insulative value and buoyancy. A heavily oiled duck at 15°C loses heat at the same rate as a normal duck does at 2°C (Hartung 1967). Ducks may be able to compensate for this heat loss by an increased metabolic rate, either by using stored reserves or by increased feed intake. Hartung (1967) estimated that oiled ducks would have to double

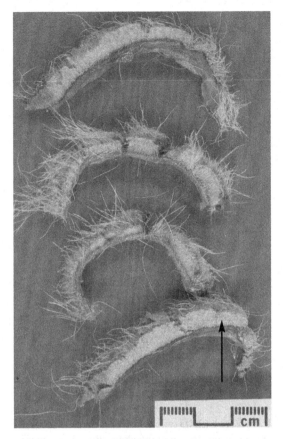

Fig. 2.4. Sections of skin from a coyote with sarcoptic mange. The thick crusts composed of inflammatory cells and proteinaceous fluid that collect on the skin surface of animals with sarcoptic mange represent one of the energetic costs of this disease. The arrow indicates the skin surface.

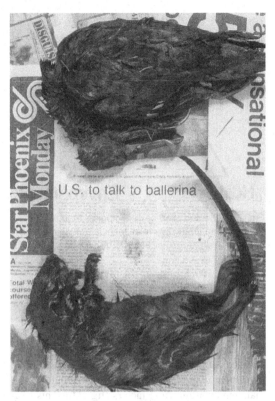

Fig. 2.5. Aquatic animals such as this muskrat and northern shoveler that have been exposed to petroleum oil have tremendous energy costs because of loss of the insulating value of their pelage or plumage.

their normal food intake to meet the demand; however, another feature of oiling is that birds fail to feed normally. In addition, the oil may destroy food materials in the environment. Birds ingest oil with food or water and through preening their soiled coats. The toxic effects of ingested oil are poorly defined but include inflammation of the intestine, potentially interfering with nutrient assimilation, and severe damage to red blood cells, resulting in anemia (deficiency in the number of circulating red blood cells). Loss of oxygen-carrying capacity in the blood as a result of anemia has dramatic energy consequences because the bird is forced to use anaerobic metabolic processes that are much less efficient than normal aerobic metabolism. Leighton (1993) described the interaction between oiling of plumage and anemia as a "sinister synergy," because both required a marked increase in metabolic rate to main-

tain normal function. Many oiled birds die of hypothermia when their energy reserves are exhausted and they can no longer maintain body temperature. Less-severe exposure to oil-contaminated food results in depressed growth in birds (Szaro 1977), probably because less energy is available for this activity.

THE AGENT:HOST:ENVIRONMENT MODEL FOR DISEASE

When disease is being considered, it is tempting to simplify it to a basic equation that resembles a chemical reaction: causative agent + animal = disease. If we combine the cause and the animal in this linear model, the inevitable result will be a dysfunction that we can label as disease. However, even in diseases in which there is only one cause and in which the disease can be reproduced by exposing the animal experimentally to that factor, the actual occurrence of the disease in the individual animal in nature and within a population is far more complex than this simple equation suggests.

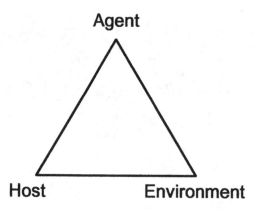

Fig. 2.6. The so-called epidemiological triangle that illustrates the interactive relationships among disease agent, animal, and other aspects of the environment.

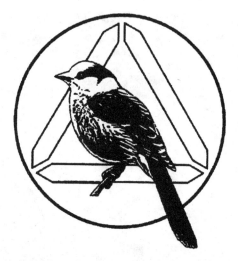

Fig. 2.7. The agent-host-environment triangle is incorporated within the logo of the Canadian Cooperative Wildlife Health Centre to symbolize the need to consider all three aspects when dealing with disease.

The relationship between agent and animal is influenced by a great variety of factors. Some of these are features of the agent, some are features of the animal, and some are not directly related to either. The latter are lumped together as environmental factors. This led to the concept that disease is the result of an interactive relationship among causative agent, animal, and environmental factors (fig. 2.6). This relationship is sometimes called the epidemiological triangle (epidemiology being the science concerned with the study of the occurrence of disease in a population). We have included the triangle within the logo of the Canadian Cooperative Wildlife Health Centre (fig. 2.7) to symbolize the importance of the concept.

Another way of portraying the relationship among the three factors is to visualize the causative agent and the animal being balanced across a fulcrum of environmental factors (fig. 2.8). This teeter-totter metaphor is useful because it suggests that the relationship is inherently unstable, with each of the three components being variable. When the balance is tipped in favor of the animal either by host factors or by the relative position of the environmental

fulcrum, relative health is enjoyed (fig. 2.8b). When the balance is in favor of the causative agent, various degrees of dysfunction or disease occur in the animal (fig. 2.8c). The term "context-dependent" that Brown et al. (2003) applied to host-parasite relationships is useful for thinking about disease in general. In certain contexts or situations, the relationship between agent and animal is benign, while it may be very harmful to the animal in other situations.

To illustrate the context-dependent nature of disease, consider a situation in which the disease agent is a worm that lives in the intestine of a grazing mammal. The life cycle of the worm is direct. Worm eggs shed with the animal's droppings hatch on the ground and the resulting larvae crawl onto vegetation. If the larvae are consumed accidentally by a suitable animal, they develop to adulthood in the animal's intestine. The relative effect of the worms, in terms of the balance above, is a function of the abil-

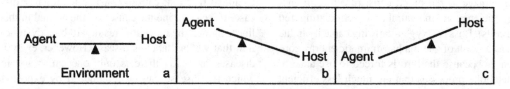

Fig. 2.8. The relationships among agent, animal, and environmental factors can also be thought of as a teeter-totter, with environmental conditions acting as a fulcrum on which the interaction between agent and animal is balanced. The relationship may be (a) relatively balanced, or favor either (b) the animal, or (c) the agent.

ity of individual worms to cause injury and the number of worms present (the intensity of the infection). The counterbalancing force is determined by the ability of the animal to resist entry of the worms into its body, expel worms from its body, repair harmful effects that the worms may produce, and meet its own and the worms' energy demands. The animal's ability to resist is determined by many factors including the animal's genotype, age, sex, nutritional condition, and prior experience with the worm. Environmental factors that serve as the fulcrum are many and can include features as diverse as weather, habitat conditions, population density of host animals, and presence of other diseases and predators.

Let us assume in the first instance that environmental conditions have been favorable for the grazing animal with warm dry weather, abundant forage, modest density of its own species, and relative freedom from other diseases, so that the animals are sleek and fat, and have a high degree of resistance to the worm. These environmental conditions also are unfavorable for transmission of the worm between host animals, because the worm's eggs and larvae are affected adversely by dry conditions. The net effect is that the animals are exposed to relatively few infective larvae and the number of worms in individual animals is small. Under such conditions, one would expect little overt evidence of dysfunction in the population, although the agent is interacting with the host. (As will be discussed in chapter 3, even under very favorable conditions a few individuals in the host population may have many worms and be affected adversely.)

Now consider the same animal and worm species at another time, in which a dense population of host animals on limited range experiences a severe winter during which the animals lose considerable weight and condition. This is followed by a cold, rainy summer in which there is limited plant growth. The animals are now "stressed" by poor nutrition as well as by social stressors associated with high population density so that their resistance to many causative agents is decreased, and one might expect to find that several types of disease are occurring. The cool damp weather is highly favorable for survival of worm eggs and larvae on the vegetation. Because vegetation is limited, the animals crop closer to the ground and, because of the high animal density, fecal contamination is abundant so that the probability of ingesting larvae with forage is increased. Under these conditions, the environmental fulcrum has shifted, with the balance now favoring the worms. One would expect to find more worms in

individual animals, more heavily infected individuals in the population, and more overt disease. A situation with these features has been documented in detail in the free-ranging Soay sheep on St. Kilda (Gulland 1992).

Combining the concept of energy as a currency with the agent-host-environment model helps to understand how environmental factors interact with or alter the relationship between an animal and disease agents. The animals in the first situation above have easy access to abundant energy (and other nutrients), reduced energy demands for thermoregulation because of mild winter weather, and low demands for energy for resisting parasites (because the level of exposure is low), so that they can store surplus energy as fat. In contrast, animals in the second situation have limited food and must expend more energy in searching for food and for thermoregulation during the cold winter. Because of the greater exposure to parasite larvae, they will expend more energy (if it is available) in resisting infection and repairing parasite-induced damage. They will have less energy for growth, reproduction, or resistance to other diseases, and some may succumb to starvation. This type of relationship between malnutrition and the effects of parasitism has been studied in snowshoe hares by Murray et al. (1997).

Reduced intake either of food in general (protein-energy malnutrition) or deficiency of specific individual nutrients such as copper, zinc, or vitamin A can have a severe effect on the ability to mount an effective defense to infectious agents. Studies of both malnourished children and experimentally induced malnutrition in animals have shown that mild to moderate levels of malnutrition diminish the ability to mount a competent immune response. Thus, disease agents may flourish in individuals that are nutritionally stressed. Wildlife pathologists are often confronted with animals found sick or dead that are emaciated and have a greater than usual number of parasites. In such situations, it is simplistic to assume either that the parasites caused the emaciation or that malnutrition allowed the parasites to flourish. The true answer likely involves some combination of the two factors acting in concert.

EXPOSURE AND RESISTANCE

Two features that are critical in determining the outcome of an interaction between a causative agent and an animal are the amount and type of *exposure* the animal has to the causative agent and the degree of *resistance* the animal has to the causative agent. The concept that exposure may vary in degree is well established in noninfectious diseases, such as those caused by contaminants and physical agents. We accept that exposure to the amount of irradiation required for an X-ray is not unduly harmful while exposure to a much larger amount, as occurred at the Chernobyl nuclear accident, is decidedly harmful. Most poisons have a dose-effect relationship, that is, the degree of disease is related to the amount of exposure. The relationship between dose and effect often is not linear, and some type of threshold phenomenon is common. An animal may deal with small amounts of an agent without detectable effect, but exposure above a critical threshold level results in disease.

The same general principle applies to disease caused by living causative agents. Although the "minimum infecting dose" is unknown for most diseases, it is clear that there are differences among agents in the number of organisms required to result in infection and disease. For example, about 10^8 *Vibrio cholerae* are required to produce the disease cholera in most humans whereas only 1–10 *Mycobacterium tuberculosis* are sufficient to produce tuberculosis (Mims et al. 2001). As a general principle, the greater the "dose" of agent to which an animal is exposed, the greater the risk of serious disease.

Resistance takes many forms. The animal may be able to prevent entry of the noxious agent into its body (e.g., intact skin is an important barrier to a wide variety of different agents). If the agent is successful in entering the body, the animal may be able to neutralize or remove it before it has an opportunity to cause significant damage. Even if the agent cannot be expelled, the animal's defenses may be able to limit the amount of damage, for example, by enclosing the damaged area and the agent in stout fibrous tissue, or compensate for the injury by replacing damaged tissue rapidly, or by increasing food intake to compensate for the effects of the agent. However, resistance or defense mechanisms are finite so that the greater the exposure the more likely that they will be overwhelmed.

Military analogies are often used to explain exposure and resistance because it is easy to visualize the animal as a fortified structure with certain defense features and a complement of defenders. The greater the number of attacking invaders and the more persistently they attack, the greater the likelihood that the walls will be breached. It is also easy to visualize that simultaneous attacks by different invaders might unintentionally improve the chances of the individual agents. Conversely, the higher the fortress walls,

the more numerous and well armed the defenders, and the more rapidly they respond to any challenge, the lower the chance that the attack will be successful. Aspergillosis, a disease that occurs commonly in birds, illustrates this principle. The causative agent, *Aspergillus fumigatus,* is ubiquitous in the environment, growing in decaying organic material. The fungus reproduces by microscopic conidia (spores) that float in the air and are inhaled by birds and other animals on a regular basis. Under normal circumstances, no disease results because defense mechanisms are adequate to deal with the inhaled conidia. Severe and often fatal aspergillosis occurs when birds inhale massive numbers of spores, for instance while consuming moldy food or occupying nests with moldy bedding, or when a bird's normal resistance is decreased so that even a "usual" level of exposure cannot be repelled. In the first situation, the birds receive exposure that overwhelms their resistance. The second occurs commonly in injured wild birds held for rehabilitation and when certain species are brought into captivity or weakened by starvation (Herman and Sladen 1958). The worst-case scenario occurs when birds with depressed resistance receive unusually large exposure to spores. Large outbreaks of aspergillosis have occurred in wild waterfowl during periods of inclement winter weather when they are forced to consume moldy food (Neff 1955; Adrian et al. 1978).

SUMMARY

- Disease means many things to different people.
- Disease is defined here as any impairment that interferes with or modifies the performance of normal functions, including responses to environmental factors such as nutrition, toxicants, and climate; infectious agents; inherent or congenital defects; or combinations of these factors.
- Disease is a relative state that occurs as part of a continuum between absolute health and death.
- Disease has many causes that may act singly or, more commonly, in combination. Wild animals are seldom exposed to just one potential disease-causing agent at a time.
- The dysfunction that constitutes disease usually results from the body's reaction to injury rather than from the injury itself.
- How diseases are named is confused and confusing. The most useful names are those that describe a recognizable feature of the condition.
- Every disease (dysfunction) has a cost to the animal, although the cost may be difficult to detect or measure.

- Sick and dead wild animals are notoriously difficult to find and are a poor indicator of the extent or cost of disease.
- Energy is a currency that can be used to aid in understanding the ecology of disease and the interaction of various factors that contribute to disease.

- Most diseases cannot be defined by a straight line model (agent + animal = disease). A three-part interactive model incorporating agent, host, and environment is more useful.
- The degree of exposure to disease-producing agents and the ability of animals to resist the effects of these agents are central to disease.

3
What Causes Disease?

The nub of epidemiology is a concern to establish causes and effects in relation to health disorders.
—M. Susser

IDENTIFYING THE CAUSE OF A DISEASE

Our understanding of what constitutes a disease goes through gradual evolution over time as we learn progressively more about its ecology. Identification of the cause is one major step in this process. Cause is used here for "that which brings about any condition or produces any effect" (Dorland 2000). Some diseases are well known for years before the cause is identified. For example, at the present time a disease called avian vacuolar myelinopathy (AVM) has been described in bald eagles and a number of other birds (Thomas et al. 1998) and reproduced experimentally (Fischer et al. 2003), but its cause is unknown. Some diseases may be prevented or controlled effectively without the cause being known. A classic example comes from human medicine. In 1854, Dr. John Snow recognized that cholera was associated with drinking water from a particular well in London. His recommendation that the pump handle be removed from the well, so that the water could not be used, controlled the disease more than four decades before its bacterial cause was discovered. In other situations, potential disease-causing agents or risk factors are known to occur in wild animals long before they are associated with any disease. This is the case for many contaminants, residues of which in wild animals have not yet been related clearly to any harmful effect.

While cause seems a perfectly adequate word, another word, "etiology" (from the Greek *aitia,* cause + *logia*, description), is used commonly when discussing disease. One definition for etiology is synonymous with cause ("the cause or origin of a dis-

ease or disorder") but a second definition ("the study of the factors that cause disease and the method of their introduction to the host") (Dorland 2000) deals to some degree with why and how a disease occurs as well as with what caused it.

New conditions often are recognized because of some peculiar clinical signs or occurrence of the condition under specific circumstances. (The term "clinical sign" is used to describe objective evidence of disease, while "symptom" is usually defined as subjective evidence, such as the sensation that a patient may experience and relate. Symptom generally is not used in describing disease in animals.) As an example, we have seen a condition in pronghorns on several occasions. It has only been seen in males during the autumn and is characterized by severe inflammation of the skin of the head and neck (fig. 3.1), and the bacterium *Arcanobacterium pyogenes* has been isolated from the lesions. This type of data may be sufficient to form a "case definition" that would allow differentiation of the condition from other diseases. For instance, cases of AVM are recognized on the basis of certain types of abnormal behavior and specific lesions in the brains of birds (Thomas et al. 1998), although the cause is unknown. At some point, a factor or agent (the "putative cause") may be suspected to be the cause of the disease, perhaps because it often occurs at the same time and place as the disease or because it is detected in animals that have features that fit the case definition. Initially, this factor is said to be associated with the disease and further evidence needs to be gathered to establish that the association is actually a cause:effect relationship.

The history of a disease in wild muskrats that I mentioned earlier is an example of this process. During the 1940s, Paul Errington, an observant biologist, described ecological features of a fatal condition in muskrats in Iowa (Errington 1946). The con-

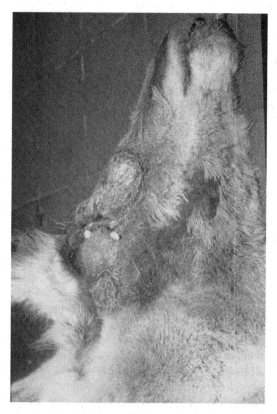

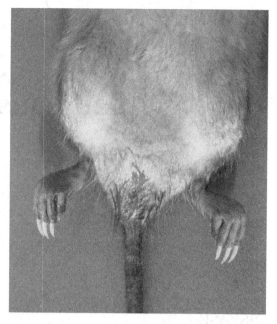

Fig. 3.2. Muskrat that died of Tyzzer's disease. The blood on the fur about the anus comes from hemorrhage into the large bowel. These changes prompted Paul Errington to call the disease hemorrhagic disease.

Fig. 3.1. Male pronghorn with severe necrotizing fasciitis. The skin below the eye is dead and pus can be seen escaping from under the dead skin in two areas. The condition is believed to result from fighting injuries among males that allow the bacterium *Arcanobacterium pyogenes* to enter the subcutaneous tissue.

dition was sufficiently different from other conditions that he had seen that he believed it to be a separate entity. He called it "hemorrhagic disease" (HD) based on the presence of blood about the anus and in internal organs of affected muskrats (fig. 3.2). Muskrats with HD were submitted to a veterinary laboratory, and pathologic features of the disease were defined. Based on the evidence available, a case definition could have been written that would have differentiated cases of HD from other diseases of muskrats. Such a case definition might have read: "HD is a disease in which muskrats are found dead without recognized signs of illness. Dead animals often have blood on the abdominal fur, hemorrhage in the wall of the cecum, and many tiny white foci of necrosis in the liver. Affected animals do not have lesions in the spleen or lymph nodes, and no pathogenic bacteria can be isolated from tissues."

It was believed that HD was caused by an infectious agent, but attempts to identify the cause were unsuccessful. HD was reported widely in western and northern North America (Errington 1963), and the name was changed informally to "Errington's disease" (ED). In 1970 (7 years after Errington's death), Karstad et al. (1971) recognized that the pathology of ED in captive muskrats matched that of Tyzzer's disease (TD) described decades earlier in laboratory mice. The distinguishing feature of TD is the presence of unusual bacteria in liver cells of affected animals. These bacteria, which were present in the muskrats and are the putative cause of TD, were called *Bacillus piliformis,* but they have not been grown on artificial media. We identified similar bacteria in dead free-living muskrats in Saskatchewan (Wobeser et al. 1978) and in archived tissues from wild muskrats found dead in 1947 by Paul Errington (Wobeser et al. 1979), confirming that HD, ED, and TD were a single entity. Disease similar to TD has now been reported in many species (Wobeser 2001). The genomic structure of the bacterium has been characterized, resulting in a name change to *Clostridium piliforme,* and host-specific strains exist (Franklin et al. 1994). Currently, we know that bacteria similar to those that occur in TD in other animals occur in liver cells of affected muskrats. It is assumed that these bacteria are the causative agent, but many aspects of the etiology (how and why the disease occurs) are unknown.

Various criteria have been proposed to test whether or not an agent is the actual cause of a disease. Often this involves exposing healthy animals experimentally to the putative cause. If the exposed animals develop disease that fits the case definition, causation is considered to be proven. Following the discovery that microscopic agents could produce disease, a set of rules (Koch's postulates) was developed for establishing the relationship between a cause and a disease. The rules are:

1. The agent must be present in every case of disease. This is usually done by "isolating" the agent in pure culture.
2. The agent must not be found in cases of other diseases.
3. The agent must reproduce the disease when introduced into experimental animals.
4. The agent must be recoverable from experimentally infected animals.

These rules are useful for defining a cause: effect relationship in diseases that involve only a single cause and in which that agent is both a necessary and sufficient cause of the disease, that is, the agent is required for the disease to occur, and the agent acting by itself results in disease. The criteria served Robert Koch well for identifying the cause of some important diseases, including anthrax and tuberculosis, because the causative bacteria could be isolated from affected animals and transmitted to experimental animals, resulting in disease.

Koch's postulates have been modified to examine the cause of some noninfectious conditions (Shepard 1998) and experimental exposure has been used for investigating cause:effect relationships related to many poisons and toxins. Production of appropriate disease in healthy animals exposed experimentally to a chemical is strong evidence of a causal relationship. However, it is often difficult to establish what constitutes a realistic exposure to a chemical in such experiments. For any chemical, even table salt, there is a threshold amount below which disease does not occur and an upper threshold amount beyond which it will cause harm. In nature, the actual dose to which wild animals are exposed is seldom known. Toxicologists often have to work from the opposite direction by identifying chemical residues in animals and then trying to define "how much of a chemical must be in the tissues of a wild animal to cause harm" (Beyer et al. 1996).

Koch's postulates are not adequate for understanding causation of many diseases of wild animals (Hanson 1969) because (a) relatively few agents are both necessary and sufficient to produce disease over a wide range of environmental conditions, (b) a single disease may require the interaction of several causes, (c) a single disease may be caused by several different factors, and (d) a single agent may cause several different diseases. A disease may have a *primary* cause (the principal factor contributing to the production of disease), *secondary* causes (that are supplemental to the primary cause), and *predisposing* causes (that render the animal more susceptible to a specific disease without actually causing it). The etiology of a disease (as distinct from the cause) might include all these factors. Changes in the agent, the animal, or other features of the environment might influence whether disease does or does not occur. The etiology of some diseases, such as the so-called lungworm-pneumonia complex of mountain sheep (Forrester 1971), involves a web of causation that may include viruses, different bacteria, lungworms, nutrition, and multiple stressors (Wobeser 1994).

Different methods for establishing causation are needed for diseases caused by two or more factors acting together, diseases caused by agents that may cause disease under some circumstances and not others, diseases in which the agent may lie latent until precipitated by some other factor, chronic diseases such as neoplasia (cancer) in which the cause may have disappeared long before the disease occurs, and diseases such as reproductive failure that may be the end result of many different processes.

Because of difficulty in fulfilling the requirements of Koch's postulates, other criteria have been developed that incorporate epidemiologic information (the way that diseases occur and are distributed in populations) together with information from experimental exposure to examine cause:effect relationships. Evans (1977) proposed a set of criteria related specifically to viruses, which Kelsey et al. (1996) used to develop the criteria shown in table 3.1. These include some elements listed by Hill (1965) for enhancing belief in association of noninfectious disease with chemical exposure.

To illustrate how a suspected cause:effect association might be examined, consider the relationship that has been suggested between calcium (Ca) deficiency and reproductive dysfunction in passerine birds (Graveland et al. 1994). The hypothesis is that in areas affected by acid precipitation and in non-acidified areas where the soil contains few minerals,

Table 3.1 Criteria Used to Test Hypotheses Related to Disease Causation

1. The putative cause should be distributed in the population in the same manner as the disease.
2. The frequency of disease should be higher in those exposed to the putative cause than in those not so exposed.
3. Exposure to the putative cause should be more frequent among those with the disease than those without the disease, when all other risk factors are held constant.
4. Temporally, the disease should follow exposure to the putative cause.
5. The greater the dose or length of exposure to the putative cause, the greater the likelihood of occurrence of the disease.
6. For some diseases, a spectrum of host responses should follow exposure to the putative cause along a logical biological gradient from mild to severe.
7. The association between the cause and the disease should be found in various populations when different methods of study are used.
8. Other explanations for the association should be ruled out.
9. Elimination or modification of the cause or of the vector carrying it should decrease or eliminate the disease.
10. Prevention or modification of the host's response on exposure to the cause should decrease or eliminate the disease.
11. Where possible, in experimental settings, the disease should occur more frequently in animals exposed appropriately to the putative agent than in animals not exposed.
12. All of the relationships should make biologic and epidemiologic sense.

Source: Modified slightly from Kelsey et al. (1996).

female birds have difficulty obtaining sufficient calcium, resulting in impaired eggshell formation, reduced nestling growth, and other signs of reproductive dysfunction. The hypothesized relationship consists of two parts: (1) that the observed disease is a result of calcium deficiency, and (2) that the deficiency of calcium is a result of inadequate calcium being available in the environment. Koch's postulates are not helpful in testing this association, but we might examine the association experimentally by feeding a calcium-deficient diet to experimental birds. This could establish if calcium deficiency can cause disease similar to that observed in the wild. We also might supply supplemental calcium in areas where the dysfunction occurs. Improved reproduction in areas with supplementation would support the hypothesis.

I am not aware that feeding trials using appropriate species have been done. Supplementation has resulted in improved reproduction in some but not all areas (Tilgar et al. 2002). The criteria proposed by Kelsey et al. (1996) could be used to examine this putative association (table 3.2).

This example demonstrates some of the problems in proving a cause:effect relationship and the need to consider the agent, the animal, and other features of the environment. While the evidence generally supports the hypothesis that reproduction of passerines is affected by low availability of calcium in the environment, the effect is different in different areas (Ramsay and Houston 1999) and in different species of bird, and the effect may vary annually depending upon food availability (Mänd and Tilgar 2003). The example also is useful for illustrating the difference between cause and etiology. Calcium deficiency may be the *proximate* cause (that which immediately precedes and produces the effect) of reproductive dysfunction in some species, while the etiology of the condition involves secondary and predisposing causative factors that influence the availability of calcium in the environment and the need for calcium by the birds.

CAUSES OF DISEASE

It is difficult to create a simple framework for discussing the many factors that cause disease because there are exceptions to every rule and because our notions of where things "fit" change as we learn more about the nature of individual diseases. The usual system for classifying disease agents has been to divide them into two broad groups: infectious and noninfectious causes. I will add an intermediate category to deal with one specific group of diseases.

The distinction between infectious and noninfectious diseases is usually made on the basis that infectious diseases are caused by living organisms that

Table 3.2 Use of Criteria to Examine an Association Between Environmental Deficiency of Calcium and Reproductive Disease in Small Birds

Criteria[1]	Relationship
1,2,3	In general, reproductive problems such as eggshell defects occur in areas with low availability of Ca in the environment; however, blue tits in a severely acidified area of Scotland with a low apparent availability of Ca did not have the disease[2].
4	Ca deficiency in the environment precedes reproductive dysfunction.
5	In general, the degree of reproductive dysfunction is related inversely to the availability of Ca in the environment. Studies found that great tits in a Ca-deficient area that had access to added Ca sources (picnic waste, chicken grit) were less severely affected than birds with no extra source of Ca[3], and that reproduction was most severely affected in years of low general food availability[4].
6	Different species were affected in different ways by an apparent deficiency of Ca[5].
7	Populations of birds in many but not all areas with acidification or poor Ca sources had similar reproductive dysfunction.
8	One possible alternate explanation for poor eggshell quality (chlorinated hydrocarbon pesticide pollution) was thought to be very unlikely.
9	In most but not all Ca-deficient areas, provision of supplemental Ca improved reproductive performance.
10	Not appropriate.
11	The experimental provision of Ca supplement improved reproduction in most but not all areas.
12	The hypothesized association between environmental Ca deficiency and reproductive dysfunction makes biological sense. Passerine birds cannot store sufficient Ca for egg production and are dependent on environmental sources of Ca. Snails and other sources of Ca are reduced markedly in acidified areas and in Ca-poor areas.

[1]Proposed by Kelsey et al. (1996) (see also, table 3.1).
[2]Ramsay and Houston (1999).
[3]Graveland and Drent (1997).
[4]Tilgar et al. (1999).
[5]Mänd and Tilgar (2003).

cause harm while residing in or on an animal's body. These living agents replicate and are involved in a trophic relationship with the animal. Noninfectious diseases are caused by factors other than living organisms that cause harm while living in or on an animal's body. (Some noninfectious diseases, such as botulism and cyanobacterial poisoning, are caused by toxins produced by living organisms but these organisms do not usually live in or on the animal.) This basic subdivision is challenged by our current knowledge about a class of diseases called the *transmissible spongiform encephalopathies* (TSE). These diseases, which include chronic wasting disease of deer and bovine spongiform encephalopathy (BSE) among others, are believed to be caused by proteinaceous agents called prions that lack nucleic acid (Prusiner 1998) and, hence, do not fit the definition of living organisms. However, the TSE are transmissible and behave like infectious agents in many re-

spects. There is no established category for the TSE, and they often are considered with infectious diseases. I believe that it is more appropriate to place them in a separate category that I have called "noninfectious transmissible diseases."

INFECTIOUS CAUSES OF DISEASE

The concept of infectious disease is not new. It was discussed by classical Greek and Roman writers, and infection caused by larger beasts such as worms and arthropods has been recognized for millennia. As early as 1546, Girolamo Fracastoro suggested that invisible animate agents were responsible for disease. Pasteur's proposal of the germ theory of disease, supported by Robert Koch's discovery of the transmissible nature of certain diseases caused by bacteria, formed the basis for a new science that studied infectious diseases. The term "infection" implies penetration and growth of organisms within an animal's body, thus, we can discuss infection of the lung by bacteria or of the intestine by nematodes. For some unknown reason, the terms "infest" and "infestation" are used to describe colonization of the outer surface of the body by larger organisms, such as fleas and lice, while colonization of the body surface by bacteria and fungi is described as an infection. However, infestations are still infectious diseases.

Infectious disease involves a trophic relationship between the causative organism and the animal, in which the organism derives benefit from the relationship while the animal is harmed in some way. This type of relationship is considered to represent parasitism and usually involves the agent obtaining nutrients and other biological necessities from the host animal while reducing the host's fitness. Parasitism is not a rare phenomenon. Some authors suggest that the majority of living organisms are parasitic at some time in their life. Every wild animal is host to many parasites. The list of infectious diseases continues to expand, and many conditions that currently are considered noninfectious or of unknown etiology will be discovered to be infectious.

Infectious agents generally are considered to include viruses, bacteria, fungi, certain algae, protozoa, helminths (worms), and arthropods. For some unknown reason and at some unclear point in time, scientists interested in parasites that cannot be seen with the naked eye (microorganisms) and those interested in larger parasites began to drift apart. Those who worked with viruses, bacteria, and fungi became known as *microbiologists* while the larger organisms (protozoa, worms, and arthropods) were called parasites and were studied by *parasitologists*. (Protozoa seem to live in a no-man's-land, some-

times belonging to parasitologists and sometimes to microbiologists; the former *Journal of Protozoology* has been renamed the *Journal of Eukaryotic Microbiology*.) The artificial division of infectious diseases persists, for example, two recent books are entitled *Infectious Diseases of Wild Mammals* (Williams and Barker 2001) and *Parasitic Diseases of Wild Mammals* (Samuel et al. 2001). However, the basic features of parasitism are common to the two groups. Ecologists have attempted to divide infectious causes of disease into two groups (microparasites and macroparasites) based on biological and population features rather than on taxonomy (Anderson and May 1979). The general features of these two groups are shown in table 3.3. In very general terms, most viruses and bacteria, and some protozoa, fit within the microparasite group, while most helminths and arthropods fit within the macroparasite group. This division is useful for thinking about how various disease agents act in populations, but some agents such as *Mycobacterium bovis*, the cause of bovine tuberculosis, don't fit particularly well. This organism is small and generation time may be relatively short, but the organism reproduces slowly within the host and infections are chronic and persistent.

Some infectious agents are *obligate* parasites, that is, infection of an animal is required for their existence. Other infectious agents are *facultative* or *opportunistic* parasites that may infect animals, but infection is not necessary for their existence or reproduction.

As scientists have become able to examine the genetic material of infectious agents more closely, it has become clear that animals with infectious diseases often are infected with more than one geno-

Table 3.3 General Features of Microparasites and Macroparasites

Feature	Microparasites	Macroparasites
Size	Small	Large
Generation time	Short	Long
Reproduction	High rate of reproduction within the host	Usually low or no direct reproduction within the host
Duration of infection	Short relative to life-span of host	Persistent, with reinfection being common
Type of disease	Short-lived, often severe	Chronic, usually sublethal, intensity of infection determines degree of injury
Immunity to reinfection	Long-lasting, reinfection uncommon	Depends upon continued presence of infection, reinfection common

type of the same agent. Thus, while we classify all of the bacteria causing a case of avian cholera in a snow goose as belonging to the species *Pasteurella multocida*, these bacteria may represent a population of different genotypes that are competing with each other for resources from their habitat (the sick goose) in exactly the same way that individual geese compete with each other for resources from a wetland. This competition among closely related infectious agents may have important implications for understanding disease (Read and Taylor 2001) but remains largely a theoretical concept at this time.

Infection, Infectious, and Disease: Differentiation

In considering infectious conditions, it is important to differentiate between the presence of an agent that has the ability to produce disease in or on an animal (infection) and the occurrence of dysfunction caused by the presence of that organism (disease). Many animals are infected without being obviously diseased. In chapter 2, I made the point that growth of an infectious agent in or on an animal has a cost to that animal, because the agent is extracting nutrients from the animal. However, the cost may be so slight that the animal is easily able to compensate for the cost and suffers no *detectable* dysfunction. (I emphasize detectable because our methods for measuring dysfunction often are insensitive, and animals may be affected in ways or to degrees that we cannot appreciate.)

An agent may cause infection without disease in one species and severe dysfunction in another species. A good example of this is ovine herpesvirus 2, which occurs very commonly in domestic sheep without causing any apparent affect but which causes severe and often fatal disease (called sheep-associated malignant catarrhal fever) in cattle, bison (Schultheiss et al. 2000), and white-tailed deer. An agent also may occur as a clinically silent infection in some individuals and cause disease in others of the same species, or an individual may be infected without disease under some circumstances and become severely diseased under other conditions.

One of the most basic factors that can influence whether an animal suffers dysfunction as a result of infection is the *intensity* of the infection (i.e., the number of organisms per infected host). Ebert et al. (2000b) observed that " the more parasites infect a host individual, the stronger are the parasite-induced effects." The relationship between intensity of infection and the degree of dysfunction that results is well recognized to occur in infections caused by macro-

parasites such as various worms and some protozoa. Individuals with few parasites are less likely to be diseased than those with many parasites. There is less information available as to whether this same principle also occurs in infections caused by microparasites. The general belief has been that, so long as the initial dose of microparasitic organisms entering an animal is sufficient to establish an infection, the organisms will give rise to a huge population that will continue to expand until they reach a certain carrying capacity (see chapter 11 for further discussion) or are limited by the animal's immune system (Ebert et al. 2000b). The actual intensity of infection with bacteria, viruses, and fungi is seldom measured, so that it is unclear if more severely diseased animals have more organisms of this type than animals with less-severe disease. However, there is good evidence that larger initial infective doses result in more rapid onset of dysfunction (perhaps because the carrying capacity is reached sooner) and may result in more severe effects under some circumstances (Ebert et al. 2000a, 2000b; Frank and Jeffrey 2000). Very small infective doses may lead to subclinical infection with development of protective immunity in some cases (Frank and Jeffrey 2000). The route by which an infection enters the body also may influence the degree of dysfunction that occurs.

It is important to distinguish between animals that are *infected* and those that are *infectious* to others. This distinction is particularly important in considering how various agents circulate and persist in a population. Not all infectious diseases are *contagious*, that is, "capable of being transmitted from one individual to another" (Dorland 2000). Tetanus and listeriosis (bacterial diseases) and aspergillosis and histoplasmosis (fungal diseases) are caused by microorganisms that reside in the soil and that may infect animals but that do not spread from animal to animal. These agents are infectious (capable of causing infection) but not contagious. Even among disease agents that are contagious, not every infected individual is capable of transmitting the infection to other animals. Some infected individuals may be in the early stages of infection before transmission can occur. For example, animals are usually infected with rabies virus for 1–3 months, but transmission "only effectively occurs during a relatively short excretion period of the virus during the final stage of the disease" (Rupprecht et al. 2001). The interval between infection and when infective stages are shed by worm parasites is referred to as the *prepatent period*. For instance, white-tailed deer are infected with the meningeal worm *Parelaphostrong-ylus tenuis* for 82–91 days before they begin to shed infective larvae in their feces (Anderson 1992). During the 3-month prepatent period, they are infected but not infectious. Many infected deer have only a single *P. tenuis* in their tissues or only worms of one sex, so that they also are infected but not infectious (Slomke et al. 1995).

Some infections enter a latent stage in which they are hidden, do not cause disease, and are not contagious. This is a feature of many herpesviruses, including anatid herpesvirus 1, which causes duck plague, and the form of herpes hominis that causes cold sores in humans. Individuals may be infected persistently, perhaps for life, with these viruses but only periodically have episodes of reactivation, viral replication, and shedding.

Some infections may not produce reproductive stages in all host species. For example, the liver fluke *Fascioloides magna* and the meningeal worm *P. tenuis* seldom produce ova in infected moose. Although moose are infected, they play no role in maintaining these agents in a region (Pybus 2001; Lankester 2002). An infectious agent also may be localized in some site in the body from which it has no exit to the external environment. This occurs in some cases of tuberculosis in which the bacteria are encapsulated in a thick-walled nodule within a lymph node. These animals react positively on various live-animal tests for tuberculosis but have little or no role in maintaining the disease in a population, compared to an animal with extensive lung involvement that is expelling bacteria with exhaled air and in which the disease is highly contagious.

Viruses

"Viruses occupy a unique position in biology. Although they possess some of the properties of living systems such as having a genome, they are actually nonliving infectious entities and should not be considered microorganisms" (van Regenmortel and Mahy 2004). Despite this assertion that they are nonliving, virus generally are considered to be infectious agents. Viruses are too small to be seen by light microscopy and contain only one type of nucleic acid, either DNA or RNA, never both.

All viruses are obligate parasites. They have no functional organelles and are totally dependent upon the host cell for energy production and synthesis of macromolecules. Outside the host cell, viruses are metabolically inert. Inside a host cell, their genome becomes integrated with that of the cell and they are metabolically active, exploiting the host cell's meta-bolic machinery to produce new copies of the viral genome, viral messenger RNA, and proteins and other constituents needed to form complete new virus particles (virions). The virion consists of nucleic acid surrounded by a protein coat called a capsid. This is surrounded in turn in some viruses by an envelope of lipoprotein that is attained when the virus particle is extruded through one of the host cell's membranes. The envelope serves to protect the nucleic acid in the external environment, and proteins associated with the envelope are important for virus attachment and entry into host cells. Taxonomy of viruses is similar to that of living organisms. The nature of the viral genome, how the virus reproduces, and structure of the virion are important taxonomic features. Classification of viruses to family, subfamily, and genus "is an easy task," whereas virus species "should be viewed as fuzzy sets with hazy boundaries" (van Regenmortel and Mahy 2004).

It is impractical to list all the viruses that have been recognized in wild birds and mammals. Every organism in the world that has been studied has yielded viruses, and it is safe to assume that every wild species is infected by a number of viruses, many of which have not been associated with disease. Virus families with selected examples of agents that are important in wild animals, either because they produce significant disease in wild animals or are transmissible to humans or domestic species in which they cause disease, are shown in table 3.4. Some viruses are highly host specific while others have very catholic tastes. For example, West Nile virus and St. Louis encephalitis virus are maintained in mosquitoes and birds but happily infect horses, people, and other mammals. This doesn't seem particularly striking until one considers that these viruses have to be sufficiently adaptable to overcome the defenses of poikilothermic invertebrates as well those of broadly divergent types of vertebrates. Similarly, San Miguel sea lion virus causes vesicles (fluid-filled blisters) on the flippers of California sea lions but also may infect domestic pigs and has been isolated from wild ocean fish. Some viruses cause little or no disease in one host but result in devastating disease in other species (e.g., the hantaviruses cause no apparent disease in their usual rodent hosts but may cause fatal disease in humans). A herpesvirus that causes no apparent disease in wildebeest (its usual host) causes fatal "wildebeest-associated" malignant catarrhal fever in cattle.

As a group, viruses are less hardy outside the an-

Table 3.4 Animal Virus Families with an Example of a Virus That Occurs in Wild Animals from Each Family

Family	Species	Principle hosts (disease)
DNA viruses		
Adenoviridae	Hemorrhagic disease of deer adenovirus	Black-tailed deer (adenovirus hemorrhagic disease of deer)
Asfarviridae	African swine fever virus	Warthog, wild boar (African swine fever)
Circoviridae	Psittacine beak and feather disease virus	Psittacine birds (psittacine beak and feather disease)
Herpesviridae	Anatid herpesvirus 1	Waterfowl (duck plague)
Papovaviridae	Cottontail rabbit papilloma virus	Cottontail rabbit (papillomatosis)
Parvoviridae	Canine parvovirus 2	Dogs, wild canids (parvovirus infection)
Poxviridae	Myxoma virus	Leporids (myxomatosis)
DNA and RNA reverse transcribing viruses		
Retroviridae	Koala retrovirus	Koala (lymphoid neoplasia)
RNA viruses		
Arenaviridae	Lassa fever virus	*Mastomys* spp. (Lassa fever in humans)
Bunyaviridae	Sin Nombre virus	*Peromyscus maniculatus* (hantavirus pulmonary syndrome in humans)
Caliciviridae	Rabbit hemorrhagic disease virus	European rabbit (rabbit hemorrhagic disease)
Coronaviridae	Feline infectious peritonitis virus	Domestic and wild felids (feline infectious peritonitis)
Filoviridae	Ebola virus	Primates, duiker (Ebola disease in humans)
Flaviviridae	Louping-ill virus	Red grouse, hares (louping ill)
Orthomyxoviridae	Influenzavirus A	Waterbirds, seals (influenza)
Paramyxoviridae	Canine distemper virus	Canids, mustelids, procyonids, some felids and seals (canine distemper)
Picornaviridae	Foot-and-mouth disease virus	Ungulates (foot-and-mouth disease)
Reoviridae	Bluetongue virus	Sheep, deer, pronghorns (bluetongue)
Rhabdoviridae	Rabies virus	Mammals (rabies)
Togoviridae	Eastern equine encephalomyelitis virus	Birds (eastern equine encephalomyelitis)

imal than bacteria or fungi. Consequently, many viral diseases are spread by intimate contact between infected and uninfected animals. However, some viruses, such as the parvoviruses, are extremely resistant in the external environment and foot-and-mouth virus has survived and spread hundreds of kilometers across oceans in air-borne droplets. Many virus infections are characterized by a short, sharp infection with recovery resulting in long-lasting immunity, as expected of a microparasite. At the opposite extreme, viruses such as the retroviruses (e.g., feline immunodeficiency virus, which infects domestic cats and wild lions [Packer et al. 1999]), persist for the lifetime of their host by integrating their genetic material into the genome of the host. Herpesviruses are notorious for lying hid-

den and latent, often within nervous tissue, as occurs with the herpesvirus that causes duck plague. These viruses may become activated and cause disease when the individual is stressed.

Bacteria

Bacteria are small (0.5 to 5 μm long), single-celled organisms with considerable morphologic diversity. Most have a rigid cell wall and multiply by binary fission. Many bacteria can be grown on inert artificial media, although two groups (rickettsia and chlamydiae) only grow in living cells. Bacteria are large enough to be seen with the light microscope and most bacteria can be separated into one of two groups based on the way that they stain when exposed to a particular stain invented by H. C. J.

Gram. Bacteria that stain blue with this stain, such as staphylococci and streptococci, are said to be gram-positive; those that stain pink, such as *Escherichia coli* and salmonellae, are said to be gram-negative. This stain often is used to identify the general type of bacteria that may be present in diseased tissue. Bacteria do not have a membrane-bound nucleus and contain a single chromosome with double-stranded DNA. There may be bits of extrachromosomal DNA (plasmids) that may encode for factors associated with disease, such as toxin production. Some bacteria are infected by viruses (bacteriophages) that may also provide genetic material that encodes for factors related to disease.

Most bacteria are free-living saprophytes utilizing organic and inorganic substrates. Some of these are facultative parasites that do not require a parasitic lifestyle, but that can take advantage of animals when the opportunity presents itself. Several bacteria in the genus *Clostridium* are examples of opportunistic disease agents. They normally live as saprophytes in the soil, but if introduced into a wound, they can grow in tissues, often causing severe injury and resulting in diseases such as gas gangrene and tetanus. A relatively small number of bacteria have become obligate parasites for at least part of their lives and a few, such as the rickettsia and chlamydiae, are only able to replicate within living host cells. Bacteria vary in their ability to persist in the external environment. Organisms of the genera *Bacillus* and *Clostridium* form highly resistant endospores that allow them to survive for years during adverse environmental conditions.

Bacteria are classified by the Linnaean system, so that species have a generic and a specific name (e.g., *Pasteurella multocida)*. There is sometimes huge variability within bacteria classified as a single species. For example, the strains or subtypes of *P. multocida* that cause avian cholera in birds are different from those that cause disease in mammals, and strains that cause the disease hemorrhagic septicemia in bison are different from those that cause pneumonia in bison. Ducks that die of avian cholera in western North America have a different type of *P. multocida* than that which causes the identical disease in common eiders on the Atlantic coast.

For practical purposes, bacteria are often arranged on the basis of what they look like rather than on a strict taxonomic basis. *Bergey's Manual of Determinative Bacteriology* (Holt et al. 1994), the ultimate source for bacterial identification, is arranged on a phenotypic basis, as this "is most useful for diagnostic purposes." Bacteria known to cause disease represent only a tiny fraction of the species described, and described species "represent only a fraction of those existing in nature" (Holt et al. 1994). The bacteria shown in table 3.5 are intended only to show the diversity of species associated with disease in wild animals.

Most bacterial infections are characterized by rapid proliferation of the bacteria in the animal's tissues followed by clearance as the host's immune response develops. Bacteria may persist in certain sites, such as the urinary tubules of the kidney or the nervous system, because the effects of the immune system are minimal there. In some chronic diseases, such as tuberculosis, bacteria may remain in localized foci for extended periods despite an immune response.

Fungi

Fungi are eukaryotes with a distinct nucleus, cell and nuclear membranes, Golgi apparatus, mitochondria, and cytoskeleton. Most fungi that cause disease in wild animals live free in the environment as saprophytes and are opportunistic parasites in debilitated animals or in animals that are exposed to the fungus in some unusual manner (table 3.6). Most fungi spread via resistant spores that can survive in the environment for an extended period. Many fungal (mycotic) diseases result from inhalation of spores that infect the lungs and then may spread secondarily to other organs. Less commonly, fungi gain entry to the body through skin wounds. Most mycotic diseases are chronic.

The most important mycotic infection in wild animals is aspergillosis, caused by infection with fungi in the genus *Aspergillus*, which occurs commonly in individual birds stressed by factors such as captivity or concurrent disease. In these birds, aspergillosis is often the proximate cause of death (fig. 3.3).

Aspergillosis occurs as an outbreak occasionally among birds feeding on feed or occupying areas in which *Aspergillus* is growing abundantly as a saprophyte (Neff 1955; Adrian et al. 1978). The underlying factors involved in some outbreaks are unknown (Zinkl et al. 1977b).

Most other fungal diseases occur sporadically in individual animals rather than as outbreaks. Infections are acquired from the environment rather than by contagion from an infected animal. *Candida albicans* is a yeast that is an inhabitant of mucous membranes, which occasionally causes disease in debilitated animals. Fungi of several genera cause a disease called *dermatophytosis* or *ringworm* that is

Table 3.5 Bacteria That Cause Specific Disease in Wild Birds and Mammals

Bacterial species	Principal animal hosts	Disease
Spirochetes		
Borrelia burgdorferi	Rodents, birds	Lyme disease in humans
Leptospira spp.	Raccoons, skunks, rodents	Leptospirosis
Gram-negative, aerobic/microaerophilic rods and cocci		
Brucella abortus	Bison, elk, cattle	Brucellosis
Francisella tularensis	Rodents, lagomorphs	Tularemia
Facultatively anaerobic gram-negative rods		
Escherichia coli	Many species	Primarily neonatal enteric infections
Salmonella spp.	Many species	Intestinal and generalized infections
Yersinia pestis	Rodents	Plague
Pasteurella multocida	Many species	Avian cholera in birds; pneumonia, hemorrhagic septicemia in mammals
Gram-negative, anaerobic, straight, curved, and helical bacteria		
Fusobacterium necrophorum	Ruminants, marsupials	Necrobacillosis
Rickettsias and chlamydias		
Ehrlichia chaffeensis	White-tailed deer	Human monocytic ehrlichiosis
Chlamydophila psittaci	Birds	Chlamydiosis
Gram-positive cocci		
Staphylococcus aureus	Many species	Skin infections, abscesses
Streptococcus spp.	Many species	Wound infections, purulent infections
Endospore-forming gram-positive rods and cocci		
Bacillus anthracis	Ungulates	Anthrax
Clostridium spp.	Various	Wound infections, gas gangrene, botulism, tetanus, Tyzzer's disease
Regular, nonsporing gram-positive rods		
Erysipelothrix rhusiopathiae	Mammals, birds	Sporadic wound infection, septicemia
Listeria monocytogenes	Many mammals	Sporadic brain or generalized infection
Irregular, nonsporing gram-positive rods		
Arcanobacterium pyogenes	Ruminants	Abscesses, purulent lesions
Mycobacteria		
Mycobacterium bovis	Bison, badger, brushtail possum, deer	Bovine tuberculosis
M. aviurn complex	Birds, incidental infection in mammals	Avian tuberculosis
M. avium paratuberculosis	Ruminants, others	Paratuberculosis (Johne's disease)
Mycoplasmas: cell wall-less bacteria		
Mycoplasma spp.	Many species	Secondary infections, pneumonia, arthritis

Note: The arrangement follows Holt et al. (1994).

an infection of the superficial layers of the skin and hair shafts. The infection results in breakage and loss of hair, with mild inflammation (fig. 3.4). The organisms that cause ringworm are unusual among fungi in that they are contagious obligate parasites that spread from infected animals to new animals through direct or indirect contact.

Protozoa

The protozoa are a large, diverse group of single-celled eukaryotic organisms, many of which have a complex life cycle. It is estimated that there may be 50,000 species, of which about 20% are parasitic in vertebrates and invertebrates. Their classification is confusing, and molecular biology is leading to

Table 3.6 Fungi Associated with Disease in Wild Birds and Mammals

Fungal species	Disease	Animals	Comments
Superficial skin infection			
Trichophyton spp., *Microsporum* spp.	Dermatophytosis (ringworm)	Sporadic cases in many mammals	Obligate parasites that spread from animal to animal
Disease of mucous membranes			
Candida albicans	Thrush	Birds, mammals	Normal inhabitant of mucous membranes
Systemic disease (opportunistic parasites)			
Aspergillus fumigatus	Aspergillosis	Birds	Important respiratory disease of birds, occasionally in outbreaks
Coccidiodes immitis	Coccidiomycosis	Sporadic cases in mammals	Restricted distribution in the New World
Blastomyces dermatitidis	Blastomycosis	Sporadic cases in mammals	Restricted distribution in North America, Middle East, Africa
Cryptococcus neoformans	Cryptococcosis	Sporadic cases in mammals	Worldwide in temperate and tropical areas
Chrysosporium spp.	Adiaspiromycosis	Fossorial (burrowing) mammals	Pulmonary infection, rarely clinical disease
Histoplasma capsulatum	Histoplasmosis	Sporadic cases in mammals	Pulmonary infection by inhalation of spores from soils enriched by bird or bat droppings

major changes. From a practical perspective, it is easier to discuss these parasites based on the part of the animal's body that is infected (table 3.7) rather than on a taxonomic basis. Some protozoa that require more than one host species to complete their life cycle occupy different niches in their different hosts. For example, parasites of the genera *Sarcocystis, Toxoplasma,* and *Frenkelia* require two different host animals (a predator and one or more prey species) to complete their life cycle. They inhabit the intestine of the predator and other body tissues of the prey host (which is usually a herbivore). Most protozoa behave like microparasites in that they are small, have a short generation time, have high rates of reproduction in the host, and tend to produce immunity to reinfection in hosts that survive.

A major feature of protozoal infections is that the severity of disease is related directly to the intensity of the infection; the more organisms that are present, the more severe the disease. The intensity of infection is usually determined by the number of infective forms that enter the animal initially (the infective dose). For example, many apparently healthy Richardson's ground squirrels in Saskatchewan have cysts in their muscles (fig. 3.5) that are one stage of a protozoan called *Sarcocystis campestris* that cycles between badgers and ground squirrels. Infection by this parasite is very widespread among ground squirrels, but there is no evidence from the wild that it causes disease (i.e., wild squirrels are not found sick or dying of this infection). However, when we experimentally infected ground squirrels with sporocysts of this parasite recovered from the intestine of a badger, most of the squirrels died, and the severity of disease was related to the number of sporocysts that the animals received (Wobeser et al. 1983). In nature, most ground squirrels likely encounter only a small number of sporocysts and suffer little ill effect from the infection. Individual squirrels that ingest many sporocysts probably succumb to the infection and die underground, or are debilitated and killed by predators, including badgers. (Producing disease in the squirrel likely enhances the probability that it will be eaten by a badger, which is to the parasite's advantage. This will be discussed more fully in chapter 5.)

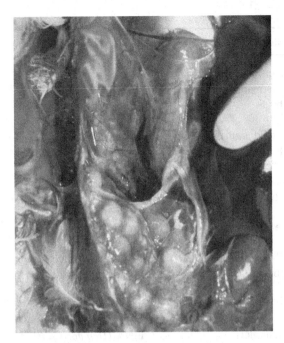

Fig. 3.3. Lesions of the disease aspergillosis in the lungs of a Canada goose. The multiple white nodules are chronic granulomas formed in response to infection with the opportunistic fungus *Aspergillus fumigatus*.

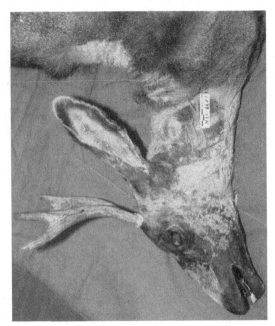

Fig 3.4. Severe dermatophytosis or ringworm in a mule deer from Saskatchewan. The animal was infected by the fungus *Trichophyton verrucosum*, which grows in the superficial layers of the skin and within hair shafts, weakening the hair so that it breaks easily at the skin surface.

Metazoa

The metazoa are an artificial and extremely diverse assemblage of multicellular animals that includes arthropods and various types of worms (helminths). These are the organisms that are usually thought of as "parasites" when different types of diseases are being discussed. In an ecological sense, most are macroparasites in that they are visible with the naked eye, are long-lived, usually do not replicate extensively within the host, result in infections that tend to be chronic, and provide short-lived immunity with reinfection occurring commonly. As with protozoa, the effect of metazoa on the host is highly dependent upon the intensity of infection. Individuals with few parasites are unlikely to have overt disease, while those with many parasites may be harmed severely. For example, moose calves that received 164 or 200 infective larvae of *Parelaphostrongylus tenuis* rapidly developed severe fatal disease, calves given 15 or 30 larvae developed moderate to severe nonresolving neurological signs, and calves given 3–10 larvae developed clinical signs that abated or disappeared (Lankester 2002).

A general feature of parasitism by metazoa is that the distribution of parasites is aggregated across the population (Shaw et al. 1998; Wilson et al. 2001).

Most members of a population have few or no parasites of a particular species, while the majority of the population of the parasite is concentrated in a few animals (fig. 3.6). This has important consequences including the following:

- Severe negative effects (detectable disease) are concentrated in the few heavily infected individuals.
- A small proportion of the host population is responsible for most of the parasite transmission.
- It is difficult to measure parasitism rates and the effects of parasitism in populations without examining large samples of animals.

Because of the diversity of taxa, lifestyles, and ecological niches filled by metazoa it is difficult to give a simple overview of the group. Table 3.8 is organized on the basis of the area of the host body inhabited by the parasite and life style.

NONINFECTIOUS TRANSMISSIBLE DISEASES

Discovery of the TSE and the importance of diseases such as chronic wasting disease of wild cervids (CWD), bovine spongiform encephalopathy (BSE), and Creutzfeldt-Jacob disease of humans

Table 3.7 Protozoa That Cause Disease in Wild Animals

Genus	Life cycle	Wild species infected	Type of disease
Parasites of the intestinal tract or other epithelial membranes			
Giardia	Cysts passed in feces are ingested from the environment.	Many mammals and birds	Often subclinical, diarrhea (*Giardiasis*)
Eimeria, Isospora, Cryptosporidium	Complex reproduction in host, oocysts passed in feces are ingested from the environment.	All wild animals likely have species of "coccidia" that are more or less host specific.	Often subclinical but diarrhea and intestinal injury may be fatal. (*Coccidiosis*)
Parasites that invade tissues			
Sarcocystis, Frenkelia, Toxoplasma, Besnoitia	Sexual replication in carnivore intestine, asexual replication in tissues of the alternate host.	Life cycle involves a predator-prey relation-ship, e.g., raptor-rodent.	Infection in carnivore seldom results in detect-able disease. Infection of the alternate host varies from subclinical to fatal.
Hepatozoon	Sexual replication in invertebrates, asexual replication with gamonts in blood cells of vertebrates.	Many vertebrates, includ-ing reptiles, birds, and mammals	Highly variable, may involve anemia or tissue injury (*Hepatozoonosis*)
Histomonas meleagridis	Infects nematode *Heter-akis* spp. in bird's intestine, carried in nematode's eggs and larvae to next bird.	Galliform birds	Intestinal and liver injury (*Histomoniasis, black-head*)
Parasites that inhabit the blood (*Hematozoa*)			
Plasmodium	Sexual replication in blood-feeding inverte-brate and asexual repli-cation in tissues of the alternate host, with para-sitism of circulating blood cells. Transmission to invertebrate occurs via ingested blood.	Many species infect wild mammals and birds.	Transmitted by mosquitoes. Often subclinical but fatal disease may occur in unusual hosts. (*Malaria*)
Trypansosoma, Leishmania		Infection widespread in wild animals in some areas	Major concern is role of wild animals as reser-voir for humans and domestic animals
Theileria, Cytauxzoon, Babesia		Various species infect wild mammals, trans-mitted by ticks	Wild animals as reservoir for diseases of humans and domestic animals
Leucocytozoon		Transmitted by blackflies (Simullidae)	Subclinical to fatal anemia (*Leucocytozoonis*)
Haemoproteus		Parasites of birds	Transmitted by biting midges (*Culicoides* spp.); usually subclinical

Note: This list is intended only to give a flavor of the thousands of protozoa that have been reported and the unknown number that wait to be described.

have confused the definition of what is an infectious or noninfectious disease. The currently accepted wisdom is that these diseases are caused by a change in structure and function of a normal host cell protein called the prion protein (PrP) (Prusiner 1998; Legname et al. 2004). Normal PrP (often called PrP^C) is found at highest concentration in nerve cells, and its biological function has not been defined. Disease is associated with accumulation of a form of the protein that is structurally different from PrP^C and that is resistant to enzymes (proteases) that break down normal proteins. This abnormal, resistant form of the protein, often called PrP^{res}, has identical amino acid sequences to PrP^C but differs in the way that the protein molecule is folded. The unique feature of the TSE is that once PrP^{res} enters a suitable animal either by some natural route or experimentally, it may promote production of PrP^{res} from PrP^C. There is good evidence that the condition can be passed from one individual to another in some TSE, particularly in CWD (Miller and Williams 2003). Although the method by which transmission occurs is unknown, deer may become affected by CWD from exposure to environments in which affected deer had lived or died previously (Miller et al. 2004b). Because of their transmissibility, various TSE may behave like an infectious disease but, because the agent has no genetic identity (no nucleic acid), the disease also might be perceived as a form of intoxication rather than an infectious disease. Miller and Williams (2003) used the

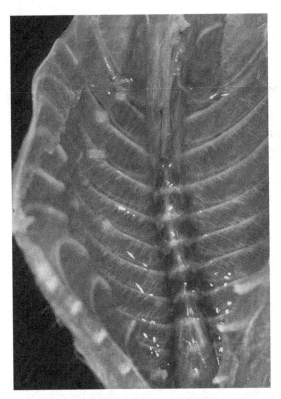

Fig 3.5. The tiny white lines visible in the muscle of this Richardson's ground squirrel are the cyst form of a protozoan parasite *Sarcocystis campestris,* which cycles between badgers and ground squirrels.

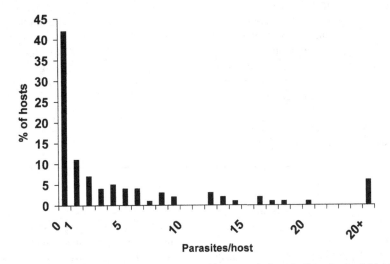

Fig. 3.6. Distribution of a hypothetical nematode parasite within a population of wild animals. A highly aggregated distribution of this type is typical of many parasites, with most animals having few or no parasites, and a few individuals having a large number of parasites.

Table 3.8 Metazoan Parasites of Wild Animals

Parasite group	Life cycle	Wild species involved	Comments
Ectoparasites			
Blood-feeding flies	Parasitic as adults only; individual flies often feed on multiple hosts.	Mammals and birds	Important for direct effects and as vectors of other disease agents
Fleas	Feed on blood as adults; larvae are free in the environment	Predominantly mammals, fewer on birds	Some species are vectors for other diseases, notably plague.
Lice	Direct life cycle, eggs laid on surface of host's skin, spread by contact	Mammals and birds	Some feed on blood, others on portions of skin; cannot survive away from host.
Mites	Obligate parasites, transferred by direct contact	Mammals and birds	Infestation with some genera (*Sarcoptes*, *Psoroptes*) cause severe skin disease.
Ticks	Some species have one host for all life cycle stages, others use different host species for different stages.	Mammals and birds	A few species cause direct disease; many are vectors for infectious agents.
Endoparasites			
Warble, bot, and flesh flies	Obligate parasites as immature stages	Predominantly rodents, leporids, and ruminants	Some inhabit the nasopharyngeal area, others inhabit subcutaneous tissues.
Nematodes (roundworms)	Extremely diverse	All species	Various species inhabit niches within all tissues of the body.
Cestodes (tapeworms)	Two-host life cycle that may involve two vertebrates or a vertebrate and an invertebrate	All species	The larval form is often more injurious than the adult tapeworm.
Trematodes (flukes)	Complex indirect life cycles that involves free-swimming stage(s) and infection of mollusk(s)	Most species	Most infections involve the digestive tract (intestine, liver, pancreas).
Acanthocephalids (thorny-headed worms)	Life cycle involves an invertebrate and a vertebrate host.	Usually aquatic species	Intestinal parasites

term "contagious prion disease." It is likely more correct to describe animals with a TSE as *affected* rather than *infected*.

Exactly how PrP^{res} produces disease is unknown, but the various conditions in different species are characterized pathologically by noninflammatory degenerative changes in the brain (encephalopathy), with cavities or spaces in specific sites that cause the brain tissue to resemble a sponge microscopically, hence, the term "spongiform" (fig. 3.7). At present, the most important TSE in wildlife is CWD that affects mule deer, white-tailed deer, and elk. A form of TSE called transmissible mink encephalopathy also has been diagnosed in ranch mink, and disease has

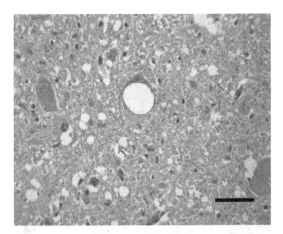

Fig. 3.7. Photomicrograph of a stained section of brain tissue from an elk with chronic wasting disease. The empty vacuoles in the brain tissue and nerve cells are typical of transmissible spongiform encephalopathy. (Bar = 50 μm)

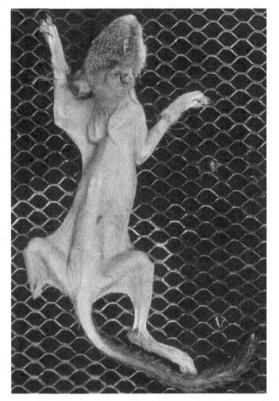

Fig. 3.8. Lack of hair (hypotrichosis) in a young Richardson's ground squirrel. The cause of this condition is unknown, but the circumstances in which the animal was found suggested an inherited condition.

occurred in certain zoo animals in association with BSE in cattle (Young and Slocombe 2003; Cunningham et al. 2004). Williams (2001) provides a review of TSE in wild animals. Collins et al. (2004) has a recent review of TSE in general, and Belay et al. (2004) discuss the potential risk from CWD for humans.

NONINFECTIOUS CAUSES OF DISEASE

The term "noninfectious disease" is a catchall for conditions not caused by living organisms that colonize the body. Included within this group are diseases caused by genetic disorders; physical agents including heat, cold, trauma, and radiation; metabolic alterations; degenerative changes; deficiency of required nutrients; and chemicals including human-made contaminants and natural toxins.

Genetic Disorders

Genetic disorders are relatively common in domestic animals as a result of inbreeding and selection for specific traits and also occur in small, closed human societies (e.g., Khoury 1985). It is unlikely that genetic disorders are common in large out-bred populations of wild animals because of negative selective pressure, although individual animals are found with conditions that are suggestive of a genetic disorder (fig. 3.8). Genetic disorders are likely to be more common in small populations and to become more important as habitats for wild animals become increasingly fragmented, resulting in isolated subpopulations in which inbreeding may occur. Inbreeding effect may be evident in some island populations.

Eldridge et al. (1999) documented reduced fecundity and increased levels of fluctuating asymmetry in an island population of wallabies and regarded this as evidence of inbreeding depression.

An important part of identifying genetic disease in humans and domestic animals is the ability to examine family trees to establish the pattern of inheritance. It is more difficult to identify genetic disorders in wild animals than in humans or domestic animals because of the difficulty in identifying individuals and establishing their genealogy. It is important to distinguish between "congenital" and inherited disorders. The term "congenital" simply means present at birth or hatching, and congenital disorders may be caused by a great variety of factors including various types of infection of the mother or the developing embryo/fetus, certain contaminants, and physical factors such as overheating or cooling of eggs. Inherited disorders are the result of a genetic abnormality, and they may be evident at birth (i.e., congenital) or develop later in life.

Physical Agents

Physical agents including cold, heat, and trauma
from natural events such as hail storms can usually
be linked to injury by association in time and space.
These stochastic events are unlikely to be important
at a population level except at the extremes of a
population's range or for very small populations.
Human-induced trauma in the form of muscle injury
(capture myopathy) is an unfortunate and to some
degree preventable side-effect of capturing and handling wild animals.

Metabolic Alterations and Degenerative Changes

Little is known about the occurrence of metabolic
disturbances such as diabetes mellitus, adrenocortical dysfunction, and pregnancy toxemia in wild animals, although such conditions undoubtedly occur.
Amyloidosis, which is the result of an accumulation
of abnormal protein in tissues, occurs in wild birds
relatively commonly. Degenerative diseases such as
dental attrition (fig. 3.9) and joint disease (fig. 3.10)
are common in aged wild animals and are a predisposing cause to mortality from starvation and
predation.

Deficiency of Required Nutrients

Food supply is one of the basic limiting factors for
wild populations. Food supply may influence both
survival and reproduction negatively, but the effects
of reduced or diminished supply are not easy to
quantify. Some wild animals die directly of starvation (loss of body condition and functions to the
point of death). Others may develop specific dysfunctions, such as the occurrence of osteoporosis in
malnourished moose calves in Norway (Ytrehus et
al. 1999), but protein-energy malnutrition often is
intertwined inextricably with predation and other
forms of disease. As discussed earlier, it may be impossible to decide if individual animals are malnourished because of the demands of parasites or if parasites have flourished because of reduced resistance
as a result of malnutrition.

It is unlikely that most wild animals within their
historic range suffer severely from deficiency of
specific factors such as essential nutrients, unless
the environment has changed in some manner so
that the nutrient becomes less available or the usual
diet of the animals changes for some reason. The
first type of alteration was discussed earlier in this
chapter (i.e., the hypothesis that acidification in
some areas has reduced availability of calcium re-

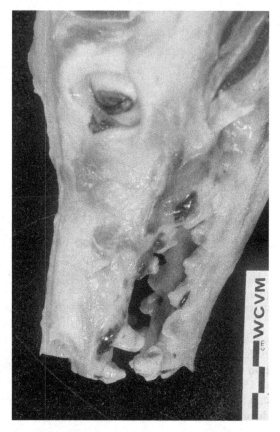

Fig. 3.9. Severe dental wear and attrition in an aged
coyote.

sulting in impaired reproduction in birds). As an example of the second type, we have observed vitamin
A deficiency, sometimes together with secondary
bacterial infection, in mallards overwintering in
western Canada (Wobeser and Kost 1992). The etiology of this condition involves the creation of
open-water areas below dams that have allowed
ducks to overwinter far to the north of their normal
range. The overwintering birds feed exclusively on
cereal grains that are deficient in beta-carotenes for
months at a time, resulting in deficiency of vitamin
A (Honour et al. 1995). Occasionally, wild animals
may experience a nutritional imbalance as a result of
a natural event. Van Pelt and Caley (1974) recognized bone defects in growing red fox pups in
Alaska that corresponded to the disease called nutritional secondary hyperparathyroidism that is well
documented in growing dogs and other carnivores
fed a diet of skeletal muscle that contains excess
phosphorus and inadequate calcium. Investigation
of prey remains about fox dens suggested that be-

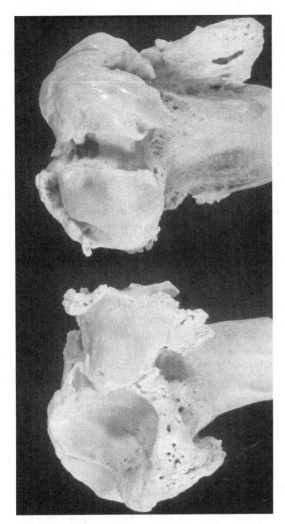

Fig. 3.10. Hind limb bones from an aged mule deer with severe degenerative joint disease.

cause of the easy availability of snowshoe hares at the peak of their cyclic abundance, fox pups were eating almost nothing but muscle.

Chemicals

There is a huge literature on the association between chemical substances and wild animals. A cause:effect relationship between exposure to the chemical and disease has been established clearly for some substances, such as those in table 3.9, but residues of many other compounds that have not been linked conclusively to a clearly defined disease are known to occur in the tissues of wild animals. Some of these chemicals may be acting as precipitating or contributing causes to other conditions, for example by modifying immune or hormonal function, but as-

sociations of this indirect type are difficult to prove conclusively or to separate from the effects of other nonspecific stressors, such as malnutrition, that might have similar effects. Effects of chemicals and contaminants usually have been considered at the individual animal level. The book *Population Ecotoxicology* (Newman 2001) is an important attempt to understand the effects of this form of noninfectious disease at the population level. Nutrients and toxicants will be discussed in more detail in chapter 9.

DISEASES OF UNKNOWN CAUSATION

There are many conditions in wild animals for which the cause is unknown, such as AVM in bald eagles and many examples of neoplasia (fig. 3.11). Such conditions are termed *idiopathic*. It is probable that many idiopathic conditions will be found to be caused by currently undiscovered infectious agents. If the suggestion that only 0.4% of extant bacterial species have been identified (Relman 1998) is correct, there is tremendous scope for discovery of new agents and new diseases.

SUMMARY

• Identifying the cause is an important step in understanding a disease.

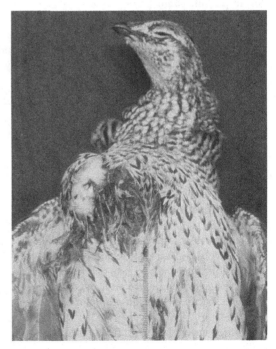

Fig. 3.11. Sharp-tailed grouse with a benign tumor (fibroma) growing from the skin.

Table 3.9 Chemical Substances That Cause Disease in Wild Animals

Substance (source for animals)	Species usually affected	Type of disease (comment)
Naturally occurring substances		
Types C and E botulinum toxin (produced by different strains of the bacterium *Clostridium botulinum* growing in decaying organic material)	Type C: freshwater ducks, American coots, shorebirds Type E: fish-eating birds	Neuroparalytic toxin (botulism)
Domoic acid (produced by certain marine algae, concentrated by shellfish)	Marine mammals and birds	Neuroparalytic toxin
Mycotoxins (secondary metabolites from fungi growing on cereal grains)	Seed-eating birds, mammals	Multiple effects, including immunosuppression
Cyanobacterial toxins (produced by blue-green algae, particularly in enriched euthrophic waters)	Birds, occasionally mammals	Lethal, sublethal effects poorly defined
Naturally occurring elements whose distribution and concentration has been altered by human activities		
Lead (lead shot, paint, mine tailings)	Birds, particularly waterbirds, with secondary poisoning of raptors	Usually chronic, anemia, paralysis.
Mercury (industrial process, fossil fuels)	Waterbirds, aquatic carnivores	Neurological
Oil (contamination of water)	Seabirds	Hypothermia, anemia
Selenium (leached from soil in irrigation drain water)	Waterbirds	Reproductive failure
Anthropogenic compounds		
Cholinesterase-inhibiting insecticides	Birds, less commonly mammals; secondary poisoning of scavengers	Usually acutely lethal
Organochlorine insecticides	Particularly birds	May be directly lethal or have sublethal effects of reproduction

- The words "cause" and "etiology" have a different meaning. Etiology includes a consideration of the factors that influence how the causative factor(s) reach or affect the animal.
- Formal criteria are available to examine putative cause:effect relationships.
- Infectious diseases are caused by living organisms involved in a trophic relationship with the animal in which the organism derives benefit and the host is harmed. Infectious agents include viruses, bacteria, fungi, algae, protozoa, and metazoa.
- Infection must be clearly differentiated from disease.
- Not all infectious diseases are contagious and not all infected individuals are infectious.
- The transmissible spongiform encephalopathies are considered to be *noninfectious transmissible diseases* caused by a structural change in a normal protein. Although not caused by a living agent, some TSE are contagious.
- Noninfectious diseases include those caused by genetic disorders, physical and chemical agents, metabolic alterations, degenerative changes, nutritional imbalances, and deficiencies.
- Idiopathic diseases are diseases currently of unknown causation.

4

How Disease Is Detected, Described, and Measured

FINDING DISEASE

Disease occurs in myriad forms and shapes. Although it is obvious that disease is present when windrows of dead ducks wash up on a lakeshore, crows fall dead from trees, skunks make unprovoked attacks on dogs, or blind elk stumble into contact with humans, this type of situation is the exception. The vast majority of disease occurrences in wild animals is invisible and unrecognized, even for those diseases that may be lethal. Disease among wild species often is likened to an iceberg in that only a tiny tip projects above the water to be visible while the bulk of disease is hidden from view. Detecting covert disease is complicated further because very few people are looking for or observing wild animals on a regular basis. Even when large conspicuous species are involved, obvious disease may go unrecognized.

In 1977, lesser snow geese (large, conspicuous white birds) were found dead near a small lake in western Saskatchewan, and we diagnosed the bacterial disease avian cholera as the cause of their death. In subsequent years, we have found snow geese dead of this disease every spring over an area of Saskatchewan that is used as a spring staging area by the birds. There never have been many dead geese at any one location, but dead birds could always be found if a day was spent visiting wetlands (fig. 4.1). However, during the more than 25 years since the first recognition of the disease, mortality of snow geese has never again been reported by a member of the public to a conservation officer in the area, perhaps because relatively few people prowl wetlands in the spring. Some of the birds died in areas where I would have expected that they might have been seen by a member of the public. As a minor test of the ability of the public to observe this type of mortality, I placed recently dead snow geese along the margins of small ephemeral ponds ("sheet water") in bare agricultural fields near well-traveled country roads. Even under these circumstances, the large, white, dead birds were never reported.

The circumstances in which diseased wild animals are most likely to be detected include:

- Mass die-offs of conspicuous species. A major factor in determining whether or not disease is recognized is the amount of use of the area by people. For example, small outbreaks of duck plague involving only a few ducks often are recognized in city parks, while very few of the thousands of ducks that die of lead poisoning are detected (Humberg et al. 1986; Stutzenbaker et al. 1986). Similarly, die-offs of passerine birds caused by infection with *Salmonella* bacteria are recognized commonly among birds at bird feeders (Daoust et al. 2000; Refsum et al. 2003), but similar-sized birds that die under other circumstances are very difficult to detect (Wobeser and Wobeser 1992).
- Individual large animals that are conspicuous because of abnormal behavior, such as bald eagles acting abnormally because of avian vacuolar myelinopathy (Thomas et al. 1998) or moose with neurologic disease caused by infection with the nematode *Parelaphostrongylus tenuis*.
- Animals with conspicuous external abnormalities that are observed at close range, for example, skin tumors in hunter-killed deer (fig. 4.2) and inflammation caused by *Mycoplasma gallisepticum* about the eyes of house finches visiting bird feeders (Hartup et al. 2001).
- Species that are the subject of intense observation or interest. Often this occurs when disease

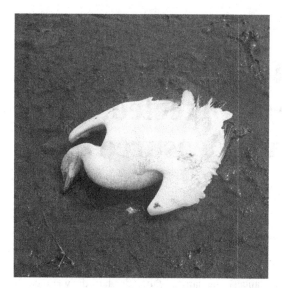

Fig. 4.1. Lesser snow goose dead of avian cholera. Even though carcasses of this type appear conspicuous, most such deaths go unrecognized and unreported.

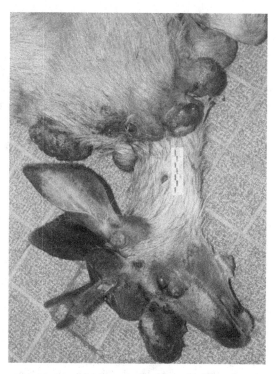

Fig. 4.2. Mule deer with numerous fibropapillomas on the skin of the head and neck. Even conspicuous lesions such as these are difficult to observe on wild animals, and hunters often are not aware of the lesions until after they have shot such an animal.

in wild animals is linked with a human health risk. For example, since 2001 many dead wild birds have been found and reported in areas where West Nile virus has been circulating in North America. Only a small proportion of the birds examined have been infected with the virus, suggesting that most of the dead birds were "background mortality" that usually went unrecognized. Individual species may be scrutinized for other reasons, for example, Sidor et al. (2003) estimated that 28% of adult common loons that died in New Hampshire over a 12 year period were recovered for necropsy. This high recovery rate was possible because the "loon population in New England is unusual in the degree of scrutiny it receives." Individual species attract different amounts of attention based on the value that people place on them. In a study of tuberculosis in birds, Smit et al. (1987) commented that "gulls become important only when several birds are found, whereas even a single dead or sick raptor always seems to be important."

In circumstances other than those described above, the presence of disease in wild animals is unlikely to be detected without some form of active, targeted surveillance even though the disease may

be occurring relatively commonly in a large, high-profile species. The recent discovery that bovine tuberculosis and chronic wasting disease (CWD) are widespread in white-tailed deer in Michigan and Wisconsin, respectively, and that the diseases likely have been present in these populations for years prior to discovery, illustrates this point. A single case of tuberculosis recognized in a hunter-killed deer in 1994 (Schmitt et al. 1997) led to targeted surveillance that identified 151 additional infected deer by 1999 (Palmer et al. 1999).

Many methods have been used to search for disease in wild populations, but these can be categorized into four basic types of surveillance:

1. Searching for sick or dead animals
2. Searching for the causative agent
3. Searching for a physiologic response to the causative agent
4. Searching for evidence of the disease or the causative agent in a species other than the primary species

SEARCHING FOR SICK OR DEAD ANIMALS

Finding animals that are sick with or that have died of a disease is the most direct evidence that disease (i.e., dysfunction) is occurring in an area or population. (The definition of population will be discussed in chapter 11. Here I will use the word only to describe a group of animals.) However, this technique has limited application and invariably results in an underestimation of the actual frequency of occurrence of disease. Sick and dead wild animals are very difficult to find. Sick animals are likely to hide, and clinical signs of disease are often ephemeral in wild animals so that there may be only a transient window of time during which a sick animal might be detected. Wild animals seem to be good at disguising illness, probably because animals with obvious dysfunction are likely to be recognized by predators and removed from the population (Moore 2002). Sick animals that die of disease or that recover also are lost to this form of surveillance.

Recent experience with CWD in wild deer is illustrative. It is believed that CWD is a progressive, invariably fatal disease. Abnormal prion can be detected in the lymphoid organs and brains of deer for months before the animals display clinical signs. Deer die soon after they begin to display clinical signs. Thus, there is only a short window of time in the course of CWD in an individual deer during which clinical illness could be detected. In Colorado and Wyoming, only 3% (4/133) of hunter-killed deer that tested positive for the presence of abnormal prion in their tissues had clinical signs of disease (Miller et al. 2000). If only the clinically affected animals had been used to estimate prevalence, the frequency of occurrence of CWD in the population would have been calculated to be 0.1%. However, 4.9% of the deer tested had abnormal prion in their tissues.

Similarly, Cavanagh et al. (2002) found that 13 of a sample of 180 voles had clinical signs compatible with vole tuberculosis (*Mycobacterium microti* infection). Based on the presence of clinically evident disease, 7% of the voles were considered to be infected. When the animals were necropsied, a further 25 voles were found to have lesions, so that at least 21% of the animals had tuberculosis. If tissues from all voles had been cultured for *M. microti,* the actual frequency of occurrence of infection undoubtedly would have been even greater, because some voles with recent infections may not have developed visible lesions. (Necropsy is the term used for the postmortem examination of animals; autopsy, from Greek *autopsiā*—seeing with one's own eyes, is usually reserved for the postmortem examination of humans.)

Searching for animals with clinical signs of disease is most applicable for those few conditions that have conspicuous external features that can be detected at a distance, such as hair loss caused by mange in coyotes and winter tick infestation in moose, and mycoplasmal conjunctivitis in house finches. Even in diseases with conspicuous abnormalities, early or mild cases will be missed. L'Heureux et al. (1996) reported that although "external lesions are readily observable" in bighorn sheep lambs infected with the viral disease contagious ecthyma, it was not possible to monitor infections at a distance, except for animals with "severe lesions and bleeding sores." The clinical signs of many diseases are not sufficiently specific or distinct so that an observer can be confident that the animals actually have the disease in question. For instance, raccoons infected with canine distemper virus act similarly to animals infected with rabies virus and the diseases cannot be reliably differentiated on the basis of clinical signs.

Carcasses of animals that have died of disease are removed rapidly by scavengers (e.g., Peterson et al. 2000) and become unavailable for detection. The rate of removal is likely to be more rapid when the animals involved are small and when only a few animals die, so that the scavengers are not satiated. Even when many carcasses are available, they may disappear rapidly. I described an experiment in chapter 2 in which we tested the persistence of small dead birds placed in an open field to simulate an ongoing disease outbreak (Wobeser and Wobeser 1992). Although 250 chicks were placed in a 1 ha area over a 5 day period and 10% of the area was searched systematically each day during the 5-day outbreak and for a further 5 days, only 1 intact chick was recovered. Scavenging was covert and we only observed the removal of 1 chick. Had this been an actual disease outbreak, we would not have recognized that it had occurred despite massive mortality (250 birds/ha) and intense surveillance. Surveillance for dead corvid birds has been used extensively during the recent incursion of West Nile virus into North America. It provides information on geographic distribution and spread of the disease and an index to regional virus activity but yields little information on the actual extent of the infection or the

consequences for the bird population. Mammal carcasses also disappear quickly. Because aborted fetuses are an important source of infection in the disease brucellosis in bison, elk, and cattle, Cook et al.
(2003) monitored the disappearance of bovine fetuses placed experimentally in habitat used by elk.
The average time for a fetus to disappear was 25.3
hours and 90% of fetuses were gone within 69.5
hours.

Searches for sick or dead animals are subject to
many forms of bias. Large animals are detected
more readily than small animals and brightly col-
ored species are found more easily than cryptic
species (Cliplef and Wobeser 1993; Philibert et al.
1993). The ease with which sick or dead animals can
be found and the rate at which carcasses are removed by scavengers are highly variable, unpredictable, and site specific.

The degree of variability that can occur is illustrated by reports of three outbreaks of rabbit hemorrhagic disease (RHD), a viral disease of European
rabbits. During the first outbreak of RHD in an area
of Spain about $55 \pm 27\%$ of the rabbit population
died over about a 1 month period, and 45 dead rabbits were collected in an intensively searched 10 ha
area (Villafuerte et al. 1994). In a park in Australia,
the initial outbreak of RHD reduced the rabbit population by about 95% over about a 1 month period.
Although a large proportion of the rabbits died underground, "there were so many carcasses that most
were left to decompose largely or completely intact"
despite vast numbers of scavenging birds (Mutze et
al. 1998). In contrast, in an area of France, a combination of myxomatosis (another viral disease) and
RHD resulted in an annual mortality rate of 88% in
adult and 99% in juvenile rabbits. Although it was
estimated that about 300 rabbits died on a small
study area during a year, only 1 dead rabbit was recovered despite intense surveys of a park where the
grass was mowed regularly (Marchandeau et al.
1998).

The use of radiotelemetry, particularly if the radios
are fitted with mortality sensors that facilitate recovery of dead animals for examination, provides a
unique window through which the actual population
effects caused by disease can be viewed. In these situations, the size of the population at risk (the marked
animals) is known and carcasses can be recovered
while suitable for necropsy. Such studies often provide a very different picture of disease occurrence
than that obtained by "passive surveillance" (waiting
for someone to report diseased animals) or even active searching for carcasses (table 4.1).

SEARCHING FOR THE CAUSATIVE AGENT

Surveying for the causative agent may provide a
more complete picture of the frequency with which
a disease occurs in the population than looking for
sick or dead animals. This is because animals are
often infected with agents, have elevated levels of
toxic substances in their tissues, or are deficient in
some required nutrient before they appear ill or die,
and because disease may be subclinical or fleetingly
clinical in many diseases. Samples can be collected
from either dead or live animals for this purpose.
Many such techniques are used in studying disease
in wild animals (table 4.2). Examination of feces for
parasitic eggs and oocysts is the most commonly
employed method of this type.

Many factors must be considered when using the
presence of a causative agent to detect or monitor
the occurrence of disease in an animal population.
Infection or contamination with residues is not synonymous with disease. Detecting the agent in an animal does not mean that the animal is currently, or
will in the future become, diseased. A second factor
is that the number of agents or the amount of residue
detected in samples may not relate directly to the intensity of infection or contamination. This is best
documented for helminth parasites in which the
number of eggs in an animal's feces may not be indicative of the number of worms present in that animal. A third factor is that not all the individuals that
are infected or that have a causative factor in their
tissue will be detected. There are a number of reasons why some animals may be missed including
the following:

1. Recently infected animals may not have eggs,
   larva, oocysts, bacteria, or virus in the tissues or
   excreta that are tested. (In the case of macroparasites, recently infected animals that have not
   yet begun to shed eggs are said to be in the
   prepatent period.)
2. Infectious agents may be present only periodically or sporadically in the tissues or excreta
   examined, for example, many helminth parasites
   produce eggs only sporadically, and birds infected with duck plague virus infection shed the
   virus infrequently.
3. The tissue distribution of agents and residues
   may vary with the length of time since exposure. For instance, the tissue distribution of lead
   varies with the time since ingestion. Lead
   residues in liver and kidney are indicative of recent exposure, and lead residues in bone are indicative of exposure in the more distant past. If

Table 4.1 Studies in Which Radiotelemetry Has Been Used to Monitor Disease

Disease	Species	Comments
Tularemia	Cottontail rabbit	During a period in which population decreased by 72%, 32% of marked rabbits died of tularemia but only one unmarked rabbit was found dead of the disease.[1]
Rabbit hemorrhagic disease	European rabbit	Radio-marked animals were used to define the beginning and end of the outbreak. Mortality was detected in marked animals for >3 weeks after the last unmarked animal was found dead.[2]
Rabies	Striped skunk	70% of marked population died of rabies, 31% of which died underground. The outbreak would have gone undetected in the area except for radio-marked animals.[3]
Hemorrhagic disease	White-tailed deer	8% of marked deer died of hemorrhagic disease over 1 month period; no mortality of deer was reported in the area and the event would have gone undetected except for radio-marked animals.[4]
Infectious diseases	Eurasian lynx	40% of marked animals died of infections vs. 18% of animals found dead opportunistically.[5]
Oiling	River otter	Carcasses of 27 otter marked with radio were recovered, only 4 of which were found in locations where they might have been found by beach searches.[6]
West Nile virus infection	American crow	68% of marked birds died of West Nile Virus infection.[7]

[1]Woolf et al. (1993).
[2]Villafuerte et al. (1994).
[3]Greenwood et al. (1997).
[4]Beringer et al. (2000).
[5]Schmidt-Posthaus et al. (2002).
[6]Bowyer et al. (2003).
[7]Yaremych et al. (2004).

only bone is examined, animals exposed recently to lead may be missed.

4. Agents may be present but latent or hidden and undetectable with most techniques. This is particularly a problem with herpesvirus infections, such as duck plague virus.

5. The tissue or excreta sampled may be inappropriate for detecting the agent. Culturing swabs of the nasal cavity has been used for many years to detect wild sheep that are carrying *Mannheimia haemolytica,* a bacterium involved in pneumonia; however, the bacterium was isolated from only 4 of 19 bighorn sheep tested by that method, compared with 18 of 19 that were detected by either tonsillar swabs or biopsy (Wild and Miller 1991).

6. The way that the samples are handled after collection may reduce the likelihood of detecting the agent. Wild and Miller (1991) recovered *M. haemolytica* from 14 of 19 tonsillar swabs cultured directly onto media versus 0 of 19 and

2 of 19 swabs stored in two different transport mediums for 24 hours before culture.

Lankester (2001) provides a thorough discussion of the various factors that influence the ability to detect a disease agent (*Parelaphostrongylus tenuis* in deer).

SEARCHING FOR A PHYSIOLOGIC RESPONSE TO THE CAUSATIVE AGENT

One of the most commonly used methods of disease surveillance is to search for some physiologic indicator of exposure to an agent. The most frequently used technique of this type is to test for evidence that the immune system has been activated. There are many tests of this type but all are based on detecting either antibody (these tests are broadly classed as serologic tests because blood serum is the usual sample) or evidence of a cell-mediated response, including elevation in substances such as cytokines produced by the immune response. (Antibody and cell-mediated immunity will be discussed

Table 4.2 Specimens Used to Survey Wild Animals for Potential Disease-Causing Agents or Factors

Specimen examined	Agent or factor sought	Disease
External body surface	Ectoparasites	Fleas, lice, mites, ticks, fly larva
	Vectorborne infectious agents in parasites	Lyme disease, plague, tularemia
Plumage and pelage	Heavy metal residues	Mercury poisoning
Feces	Antigens (coproantigens)	*Echinococcus multilocularis* infection
	Bacteria	Salmonellosis, yersiniosis, paratuberculosis
	Parasite ova and oocysts	Many helminth and protozoa
	Sediment	Lead poisoning from sediment
	Viruses	Parvoviruses
Urine	Bacteria	Leptospirosis
	Parasitic ova, oocysts	*Dioctophyma renale*, renal coccidiosis
Blood	Antibody	Many infectious agents
	Bacteria	Many
	Contaminant residues	Many
	Enzyme activity	Lead, insecticide poisoning
	Helminth larvae	*Elaeophora schneideri*, *Dirofilaria* spp.
	Hematozoa	Malaria, leucocytozoonosis, babesiosis
	Viruses	Many
Soft tissues	Bacteria, viruses, protozoan and helminth parasites	Many
	Contaminant residues	Many
	Enzyme activity	Insecticide poisoning (brain)
	Prions	Chronic wasting disease
	Trace minerals	Copper, molybdenum
Bone	Contaminants	Lead, fluoride poisoning

in detail in chapter 6.) Exposure to some noxious substances can be detected by measuring physiological indicators often called *biomarkers*. Examples of the use of biomarkers include measuring the level of activity of specific enzymes that may be affected by a contaminant such as depression of brain or blood cholinesterase activity by organophosphorous and carbamate insecticides, depression of delta aminolevulinic acid dehydratase activity in blood by lead, and activation of liver enzymes by many compounds such as polyaromatic hydrocarbons. Other examples are measurement of the alteration of retinoids and thyroid hormones caused by polyhalogenated aromatic hydrocarbons and the accumulation of metabolic substances in blood or tissue such as the protoporphyrin that accumulates in red blood cells of birds exposed to lead.

Several factors must be considered when interpreting the results of tests that measure a physiologic response:

1. *Recent exposure and test results.* Animals exposed recently to the causative agent may not have had sufficient time to respond and will test negative. For instance, antibodies are usually not detectable in serum until about a week after first exposure to an agent.

2. *Exposure versus infection.* The presence of an immune response indicates that the animal has been *exposed* to an agent at some point in time. It does not necessarily indicate that the animal is infected when the sample was taken. In many diseases, appearance of high levels of antibody in serum coincides with clearing of the infection. Less commonly, such as in herpesvirus infections and tuberculosis, infection may persist despite high levels of antibody.

3. *Exposure response and level of detection.* Animals may have responded in the past to exposure to an agent but the response has waned below the level of detection of the test. We do

not know how long physiologic responses to many diseases persist at detectable levels in wild animals. For example, a troubling feature of tuberculosis in ungulates is that some animals with advanced disease fail to react in tests of cell-mediated immunity used to identify infected animals. These animals may be highly infectious but go undetected.

4. *Antibodies in young animals.* Young animals may have antibody acquired passively from their mothers. Presence of this antibody indicates that the mother and not the offspring was exposed to the agent.

5. *Generic versus specific responses.* Many physiological responses are generic rather than specific. This is a problem with some biomarkers such as activation of hepatic detoxifying enzymes that may be elevated after exposure to several types of compound. So-called cross-reaction with other organisms also occurs in some serological tests.

6. *Exposure response and disease development.* A physiological response may indicate exposure to an agent but provides no indication if the animal developed disease as a result of that exposure.

7. *Responses by different species.* The response by different species to an agent may be substantially different so that tests that are useful in one species may be worthless in another species. For example, the presence of antibody is useful for recognizing tuberculosis in most species of waterfowl but not in whistling ducks (Cromie et al. 2000).

8. *Response and energy demands.* The ability of individual animals to respond to an agent is dependent upon the conditions at the time of exposure and is subject to trade-offs with other demands for energy. Animals may be exposed to the agent but may not produce a detectable response. For instance, animals that are nutritionally stressed may not produce antibodies in response to a disease agent.

SEARCHING FOR EVIDENCE OF DISEASE IN SPECIES OTHER THAN THE PRIMARY SPECIES

It may be more convenient or practical to look for evidence of a disease in a species other than the one that is affected by the disease or that is important in its maintenance or perpetuation. Often this technique takes advantage of a trophic relationship in which predators or scavengers are examined for evidence of a disease that occurs in their prey. The method is effective because predators and scavengers examine or "screen" a large sample of prey animals, and because predators are generally longer-lived than prey. Plague (*Yersinia pestis* infection) is primarily a disease of rodents, but carnivores including coyotes, dogs, badgers, and bobcats have been used to monitor plague activity in the western United States. Gage and Montenieri (1994) estimated that hundreds of rodents would have to be sampled to yield equivalent information to that obtained using a small number of predators. Leighton et al. (2001) tested farm dogs and cats in an area of western Canada for antibodies to several disease that are associated with rodents. Antibodies to all of the diseases were detected in dogs or cats, including antibodies to plague a disease that had never been detected in rodents in the area. Feral pigs (that are active scavengers) have been proposed as a suitable sentinel species to monitor the success of a program to eradicate bovine tuberculosis from wild brushtail possums in New Zealand (Nugent et al. 2002). This is because of the difficulty in detecting tuberculosis directly in possums when the frequency of occurrence of the disease is extremely low.

SAMPLING TO DETECT DISEASE

All types of sampling used to detect or monitor disease are potentially compromised by several basic problems, and these often are more profound and difficult to deal with in wild animals than in either humans or domestic animals. These will not be dealt with in detail here, but anyone contemplating a disease survey should be aware of the basic concerns and try to address those relevant to their situation.

BIAS

If inferences are to be drawn about the frequency of occurrence, distribution, or significance of a disease in a group of animals, any sample of animals that is examined must be representative of the group. Sampling theory dictates that samples should be selected randomly from the population, but this is probably never actually possible when dealing with wild animals because the methods for obtaining samples are inherently guilty of some form of *selection bias*. There is abundant literature documenting that animals collected by various forms of trapping, hunting, and capture and those submitted to laboratories for diagnosis are more or less likely to have any particular disease than the general population from which they were drawn (e.g., Conner et al. 2000). Often, the best that one can do is to compare samples collected by different methods and identify the direction, if not the extent, of the bias. A second type of bias, called *measurement bias*, relates to the actual test that is used to detect disease and how it might lead to a systematic error. Techniques often are used without considering this factor. For example, examination of blood smears from birds for protozoan parasites has been used widely to study the effects of infection on reproduction and survival. However, Holmstad et al. (2003) found that examination of peripheral blood smears from willow ptarmigan led to systematic underestimation of the occurrence of certain types of blood parasites, confounding any assessment of the significance of the different parasites for health of the birds.

SAMPLE SIZE

Sampling often is done to answer two basic questions about a disease:

1. Is the disease present in the population?
2. How common is the disease in the population?

Although the questions appear simple, obtaining a useful answer is not a simple task. For both questions, the confidence one can have in the answer depends upon the number of animals examined (sample size) and the accuracy (validity) of the test that has been used. DiGiacomo and Koepsell (1986) provide a brief explanation of the sampling theory related to these questions as well as useful reference tables indicating the approximate number of animals needed to have statistical confidence in the results.

A basic fact that often is not recognized is that the more rarely a disease occurs in the population, the larger the sample that is needed to answer either question adequately. Determining whether or not a disease is present in wild animals is a particularly perplexing problem, especially when the disease in question affects humans or domestic animals and there is pressure for an absolute *yes* or *no* answer.

One can state unequivocally that the disease is present if even a single animal with the disease is found, but how confident can one be that the disease is not present if no diseased animals are detected? A useful rule of thumb when confronted with this question is the "rule of three" (Hanley and Lippman-Hand 1983), which is based on the observation that "if none of n patients shows the event about which we are concerned, we can be 95% confident that the chance of the event is at most 3 in n (i.e., 3/n)." For example, assume that 40 elk (n = 40) from a large population have been tested for tuberculosis and all were negative. Based on this sample of 40 animals, how confident can we be that the population is actually free of tuberculosis? Assuming that the test is 100% accurate (which is highly unlikely) and that the sample is representative of the population (also highly unlikely), the answer is that we can be confident, at the 95% level, that the prevalence of tuberculosis in the population is not greater than about 3/40 or 7.5%. This is a very long way from being certain that the population is free of the disease!

The formula can be rewritten n = 3/p to give a rough estimate of an approximate sample size needed to detect a particular prevalence (p) of disease. If we wished to be 95% confident that the prevalence was not greater than 1%, we would have to find no positive animals in a sample of 3/.01 = 300 animals. (If it were necessary to be absolutely certain that the disease was not present, every single animal in the entire population would have to be tested with a test that was 100% sensitive [see below]). Diefenbach et al. (2004) analyzed the probability of detecting CWD in samples of hunter-killed animals from an adult population of about one million white-tailed deer in Pennsylvania. Based on computer simulations, >25,000 deer would have to be tested at a cost of >$1.4 million to have a >50% probability of detecting the disease when it occurred in 0.1% of the deer.

VALIDITY OF TESTS

When the term "test" is used, the usual assumption is that some type of sample such as blood, urine, or hair has been collected and analyzed in a laboratory. However, any method used to look for evidence of disease, including a visual survey of wild sheep or postmortem examination of dead animals, is a test. When a group of animals is examined for disease by any method, we hope that we will detect all of the individuals that have the disease and that we will not wrongly identify any animal that does not have the disease as being affected. The *validity* of a test is defined as the ability to distinguish between those that have the disease and those that do not.

Validity includes two components: *sensitivity* and *specificity*. Sensitivity describes the ability of a test to correctly identify those with the disease and is expressed as the proportion of affected animals that is identified as positive by the test. Specificity is the ability of the test to correctly identify those that do not have the disease and is expressed as the proportion of animals that do not have the disease that are identified as negative. In order to calculate the specificity and sensitivity of a test, we obviously must know which animals actually do have the disease.

Table 4.3 Hypothetical Test for Disease

	Diseased	Not diseased	Total
Test positive	81	100	181
Test negative	37	782	819
Total	118	882	1000

Note: Data from a hypothetical situation in which 1000 animals were tested. On the basis of another "gold standard" test, 118 of the animals were considered to be diseased and 882 were considered to not have the disease. The sensitivity of the test is the proportion of the diseased animals that was correctly identified (81/118 = 68.5%), the specificity of the test is the proportion of the animals that were not diseased that tested negative (782/882 = 88.7%).

This usually is done by comparing the test results with the results of some so-called gold standard. For instance, the gold standard for tuberculosis is isolation of the causative bacteria from specific tissues following detailed necropsy. The methods used and the tissues to be cultured are rigidly defined, and if bacteria are not isolated, the animal is considered to have been free of the disease. It is very important to realize that while gold standards are the best evidence available, they are not infallible. In the case of tuberculosis, bacteria cannot be isolated from a small proportion of animals that are known on other grounds to be infected. The method used to determine sensitivity and specificity is shown in table 4.3.

To see how sensitivity and specificity affect the use of a test, let us assume that the test described in table 4.3 (sensitivity = 68.5%, specificity = 88.7%) is to be used as the basis for removing bison from a wild herd in which about 40% of the animals are infected. Every animal that tests positive will be removed from the herd (culled) in an attempt to control the disease. We can predict that if 1000 bison are tested, about 400 of them actually will be infected. Since the test is 68.5% sensitive, it will detect 274 bison that have tuberculosis (these are *true positives*) but it will miss 126 infected animals (*false negatives*) that would remain in the herd. The other side of the test is that 600 of the 1000 bison are not diseased. Because the specificity is 88.7%, 532 of these will test negative (*true negatives*) but 68 will test positive (*false positives*) and these will be culled in error.

We might conclude that this test is not a very good method on which to base a disease control program, but a test very similar to that just described has been used to eradicate tuberculosis in domestic cattle. However, the test is used in a different manner in

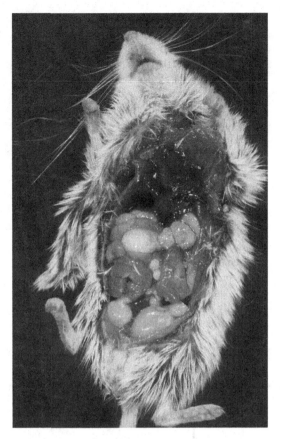

Fig. 4.3. Larval cysts of the tapeworm *Echinococcus multilocularis* in the liver and abdomen of a white-footed mouse.

cattle than the one described for bison. Although the test has relatively poor ability to detect *individual* infected animals, it has been useful in detecting infected *herds*. If an animal in a herd tests positive, the entire cattle herd including many noninfected animals has been depopulated.

In some tests, animals can only be positive or negative. For instance, if we examined dead mice for the larval stage of the tapeworm *Echinococcus multilocularis* (fig. 4.3), animals either do or do not have visible cysts. But even in this disease, there is some likelihood that very early infections in which the larvae are minute and buried deep in the liver parenchyma will be mistakenly classed as not being infected, so the sensitivity of this simple test is likely to be <100%. Animals misidentified in this way are false negatives and result in underestimation of the actual frequency of occurrence of *E. multilocularis*. Larval cysts of other tapeworms might be wrongly identified as *E. multilocularis* so that the specificity might be <100%, resulting in false positives and overestimation of the abundance of *E. multilocularis*. (The sensitivity and specificity of this test could be improved by thorough dissection of the liver to detect small cysts and by microscopic examination of the cyst contents to confirm their identity.)

The potential for making mistakes in identification of affected and nonaffected animals is much greater for most tests than in the test just described for *E. multilocularis*. In most serological tests and residue analyses, the results occur across a continuous spectrum rather than in a yes/no distribution. Often there is overlap of values between affected and nonaffected animals. The scientist developing such a test has to choose a value (often called a "cutoff" or "threshold") that will be used to differentiate between affected and nonaffected animals.

The problem in choosing an appropriate cutoff value is illustrated in figure 4.4. The sensitivity and specificity of the test depend upon the cutoff value that is chosen. In the situation shown in figure 4.4, if the cutoff is set at 3.5 ppm, all the exposed animals are identified correctly (sensitivity = 100%) but four animals are identified incorrectly as positive (specificity = 85%). If the cutoff is set at 10.5 ppm, all unexposed animals are identified correctly (specificity = 100%) but only 50% of exposed animals are identified correctly. At an intermediate cutoff of 6.5 ppm, the sensitivity = 85% and the specificity = 96%. The cutoff level used in any test is critical, and it needs to be established on the basis of results from a large sample of animals known to have and not to have the disease in question. This process is called test validation. The cutoff value used can be adjusted depending on the purpose of the test. For instance, if a test is to be used to identify animals that should be removed from the population to control or eradicate a disease (such as the bison described above), a cutoff that had a very high sensitivity would be desirable so that the likelihood of missing diseased animals would be minimal. However, this would result in culling many nondiseased animals that tested false positive. In some circumstances, two different cutoff values may be used for a test to meet different objectives (e.g., Mazet et al. 1992).

One method for dealing with the relative sensitivity/specificity deficiency of tests is to use two different tests in combination. A cheap, easily applied test with high sensitivity (often called a *screening test*) might be used first to identify all of

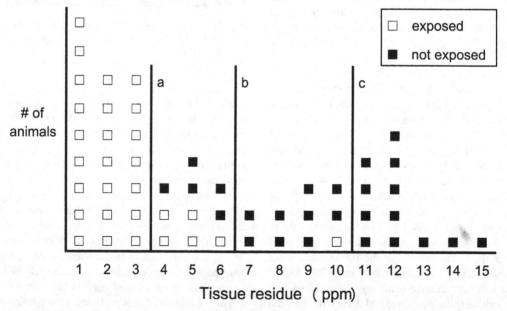

Fig. 4.4. Hypothetical data set showing the concentration of a contaminant in tissues of a group of animals. Some of the animals were exposed to the contaminant experimentally. The data are to be used to establish a cutoff value for screening samples from wild animals. Three possible cutoff points (a, b, c) for distinguishing between exposed and nonexposed animals are shown. If cutoff value a is used, all exposed animals would be identified correctly; if cutoff c is used all nonexposed animals would be identified correctly. Cutoff b is a compromise with sensitivity of 85% and specificity of 96%.

the animals that might be affected. This is done in the knowledge that there will be many false positives. As the second step, all animals that were positive on the first test are reexamined using a second test (the *confirmatory test*), which has high specificity but might have lower sensitivity. In this way, the best features of the two tests can be exploited and the number of animals subjected to the more-specific test is reduced.

Proper validation of tests is difficult. Unfortunately, many tests that have been used in wild animals have not been validated adequately, and there is real doubt about what some of these tests are actually telling us. Many tests developed for use in humans, domestic animals, or other wild species have been applied directly to wild animals without adequate testing to determine whether the methodology or cutoff values used for these other species are appropriate for the wild animal being tested.

In the past, a major concern has been that many tests lacked adequate sensitivity. Technical developments have made it possible to detect diminishingly small amounts of agents of disease and the physiologic responses to these factors. Some tests are now so sensitive that possible contamination of samples in the field or laboratory has become a problem, and the significance of positive results is becoming questionable. For example, molecular techniques have made it possible to detect minute amounts of residual nucleic acid for extended periods after intact viable microbes can no longer be isolated from animals. This raises the question of whether animals should be considered infected, infectious, or simply carrying remnants of exposure that occurred at some unknown time. As an example of the sensitivity of molecular tests, Rothschild et al. (2001) detected DNA of *Mycobacterium tuberculosis* complex bacteria in bones of an extinct species of bison that died out about 17,000 years ago. The same problem of extreme sensitivity is true for many contaminants for which the ability to detect nanogram or picogram amounts of residue has not been matched by an ability to relate the residues to an effect on the animal.

TERMS USED TO DESCRIBE DISEASE

In common with other scientific disciplines, those concerned with disease have developed a vocabulary of which some is jargon, some is archaic, and some is useful, if used appropriately. As an example, a disease of bighorn sheep might be described as *enzootic, subacute, verminous pneumonia of moderate pathogenicity, with high morbidity and low mortality*. While this is a mouthful, it encapsulates how the disease occurs in the population over time (enzootic), the usual duration and severity of clinical disease in the individual sheep (subacute, moderate pathogenicity), the usual or expected occurrence and outcome among affected animals (high morbidity, low mortality), the cause (verminous), and the organ and the pathology that are primarily involved (pneumonia). If we were to rewrite the description in nontechnical terms, it would be something like *a disease characterized by filling of the lungs with red and white blood cells and fluid, caused by infection with parasitic worms. There is moderate injury to the lungs and the resulting illness extends over a period of several days to a few weeks in affected sheep. The disease has occurred with predictable regularity and at a predictable rate in the population in the past. Within the population, a large proportion of animals becomes sick but relatively few die as a result of the disease.*

At various points, I will introduce a small number of terms that are important for those working with disease on a day-to-day basis. In this chapter, I will describe some terms that are used for describing the pattern of occurrence of disease within a population. This is part of the vocabulary of the branch of medical science known as epidemiology. Elsewhere, I will deal with terms that describe the effect of disease on animals (the vocabulary of clinical medicine and the pathologist).

MEASURES OF FREQUENCY OF OCCURRENCE

One of the basic features considered in investigating any disease is its pattern of occurrence within the population or group. By necessity, this requires quantification of the number affected as a proportion of the total group. There are different ways to approach counting a disease, but any enumeration must be approached with the knowledge that disease and populations are not static. While we are doing the count (particularly if this takes some time), new animals will enter the population, some will become affected, others may recover, some may leave, and some may die. Thus, there is a good deal of coming and going in and out of the diseased state (the numerator) and the population (the denominator), which complicates our counts and calculations.

Two measures, *incidence* and *prevalence*, are used to describe the frequency of occurrence of disease in a population. They are not synonymous and they are often misused. Incidence is defined as the number of *new* cases of disease occurring during a *fixed period of time* divided by the number of animals *at risk* of developing the disease during that time. The important parts of the definition are that:

1. incidence deals only with new cases of disease and is a measure of risk.
2. only animals that have the potential to develop the disease (i.e., that are at risk) are considered in the population denominator. Animals may be excluded from risk for many reasons: innate resistance, acquired immunity, lack of exposure to the cause, or because they were already affected when the study period began.

Figure 4.5 illustrates a hypothetical situation in which 10 animals within a group of 200 tested positive for disease X at some time during the year. (Only the 10 positive animals are shown.) Of the 10 animals that tested positive, only animals 2, 4, 6, 8, 9, and 10 developed the disease *during* the year so that the appropriate numerator of new cases for calculating incidence is 6. Within the population, 37 animals were resistant to infection (because of prior exposure and resulting immunity) at the start of the year and were not at risk. Animals 1, 3, 5, and 7 had the disease at the beginning of the year, so they also

were not at risk of developing the disease during the year. Thus, the appropriate denominator (population at risk) is 200 - (37 + 4) = 159 and the annual incidence is 6/159 or 3.8 cases per 100 animals in the population for the year. The period of time used to calculate incidence can be of any duration but it must be specified. Incidence is very difficult to measure in wild animals, because of the difficulty in following individual animals over a period of time, so that incidence has seldom been measured, although it is the best measure of risk.

Prevalence is a measure of how many animals have the disease *at a point in time* and is defined as the number of affected animals divided by the number of animals in the population at that time. Prevalence should be thought of as a snapshot of the population in which those who have the disease and those who do not have the disease are identified. Prevalence is not concerned with when the disease developed in these individuals. In chronic diseases, such as tuberculosis or brucellosis in bison, some of the individuals that test positive on a particular day may have become infected recently, some may have been infected for months, and others may have been infected for years. Because the numerator includes animals with a mix of disease duration, it does not

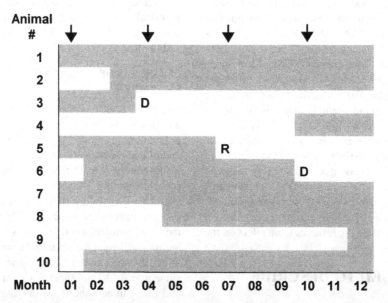

Fig. 4.5. Hypothetical disease history of 10 animals within a group of 200 that was tested for disease X each month for a year. At the beginning of the year, 37 animals had antibodies and were resistant to infection with the disease. Shading indicates that an animal tested positive in that month. Some animals died (D) and some recovered (R). It is assumed that no recruitment of new individuals or mortality from causes other than disease X occurred. Arrows indicate dates on which the prevalence was calculated. (See text for discussion of the calculation of incidence and prevalence for disease X.)

provide a measure of risk. We can calculate the prevalence of disease X at different points during the year from the data in figure 4.5. On January 1, the prevalence was 4/ 200 or 2%. By April 1, an animal had died, so the prevalence was 6/199 or 3%. In July, it was 6/199 = 3%, and in October it was 6/198 = 3% (two animals had died).

The hypothetical occurrence of disease Y (fig. 4.6) illustrates how measurement of incidence and prevalence can give very different pictures of a disease. This group of animals contained 100 animals at the beginning of the year, all of whom were naive, never having experienced the disease previously, so that all were at risk. (Occurrence of a disease in a naive population is sometimes called a "virgin ground" outbreak [Plowright 1982].) Disease Y has a rapid course in individuals, with animals either dying or recovering within 2 weeks (as might occur with a disease such as canine distemper). During the year, 25 animals developed disease, so the annual incidence = 25/100 or 25%. The prevalence of disease on January 1 was 0/100, on April 1 it was 0/98 (the population had been reduced by 2 deaths), on July 1 the prevalence was 4/94 = 4.3%, and on October 1 it again was 0 (0/88). It is obvious that periodic cross-sectional sampling of the population suggested a rather minor occurrence of disease Y with a maximum prevalence of 4.3%, while the actual risk and the number of animals affected were substantial. With a very chronic disease, the reverse situation may occur in which the prevalence is substantial but the number of new cases and the incidence are quite low. This could be very important in trying to evaluate the effectiveness of a program to control a chronic disease such as tuberculosis. Even if the management is effective in preventing the occurrence of new cases, the prevalence in the population will decline slowly and it may be difficult to detect that progress is being made.

The *mortality rate* (the number dying per unit of time divided by number in the group) is analogous to incidence but measures deaths rather than illness. The annual mortality rate from disease X was 2% while that from disease Y was 12%. The *case fatality rate* (the number dying of the disease divided by the total number with the disease) is a measure of the severity of a disease. The case fatality rate was 2/10 or 0.2 for disease X and 12/25 or 0.48 for disease Y.

In reality, it is very difficult to accurately define the number of wild animals affected with a particular disease (i.e., to determine an accurate numerator), and usually it is even more difficult to define the total size of the population or more specifically the population at risk. Consequently, in many disease situations, various rates are speculative at best and *dangling numerators* (i.e., numerators with no denominator), such as the number of dead birds picked up during an outbreak, may be the only quantitative data available.

PATTERNS OF DISEASE OCCURRENCE IN POPULATIONS

In addition to the number of animals affected, it is important to understand other features of how a disease is occurring within a group of animals. This might involve determining if it is a new disease or one that has been present in the past and if it is expanding in geographic range or prevalence. Two

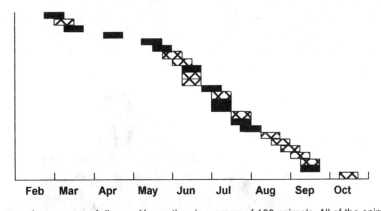

Fig. 4.6. Distribution of new cases of disease Y over time in a group of 100 animals. All of the animals were susceptible at the beginning of the "outbreak." The duration of the disease in individual animals was 2 weeks, and animals either died (dark boxes) or recovered (cross-hatched boxes). No recruitment or deaths from causes other than disease Y occurred.

terms are used to describe the way that diseases occur in a population. These are based on the number of cases that occur over a time period relative to the number of cases that would be expected or that would "normally" occur during that period.

A disease is said to be *enzootic* (endemic) if it occurs at a regular, predictable, or expected rate in a population or area. An *epizootic* (epidemic) occurs when a disease occurs at a time or place where it is not expected or at a rate substantially greater than expected based on past experience. (Enzootic and epizootic have been used for disease in animals, while endemic and epidemic are used for human populations.) Classification of a disease as enzootic or epizootic depends upon prior knowledge of its occurrence. All newly discovered diseases are epizootic by definition, because they occur at a time or place where they are not expected. This may change if on further investigation it is discovered that the disease occurs predictably in the area. Hantavirus infection was regarded as epizootic when first discovered in North America, but it is now known that Sin Nombre virus is very widespread in deer mice and that it has been causing sporadic disease in humans for many years. However, the prevalence in mice can change dramatically from year to year so this disease might be considered enzootic with sporadic epizootic flare-ups.

The pattern with which a disease occurs may differ in different areas. Hemorrhagic disease in deer, caused by oribivirus infection, is constantly present and occurs in an enzootic pattern in Texas. It occurs as frequent and repeated epizootics in the southeastern United States and as infrequent epizootics in northern states and southern Canada (Stallknecht et al. 1996; Gaydos et al. 2002a). The classification of a disease as enzootic or epizootic is not related to the absolute numbers of cases that occur or to the severity of the disease in individual animals. Rabies, which is usually fatal, occurs at a high but predictable incidence and is considered enzootic in many parts of the world.

A technique that often is used to aid in understanding disease pattern is to plot the occurrence of new cases over time. The epizootic curve (fig. 4.7) may be helpful in relating the occurrence of disease in time to natural events such as weather or human activity that may be associated with the disease.

The term "emerging disease" (and "reemerging disease") has become fashionable recently to describe infectious diseases of humans "that have newly appeared in a population or have existed but are rapidly increasing in incidence or geographic range" (Morse 1995). Lashley and Durham (2002) said "this interest followed decades of complacency . . . and a trust in the ability of medical science to conquer infectious diseases." The term has begun to appear in reference to diseases of wild animals, although "infections have been emerging since the first microbe tried to climb the food chain ladder, preying on the protoalgae who were the primary producers of photosynthate" (Lederberg 1997). Those who deal with wildlife diseases have never been complacent about or confident of their ability to deal with infectious diseases. The term has no particular value except perhaps to make a grant application or presentation appear more topical.

SUMMARY

- Disease is difficult to detect and measure in wild animals.
- Surveillance for disease can involve looking for sick or dead animals, looking for the causative agent, looking for a physiologic response to the causative agent, or using another species as a sentinel for the disease.
- Sick and dead animals are hard to find and are removed rapidly by predators and scavengers.

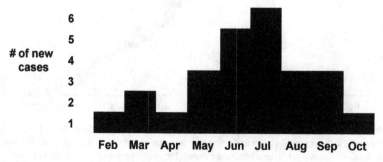

Fig. 4.7. Epizootic curve (number of new cases/month) of disease Y (data from fig. 4.6).

- Counts based on sick or dead animals always underestimate the actual frequency of occurrence of disease.
- Presence of a causative agent is not synonymous with occurrence of disease.
- Physiologic responses such as production of antibody and concentration of various biomarkers are used widely to measure exposure to disease agents.
- Predatory and scavenging species may be efficient sentinels for the occurrence of some diseases in other species.
- All forms of surveillance are subject to sampling bias.
- The number of animals that must be examined to provide credible information about a disease is usually larger than expected, particularly for diseases that occur at low frequency.
- The validity of a test is a measure of its ability to distinguish between those individuals that have the disease and those that do not. Validity has two components: sensitivity (the ability of a test to correctly identify those with the disease) and specificity (the ability to correctly identify those who do not have the disease).
- Most tests that have been used in wild animals have not been validated adequately.
- The frequency of occurrence of disease in groups of animals is described by two measures: *incidence* is a measure of the number of new cases that occur over a period of time, *prevalence* is a measure of the number of cases present at a particular time. The terms are not synonymous.
- Incidence is very difficult to measure in wild animals, because of the difficulty in following individuals over time.
- Effective measurement of both the number of individuals affected and the population size is required for determining the significance of a disease.
- The pattern of occurrence of a disease in a population is described by two terms: *enzootic* and *epizootic*, both of which are defined on the basis of the past history of the disease in the population.

5
Damage, Pathogenicity, and Virulence

The fundamental feature of disease, regardless of cause, is that there is dysfunction that causes harm or cost to the affected animal. The harm may range from effects that are so mild that they are undetectable with most measures that we use commonly (but not necessarily insignificant biologically) to conditions that are acutely lethal to the individual.

A term is needed that expresses the relative propensity of an agent to injure the animal so that different diseases can be discussed and compared. Two candidate words are in common usage: *virulence* and *pathogenicity*, both of which have been used primarily to describe disease caused by infectious agents. Virulence is derived from Latin *virulentus* (poisonous) and pathogenesis is derived from Greek *pathos* (suffering) + *genesis* (generation or creation), hence, creation of suffering. Virulence is defined in a medical dictionary as "the degree of pathogenicity of a microorganism as indicated by case fatality rates and/or its ability to invade the tissues of the host" (Dorland 2000). Pathogenicity is defined as "the ability of a microorganism to produce disease." The word "virulence" also has been used to describe "the ability to cause disease" and virulent as "actively poisonous, intensely noxious, venomous," suggesting that on an etymological basis, virulence should be equally applicable to noninfectious and infectious causes of disease.

Virulence will be used here as a measure of the ability of an agent to cause harm. The degree of injury will not be limited to increased mortality of affected animals. This definition of virulence is similar to "the harm done to hosts following infection" used by Read et al. (1999). Hochberg and van Baalen (2000) described two types of virulence that occur in infectious diseases. Type 1 is related to the compatibility of a parasite for a specific host and the evasion or manipulation of the host's defenses during the sequential stages of infection, development,

and transmission from the host. Type 2 deals with the effects of infection on host fitness in terms of increased probability of mortality, reduced levels of reproduction, alterations in host life history, and homeostasis. Only type 2 virulence will be dealt with here. In human and veterinary medicine, virulence usually is considered at the level of the individual person or animal. For wild animals, effects on the individual animal are important primarily for their consequences for host life span and fecundity and for how these influence host fitness and population density, so we must consider virulence in that context. Schall (2002) considered that, from the host animal's perspective, virulence is any consequence of infection that reduces the host's lifetime reproductive success.

Two features that we would like to understand about any disease are *how* and *why* injury occurs as a result of the interaction between the animal and the causal agent(s). How injury occurs is primarily a question of the physiological and immunological mechanisms that result in harm. These will be discussed later when we deal with the effects of disease on the individual animal. In this chapter, I will deal with why harm occurs and why marked differences in virulence can be observed in different situations, that is, why a disease agent may be very harmful in one situation and essentially harmless in another. Why virulence occurs is of more than academic interest because it is important to understand how environmental change and measures designed to manage and control disease might influence the ability of agents to cause injury.

Ebert (1999) proposed three possible explanations for why virulence occurs and how it may have evolved:

1. Virulence is a coincidental by-product of parasitism.

2. Virulence is adaptive or beneficial for the parasite.

3. Virulence is a result of coevolution of the causal agent and the host.

Although these explanations were developed specifically in relation to parasites, I believe that they provide a framework that is useful for understanding virulence in general, and that the explanations can be stretched to accommodate agents other than parasites including some noninfectious diseases.

VIRULENCE IS A COINCIDENTAL BY-PRODUCT OF THE ASSOCIATION BETWEEN AN AGENT AND AN ANIMAL.

The basic feature of this explanation for virulence is that injury to the animal offers no particular advantage to the causative agent. Many noninfectious diseases, such as poisoning of wild animals by various contaminants and traumatic injury from physical agents, are examples of coincidental virulence. When lead shot is used to hunt birds, the intent is not to poison ducks that might consume spent pellets from the bottom of ponds or to poison eagles that ingest lead pellets embedded in the tissues of waterfowl. The lead pellets do not benefit from causing disease; however, lead poisoning is a coincidental virulence effect that has killed millions of birds. Cyanobacteria (blue-green algae) likely synthesize potent toxins to ward off attack by fellow planktonic species (Carmichael 1994). It is coincidental and of no advantage to the bacteria that the toxins also kill wild and domestic animals that drink water containing the organisms. Cyanobacterial toxins resemble many man-made pesticides in that a poisonous property that is useful in one situation has undesirable coincidental effects in other situations.

The transmissible spongiform encephalopathies including chronic wasting disease of deer and elk (CWD) also may be examples of coincidental virulence. It appears that the cause of CWD is conformational change in a specific natural protein to a form that is resistant to normal proteolysis. This abnormal prion protein accumulates within the nervous system causing irreversible and fatal disease. Because the abnormal protein lacks nucleic acid and is not a living entity, there is no advantage to it in propagating itself and causing disease.

Coincidental virulence may occur in unusual and often new or novel host-parasite interactions (Ebert 1999). In these situations, the genes responsible for virulence evolved in the agent in different circum-

stances than are found in the novel host or situation. There are many examples of this type of disease in wild animals (table 5.1) including a number of parasitic worms in wild ungulates.

One of the best studied of these is the meningeal worm *Parelaphostrongylus tenuis,* which is common in white-tailed deer in eastern North America. Infection in white-tailed deer is generally clinically silent, even though the worms migrate through the deer's central nervous system during development. The worm is highly virulent in other ungulates including moose, elk, mule deer, caribou, bighorn sheep, pronghorn, domestic sheep, goats, and llamas in which it often causes fatal neurological disease. The harm caused these novel hosts is a result of abnormal growth and behavior of worm larvae within their nervous system as well as marked inflammatory response by the host. *Parelaphostrongylus tenuis* is particularly virulent in caribou, and infected white-tailed deer and caribou likely cannot coexist in an area where *P. tenuis* is present.

Another nematode *Elaeophora schneideri* occurs in mule deer in areas of western North America (Hibler and Adcock 1971). The adult worms live in major arteries, particularly of the head and neck, without causing apparent disease in mule deer. The parasite is transmitted between deer by large blood-feeding horseflies that become infected by ingesting microscopic larvae circulating in a mule deer's blood or in its skin. Larvae develop within the fly and are transmitted when the fly feeds on another animal. If an infected horsefly feeds on an elk instead of a mule deer, the result for the elk may be severe disease including blindness, brain hemorrhage, and death. This results because of reduced blood flow to parts of the body nourished by large arteries of the head and neck including the ears, nose, and antlers. Injury occurs because the worms behave differently in elk than in mule deer, perhaps because the cues from the host are different or "indecipherable" by the worm, and because elk respond to developing worms with an exaggerated inflammatory response that may result in obstruction of blood flow through arteries. *Elaeophora schneideri* also causes disease in other novel hosts including domestic sheep (Kemper 1938), moose (Worley et al. 1972), sika deer (Robinson et al. 1978), white-tailed deer (Couvillion et al. 1986), and bighorn sheep (Boyce et al. 1999).

In white-tailed deer and elk, adults of the North American liver fluke *Fascioloides magna* mature as pairs or groups in thin-walled cysts within the liver (Pybus 2001). The cysts communicate with bile

Table 5.1 Coincidental Virulence Caused by an Infectious Agent in a Species Other Than the Usual Host

Agent	Usual host	Abnormal host	Type of injury
Hantaviruses	Various rodents	Humans	Hemorrhagic fever with renal syndrome, hantavirus pulmonary syndrome[1]
Alcelaphine herpesvirus 1	Wildebeest	Cattle, other bovids, cervids	Malignant catarrhal fever[2]
Herpesvirus simiae (virus B)	Asian macaques	Humans	Paralysis, death[3]
Brucella abortus	Cattle, bison, elk	Moose	Septicemia[4]
Plasmodium spp.	Indigenous passerines	Penguins	Malaria[5]
	Introduced passerines	Endemic Hawaiian birds	Malaria[6]
Cytauxzoon felis	Bobcat	Domestic cat	Anemia, icterus, often fatal[7]
Parelaphostrongylus tenuis	White-tailed deer	Moose, elk, mule deer, pronghorns, bighorn sheep, caribou	Neurological disease, often fatal[8]
Elaeophora schneideri	Mule and black-tailed deer	Domestic sheep	Dermatitis (sorehead)
		Elk, moose	Vascular injury, occlusion, tissue infarction[9]
		Sika deer	Tumorlike growths on head[10]
Fascioloides magna	White-tailed deer, elk, caribou	Moose, bison, cattle	Severe hepatic fibrosis.
		Domestic sheep, bighorn sheep, roe deer	Severe, and often fatal liver injury caused by failure to encapsulate and contain fluke movement.[11]

[1] Mills and Childs (2001).
[2] Heuschle and Reid (2001).
[3] King (2001).
[4] Forbes et al. (1996).
[5] Fix et al. (1988).
[6] van Riper et al. (1986).
[7] Kocan (2001).
[8] Lankester (2001).
[9] Kemper (1938); Hibler and Adcock (1971).
[10] Robinson et al. (1978).
[11] Pybus (2001).

ducts so that fluke eggs can enter the intestine with the bile and pass to the external environment. White-tailed deer and elk suffer relatively little injury from the infection unless the number of worms is very large. In the external environment, the eggs hatch in water, and there are several life cycle stages that result in infective larvae becoming encysted on vegetation. If larva are eaten by a moose, bison, or domestic cow, the developing flukes reach the liver, but these hosts react intensely to the parasite with severe inflammation and fibrosis (fig. 5.1). The flukes seldom mature or are able to find each other in these animals, and any eggs produced usually do not reach the intestine. The result is much different if a domes-

tic or bighorn sheep becomes infected. In these "abnormal" hosts, the larval flukes continue to migrate through the liver causing severe and often fatal damage, so that both the host and the parasites may die.

The injury that occurs to humans when they become infected with many infectious agents acquired from wildlife also is an example of coincidental virulence as a result of a novel host-parasite interaction. Examples include infection with viruses that usually cycle between mosquitoes and wild birds, such as West Nile virus and eastern equine encephalitis virus, viruses usually found in rodents, such as hantaviruses and arenaviruses, and *Baylisascaris procyonis* (a roundworm of raccoons).

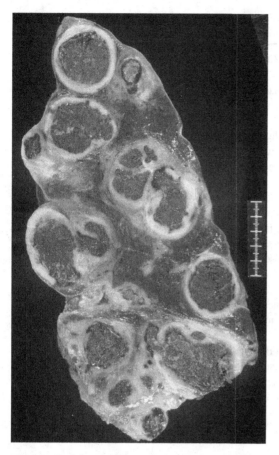

Fig. 5.1. Liver from a moose infected with the North American liver fluke *(Fascioloides magna)*. There is severe reaction to this parasite in moose with extensive fibrosis of the liver.

A feature of coincidental virulence is that high virulence in the novel host is not associated with high or successful parasite transmission (Ebert 1999). In many instances, such as in moose infected with *P. tenuis* or *F. magna*, no transmission occurs, and infection of the novel host is a dead-end from the agent's perspective. This type of "accidental" infection has limited significance for the evolution of either the disease agent or the host animal (Schall 2002).

Disease that results from infections caused by opportunistic bacteria and fungi that usually live independent of the animal as saprophytes in the external environment also is an example of coincidental virulence. The fungus *Aspergillus fumigatus* is an ubiquitous environmental saprophyte that, under certain conditions, can invade the lungs and air sacs of birds, causing the severe disease aspergillosis (fig.

3.3). The bacterium *Clostridium tetani* is a soil saprophyte that can invade skin wounds, grow very locally there, and produce a potent toxin that causes the paralytic disease tetanus. Causing disease is usually thought of as having no advantage for *A. fumigatus* or *C. tetani,* as animal infection is not required for their reproduction, although Mims et al. (2001) speculated that a "dead putrefying corpse is a fine growth medium" for *C. tetani.*

Injury that occurs when organisms that normally live as commensals on the body's surfaces invade more deeply into other parts of the body is more difficult to categorize. (A commensal is an organism that derives nourishment from the host but is neither harmful nor beneficial.) Infection of the "wrong" tissue may be similar to infection in a novel host, and some of the damage that results is likely coincidental virulence. Several important infectious diseases of wild animals are the result of tissue invasion by commensals (table 5.2). In these situations, adaptations that the agent developed for living in one site may result in severe injury when it grows in another site. For example, adhesins developed by the bacterium *Escherichia coli* to assist it in colonizing the intestine are responsible for the severe inflammation that results when this bacterium infects the urinary tract opportunistically (Levin and Svanborg-Eden 1990). There seems to be little advantage to the agent in many such situations. For example, *Mannheimia haemolytica* and *Pasteurella trehalosi* can live in the upper respiratory tract of sheep without causing disease but cause severe pneumonia that may decimate populations of bighorn sheep. When this occurs, the bacteria die with the sheep. A possibility that has not been explored widely is that the organisms that are highly virulent in abnormal tissues are specific strains that may or may not be a subset of those living as commensals on the body's surfaces. Some such excursions by agents into unfamiliar territory may represent so-called short-sighted adaptation that is described more fully below.

VIRULENCE IS ADAPTIVE OR BENEFICIAL FOR THE AGENT.

The basic assumptions underlying this hypothesis are that injury to the animal increases the agent's fitness in some way and that evolution of virulence is agent driven. Host evolution in these situations is "considered to be too slow to be important" (Ebert 1999). Obviously, this explanation does not apply to most noninfectious diseases in which the causative agent has no ability to adapt or evolve and fitness is

Table 5.2 Bacteria That Behave As Commensals at One Site in the Body But Have High Virulence When They Penetrate into Other Tissues

Organism	Wild animals affected	Site where live as commensals	Site where produce severe disease	Disease
Pasteurella multocida	Wild birds	Upper respiratory(?)	Generalized (septicemia)	Avian cholera
Mannheimia hemolytica, Pasteurella trehalosi	Wild sheep	Upper respiratory	Lung	Pneumonia
Fusobacterium necrophorum	Ruminants	Digestive tract	Deeper tissues of oral cavity, feet, liver	Necrobacillosis
Staphylococcus aureus	Many species	Skin	Many tissues	Abscesses, fasciitis, pyemia
Clostridium piliforme	Muskrats	Intestine(?)	Liver	Tyzzer's disease
Actinomyces bovis	Ruminants	Oral mucosa	Mandible	Osteomyelitis (lumpy jaw)
Arcanobacterium pyogenes	Ungulates	Mucosal surfaces	Many tissues	Abscesses and purulent lesions
Haemophilus somnus	Bison, cattle	Mucosal surfaces	Brain, lung, joints	Encephalitis, arthritis, pneumonia

an irrelevant concept. (There are a few exceptional circumstances in which virulence might confer an advantage to the causative agent of a noninfectious disease. These will be discussed later.) Ebert (1999) subdivided this general hypothesis into three subtypes: the benefit of virulence hypothesis, the cost of virulence (trade-off) hypothesis, and the shortsighted evolution hypothesis.

THE BENEFIT OF VIRULENCE HYPOTHESIS

It might be advantageous for a disease agent to be virulent if injury to the host allows the agent to extract resources that otherwise would not be available. I will use two human diseases to illustrate this hypothesis, but similar situations undoubtedly occur in wild animals. Iron often is a limiting nutrient for bacteria growing in the body because although the body contains abundant iron, it is bound up within cells and unavailable to bacteria. One method of gaining access to intracellular iron is to kill host cells releasing the iron. The bacterium *Corynebacterium diphtheriae,* which causes diphtheria in humans, grows on the mucosal surface of the pharynx and does not penetrate deeply into tissues. However, the bacterium, directed by a virus (bacteriophage) that provides the gene for toxin production, produces a toxin that kills tissue in the pharynx, providing access to iron. High levels of toxin only are produced when the bacterium runs out of iron. The

toxin not only affects cells of the nasopharynx where it is useful to the bacterium, it also damages many other host cells including in the heart. Thus, in diphtheria, part of the virulence is beneficial to the bacterium and part is a coincidental by-product that may harm the bacterium if the human dies because of damage to the heart.

Vibrio cholerae, the cause of cholera in humans, also uses toxin to cause damage that is to its advantage. This bacterium is adapted to live in brackish coastal waters. Humans become infected primarily through drinking contaminated water or eating shellfish containing the bacterium. If the bacteria survive passage through the acid environment of the stomach, they attach to the lining of the small intestine and produce a toxin that turns off sodium absorption and promotes sodium secretion by the epithelial cells. The result is a "salty flood" (Ewald 1994) into the intestine that favors growth of *V. cholerae* over that of other intestinal bacteria. The resulting diarrhea flushes other bacteria from the intestine, together with massive numbers of *V. cholerae* that have been produced in the favorable environment. It is thought that the diarrhea, which may cause fatal dehydration and shock in the human, favors transmission of the bacteria (Mims et al. 2001). Diarrhea resulting in increased contamination of the external environment may also facilitate transmission of other bacteria such as *Salmonella*. In a simi-

lar manner, stimulating a cough response may benefit spread of some respiratory infections.

Many other bacteria produce toxins that are responsible for disease. Schlessinger and Schaechter
(1993) suggested that although the benefits to the
bacterium of producing toxin often are unknown,
this is a reflection of our ignorance "for it must be
true that toxins help bacteria grow and survive." Not
all toxins are beneficial to the bacterium. Endotoxin,
a lipopolysaccharide component of the cell wall of
gram-negative bacteria, is probably a coincidental
cause of severe virulence in many bacterial diseases
including such important diseases of wild animals as
avian cholera, tularemia, plague, and brucellosis.

Fitness of infectious agents is determined by their
reproductive success. Success is measured by the
number of new infections that result from an existing infection in microparasites and by the number of
female offspring that live to reproduce in macroparasites. The rate of transmission to new hosts is central to fitness in both types of agent. There are many
infectious diseases in which virulence enhances the
probability of transmission to new hosts. Schall
(2002) applied the term "transmission-opportunity
hypothesis" to this explanation for the evolution of
virulence. For instance, infection of the brain resulting in aggressive behavior enhances the transmission of rabies virus among foxes because the virus is
transmitted primarily through saliva and biting. (The
same virulence is coincidental when a rabid fox
bites a human or a cow, because these are a dead end
for the virus.)

The disease anthrax, caused by infection with the
bacterium *Bacillus anthracis,* is an extreme example
of this strategy: "The basic fact to remember about
B. anthracis is that it survives by killing" (Hugh-
Jones and de Vos 2002). It is believed that vegetative
growth and multiplication only occur when *B. anthracis* infects an animal. Bacterial multiplication is
rapid, killing the animal. Living infected animals do
not spread the disease; an animal only becomes a
source of infection when it dies (Furniss and Hahn
1981). After the animal dies and conditions are no
longer suitable for vegetative growth, the bacteria
form very resistant spores. Oxygen is needed for
sporulation so that sporulation occurs primarily after
a recently dead carcass is opened by scavengers. The
spores are extremely long-lived in soil under suitable conditions where they sit in wait for another animal in which they can reproduce.

The clearest examples of virulence that benefit an
agent occur among protozoan and metazoan parasites that require two different species as hosts to
complete their life cycle and in which the final host

becomes infected by eating the intermediate host. In
such a life cycle, the intermediate host must die for
the parasite to be transmitted. Many parasites of this
type alter the intermediate host in a manner that increases the chance that it will be eaten by a suitable
final host. This has been called "parasite increased
trophic transmission" (PITT), and Lafferty (1999)
suggested that it is useful to think of the intermediate host as the "vehicle" and the final host as the
"destination" for the parasite in such infections. The
intermediate host may be manipulated in different
ways, most commonly by changing its behavior or
appearance so that it is more easily detected by the
predator or by impairing its ability to escape when
detected. A classic example of alteration of behavior
of an intermediate host by a parasite comes from the
study of the acanthocephalid *Polymorphus paradoxus* by Bethel and Holmes (1973, 1974). The am-
phipod *Gammarus lacustris* is an intermediate host
and ducks are the final host for this parasite. Gammarids that are not infected are strongly photopho-
bic and respond to disturbance by diving deeper into
the water. Gammarids infected with *P. paradoxus*
are attracted to light, and when disturbed "skim"
along the surface "creating an obvious surface disturbance" or cling persistently to surface material.
This alteration in behavior coincides with the exact
stage of development of the parasite that is infective
to ducks.

An arthropod is the final host in which sexual reproduction of some parasitic protozoa occurs.
Parasites of this type may alter a vertebrate's behavior to facilitate transmission. For instance, mice infected with malarial parasites of the genus
Plasmodium have reduced antimosquito behavior at
precisely the time at which the *Plasmodium* life
cycle stages in the mice are most infective for mosquitoes (Day and Edman 1983). Malarial parasites
also may induce a behavioral change in mosquitoes
so that they are more tenacious in obtaining a blood
meal (Koella and Packer 1996).

Most examples of PITT that have been well documented involve small animals that can be studied in
the laboratory (table 5.3), but the phenomenon
seems to be so widespread that it is likely a feature
of many parasites with a predator-prey life cycle. In
some situations in wild animals, parasitized individuals are known to be more vulnerable to predation
than their unparasitized colleagues, but the actual
mechanism resulting in increased vulnerability is
unknown. For example, rodents infected with protozoa of the genera *Sarcocystis* and *Frenkelia* are more
susceptible than uninfected animals to predation by
raptorial birds that are potential final hosts for these

Table 5.3 Parasitic Infections in Which Intermediate Host Is Manipulated to Increase the Likelihood of Being Eaten by Appropriate Final Host

Parasite	Intermediate host	Final host	Type of manipulation
Euhaplorchis californiensis (trematode)	Fish	Fish-eating birds	Abnormal behavior[1]
Hymenolepis diminutata (cestode)	Beetle	Rat	Abnormal behavior[2]
Raillientina cesticillus (cestode)	Beetle	Chicken	Abnormal behavior[3]
Curtureria australis (trematode)	Cockle	Shorebirds	Reduced growth of foot, impaired burrowing ability[4]
Pompyrhynchus laevis (acanthocephalid)	*Gammarus pulex*	Fish	Abnormal coloration[5]
Toxoplasma gondii (protozoan)	Rat	Cat	Abnormal behavior[6]
Dicrocoeliium dendriticum (tapeworm)	Ant	Ruminants	Abnormal behavior[7]
Eustrongylides ignotus (nematode)	Fish	Predatory fish	Abnormal behavior[8]
Plasmodium spp. (protozoan)	Mouse	Mosquito	Reduced antimosquito behavior[9]

[1] Lafferty and Morris (1996).
[2] Hurd and Fugo (1991).
[3] Graham (1966).
[4] Thomas and Poulin (1998).
[5] Bakker et al. (1997).
[6] Berdoy et al. (1995).
[7] Carney (1969).
[8] Coyner et al. (2001).
[9] Day and Edman (1983).

parasites (Hoogenbloom and Dikstra 1987; Vŏrišek et al. 1998). It has been suggested that moose infected with the tapeworm *Echinococcus granulosus* (fig. 5.2) are more susceptible to human hunters and may be more susceptible to wolf predation than uninfected moose, perhaps because of reduced endurance and ability to escape (Rau and Caron 1979). Timing of infection may be important in the effect. Only voles infected at a young age with larval *Echinococcus multilocularis* are likely to be debilitated by the parasite, because the developmental period of the parasite (about 3 months) is similar to the expected life span of most voles (6 months) (Hansen et al. 2004).

Not all instances of parasite-induced susceptibility to predators represent PITT. Some may be a coincidental effect. Mice infected with the intestinal coccidium *Eimeria vermiformes* have reduced avoidance behavior toward cats. Being eaten by a cat does not benefit this parasite, because its life cycle involves direct transmission from mouse to mouse. However, the same altered behavioral pattern that facilitates cat predation also facilitates interaction and transmission between infected and uninfected mice (Kavaliers and Colwell 1995a). Another possible explanation is that parasitism reduces resources that could have been used for pred-

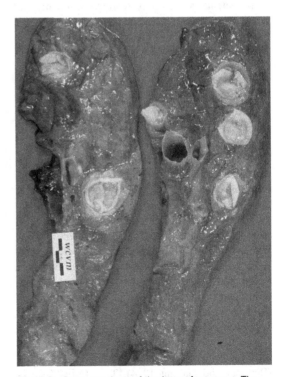

Fig. 5.2. Cross-sections of the lung of a moose. The large white structures are opened hydatid cysts of *Echinococcus granulosus*. The adult of this tapeworm occurs in the intestine of wolves and dogs.

ator avoidance behavior. Some years ago, I observed that ducks killed by a hunter using a falcon were much more often infected by renal coccidia than were ducks of the same species and age shot in the area. Because raptors play no role in the life cycle of renal coccidia, this probably was an instance in which some subtle debilitation by the parasite made infected ducks more vulnerable to predation.

In relationships characterized by PITT, virulence is distributed asymmetrically. Virulence is high in the intermediate host and low in the predator. This makes good sense from the agent's perspective. The predatory final host needs to remain active and mobile so that it can catch prey and spread the parasite's eggs or oocysts widely, hence, it should suffer relatively little injury. The intermediate host can be injured more severely because injury increases the probability of transmission. PITT may be a feature that allows populations of parasites to persist in carnivore populations at very low density (Apanius and Schad 1994). It is interesting to speculate why predators have not developed avoidance behavior to prevent becoming infected with this type of parasite since avoidance of other diseases is common (Moore 2002). It is likely that the trade-off between easy access to nutrients outweighs the minor costs of parasitism, as in "it is worthwhile eating this mouse now because it is so nutritious even though I may have a mild belly ache later from the parasites I might receive" !

The injury that occurs in most noninfectious diseases is coincidental and does not benefit the causative agent. Levin (1996) and Ebert (1999) used botulism as an example of a disease in which virulence is coincidental, and Levin stated, "It would be difficult to account for the evolution of botulism toxin by selection favoring *Clostridium botulinum* that kill people who eat improperly canned food." However, Mims et al. (2001) suggested that toxin could be useful to *C. botulinum* as a means of providing growth medium for these saprophytic organisms. This is particularly applicable to the type of botulism that occurs in wild ducks in which virulence does appear to benefit the agent. Botulism in waterfowl is caused by a strain of *C. botulinum* that produces a toxin called type C_1. Decaying carcasses are optimal habitat for growth of this strain of *C. botulinum*, because of their high protein content and because the temperature within a decaying carcass is ideal for bacterial replication and toxin production (Wobeser and Galmut 1984). Type C botulism is unique among poisonings in that birds killed by the toxin become habitat for proliferation of the next

generation of bacteria and toxin production. Thus, killing birds is advantageous for the bacterium (and for the viral phage that provides the gene for toxin production) because the carcass provides them with new habitat. Toxin produced in carcasses is ingested by fly maggots, and ducks that eat these maggots die of botulism, creating a carcass-maggot cycle that leads to the explosive mortality typical of this disease.

COST OF VIRULENCE HYPOTHESIS (THE TRADE-OFF HYPOTHESIS)

This hypothesis has received a great deal of attention since Anderson and May (1982) began modeling how virulence might evolve in parasites. In the benefit of virulence hypothesis described above, virulence benefits the agent. In the trade-off hypothesis, it is assumed that virulence (as measured by host survival) is a cost to the agent and an unavoidable consequence of reproduction in the host. However, virulence may be coupled with some other trait that has positive value for the agent. This creates a situation in which a trade-off may exist between virulence (a cost) and that other feature (a benefit). The feature that has been identified as a positive trade-off is parasite fitness, as determined by survival, reproduction, and transmission. Models predict that if virulence is not related to the agent's transmission or to the rate at which the host recovers from the infection, evolution should proceed toward benign coexistence, that is, the causative agent should become less damaging over time. Similarly, if virulence limits transmission, for example, by premature death of the host animal, so that there is limited time for growth or reproduction by the agent, or because severe reaction by the host reduces the agent's viability or fecundity, evolution also should be toward a benign state. However, if virulence improves the agent's fitness, some level of virulence is favored. In the trade-off model, the optimal solution for the disease agent is to balance virulence and within-host reproduction and growth so that transmission success is maximal during the lifetime of the infection (Ebert and Bull 2003).

This hypothesis gives another perspective from which to look at examples of PITT. The tapeworm *Echinococcus granulosus* cycles between wolves and moose where these species coexist. In the wolf, virulence would be very costly for the tapeworm if it limited egg production or impaired the wolf's mobility so that it could not spread the worm's eggs widely in the environment or catch moose. Virulence in the moose is not costly for the tapeworm, because it is coupled with enhanced transmission by rendering the moose more easily caught by a wolf. Thus, the trade-off for *E. granulosus* is much different in the two species, favoring virulence in the moose and favoring a benign relationship with the wolf.

The trade-off hypothesis has spawned a huge amount of intellectual activity among evolutionary ecologists. It is helpful in understanding why a disease such as rabies can persist even though the virus is almost uniformly fatal to its hosts. (In rabies, transmission is favored by a particular form of virulence.) The notion of trade-offs has led to the concept that some intermediate level of virulence may be favored in many infectious diseases (Claessen and Roos 1995). It also has been at least partially responsible for other concepts, including that of coevolution of host and parasite as an "arms race" (Ewald 1995) that will be discussed shortly. The idea of trade-offs also has provided some explanation for why certain methods of disease transmission are associated with a particular level of virulence. Transmission from mother to offspring (vertical transmission) usually is associated with low virulence, perhaps because transmission is dependent upon the mother remaining healthy and fecund. Diseases transmitted by arthropod *vectors* often are highly virulent, perhaps because sickness and immobility of the vertebrate host enhance the probability of being fed upon by arthropods.

The relationship in hypothesized trade-offs is complex, and the direction of natural selection related to virulence in any given host-agent relationship "depends to a great extent on the life-history of the parasite—the mode of transmission, the way it uses host resources, the longevity, and reproductive schedule of host and parasite" (Moore 2002).

THE SHORT-SIGHTED EVOLUTION HYPOTHESIS

Improved molecular techniques have revealed that diseased animals often are infected by more than one genotype of the same agent (Read and Taylor 2001). The worms infecting the gut of a deer may not be identical members of a clone but may represent a population of slightly dissimilar individuals occupying a particular patch of habitat. This has led to the notion that competition among genotypes of an agent within a host might lead to high virulence without enhanced transmission to other hosts. Mutants or genotypes that have a high growth rate (and associated high virulence) may be able to replace more slow-growing strains of the organism

and gain dominance within the entire host or some part of the host even though they may or may not be able to be transmitted to a new host. This explanation might apply in part to some of the diseases shown in table 5.2, in which organisms that normally live without causing harm in one area of the body invade new areas of the host. The virulence is short-sighted in the individual animal because the organisms may die along with the host, but a high rate of mutation that results in this type of dispersion out of the normal range might be adaptive in the overall evolutionary arms race between the host's defenses and the agent. Recent information suggests that both the host genotype (de Roode et al. 2004) and the mechanisms of competition among agents (Massey et al. 2004) may influence the resulting virulence of an infection.

COEVOLUTION

The hypotheses discussed thus far have dealt with the advantages that may accrue to the disease agent by causing injury to the host animal, and they largely ignored adaptations that might occur in the host. Evolution of the relationship between a disease agent and an animal species might take one of three courses over time.

If an animal species is unable to evolve in response to injury or if its response is so slow as to be insignificant, the agent would be expected to adapt to extract an optimal amount of resources from the animal and the most favorable outcome for the agent might be severe disease (high virulence).

If the animal species can adapt to counter the effects of the agent and the agent cannot change, selection in the host should reduce harmful effects (virulence) to a minimum over time. This is the evolutionary direction that one would expect to occur in certain noninfectious diseases, such as those caused by contaminants, in which the agent has no ability to evolve. Acquired resistance at the population level to chemicals and drugs is well known in bacteria and invertebrates and constitutes a serious problem in the widespread use of antibiotics, anthelmintics, and pesticides to control disease in humans and livestock.

There are few well-documented examples of acquired resistance to noxious substances in wild animals, but experience with some pesticides illustrates that populations can develop genetic resistance. Pine mice from an area where the pesticide endrin was used for 11 years had 12-fold greater tolerance to the chemical than mice from an area where the chemical had not been used (Webb and Horsfall

1976). Populations of rats and mice in many areas of the world became resistant to the anticoagulant warfarin within a decade of its first use (Jackson and Ashton 1986). If there is an advantage in being resistant to a poison and exposure to the poison is widespread, there should be an increase in resistance over time within the population and the average virulence of the poison should decrease. Unfortunately, populations of birds do not seem to have become noticeably more resistant to contaminants, such as carbamate insecticides or lead, perhaps because there has been inadequate time or selection pressure by these chemicals on populations to result in an obvious change in resistance. It is interesting to speculate whether waterfowl have developed resistance to type C botulinum toxin to which they have been exposed for centuries. To my knowledge, no one has determined if ducks in western North America (where botulism occurs frequently) are more resistant to botulism than ducks in eastern North America (where exposure to botulinum toxins is uncommon). Turkey vultures are resistant to botulinum toxin, perhaps because they "through their feeding habits have for ages been thrown in intimate contact with the toxin elaborated by *C. botulinum*" (Kalmbach 1939).

Development of resistance represents a trade-off for the animal. Resistance is costly in resources that could be used for maintenance, growth, or reproduction, so that an animal should choose a level of resistance that maximizes its fitness (Sheldon and Verhuist 1996). In some circumstances, individuals that commit resources to resistance may have a selective advantage, although they may, for example, grow more slowly. In other circumstances, it may be advantageous for the individual to suffer (tolerate?) some degree of harm from disease if resources used for growth or reproduction, rather than resistance, result in greater fitness.

The third alternative course is that both the agent and the animal adapt. In diseases caused by living agents, both host and agent have the ability to adapt (although the rate of adaptation may be radically different) and the "equilibrial" level of virulence is likely somewhere between the optima for the host and that for the agent, because of their opposing needs. The traditional view of host-parasite evolution was that it proceeded inevitably toward a benign state (commensalism). This was based on the concept that disease agents that harm their host also are likely to harm themselves. Thus, agents should not imperil their own survival by compromising the survival of the host; the agent should be prudent in

its demands on the host. This view held that "successful parasite species evolve to be harmless to their host" (Anderson and May 1982), and that old relationships are characterized by limited or no virulence. By extension, it was thought that severe disease represented a lack of coadaptation between host and agent (Ewald 1983), and that "mildness is a sign that a host is a natural host" (Ewald 1995). Many observations on disease (particularly of new or emergent diseases) seem to be consistent with this "conventional wisdom" about coevolution. But, beginning with Ball (1943), parasitologists and evolutionary ecologists have demonstrated that the conventional wisdom has both theoretical and empirical weaknesses. The weaknesses were stated most clearly by Anderson and May (1982).

An alternative view of evolution of host-parasite relationships is that it involves stepwise adaptation-counteradaptation in the form of an "arms race" (Barnard 1984). In this arms race, adaptation by the parasite to extract more from the host is followed by counteradaptation by the host, which in turn is followed by further adaptation of the parasite, and so forth. Mocarski (2002) termed this a "battle of genetic one-upmanship." Over time, oscillations favoring one or the other antagonist become progressively damped around a point of optimal fitness for each that allows optimal replication of each gene lineage (Wakelin 1994).

During the past two decades, the "prudent parasite" hypothesis has been replaced by a series of hypotheses in which natural selection could favor a range of outcomes from development or maintenance of virulence to progression to commensalism, with selection favoring a level of virulence that maximizes the rate of parasite increase. In many cases, selection appears to favor an intermediate level of virulence. There is no single hypothesis that explains all situations. Lenski and May (1994) reviewed the evidence for the two opposing hypotheses (i.e., evolution to avirulence, evolution to an intermediate level of virulence) and concluded that the ideas are not incompatible and that most models suggest evolution toward reduced (but not zero) virulence.

The most completely studied example of the coevolution of a disease agent and a wild animal is the disease myxomatosis in wild rabbits in Australia and Europe. Myxomatosis is caused by myxoma virus (a poxvirus) of which two strains are found naturally in two species of the genus *Sylvilagus*. In the jungle rabbit (*S. brasiliensis*) in Central and South America and the brush rabbit (*S. bachmani*) in California, myxoma causes a localized wartlike skin tumor called a fibroma, but in the European rabbit, the virus causes severe and often fatal generalized disease. The virus is transmitted primarily on the mouthparts of blood-feeding arthropods (mosquitoes, fleas) feeding on live rabbits. The virus does not infect or multiply in the arthropod, it is simply carried on the mouthparts as the arthropod moves from one rabbit to the next.

In 1950, a South American strain of myxoma virus was released intentionally in Australia to control European rabbits. In 1952, another strain of myxoma virus of South American origin was introduced in France and spread throughout Europe. When first released, the disease in each area was devastating, killing virtually every rabbit that became infected (>99% mortality with a mean survival of <13 days). In Europe and Australia, strains of virus emerged within 1 to 2 years that allowed some rabbits to survive (Kerr and Best 1998). Within a decade, the fully virulent virus had almost disappeared and had been replaced by less-virulent strains. The majority of viruses recovered from wild rabbits at this time were of intermediate virulence (70–95% mortality, survival time 17–28 days, as measured in fully susceptible, laboratory-reared rabbits). To that point in time, the evolutionary trajectory of the disease seemed to follow conventional wisdom (i.e., toward avirulence). However, over the next decade, the virus did not continue to become less virulent. Instead, virulence stabilized, and in both Great Britain and Australia, the circulating viruses actually became somewhat more virulent (Kerr and Best 1998).

Interpretation of the myxomatosis example has been that evolution of this disease is driven by a trade-off between virulence and transmission. Transmission among rabbits depends upon arthropods picking up virus on their mouthparts as they probe through the rabbit's skin. Hence, the amount of virus present in the skin of infected rabbits and the length of time that this virus is available to arthropods are very important. The minimum threshold of virus for rendering mosquitoes infective is about 10 million infectious viral particles per gram of skin (Kerr and Best 1998). Rabbits that survive for 18–27 days yield the highest proportion of infective fleas (Ross 1982). Strains of virus with somewhat reduced virulence are thought to have replaced fully virulent strains because they provided more opportunity for transmission. These moderately virulent strains produced large amounts of virus in the skin of rabbits and the infected rabbits

survived for longer than those infected with the fully virulent virus. Strains of virus that were even less virulent produced relatively small amounts of virus in the skin, so that even though rabbits infected with these mild strains survived for an extended period, less virus was transmitted by arthropods (Ross 1982). Thus, viruses of moderate virulence were selected for because they provided optimal conditions for transmission. Ross (1982) noted that transmission in Australia and France is mainly by mosquitoes, while transmission in Great Britain is by fleas. He attributed further progression toward a less-virulent state in Australia and France to greater ability of mosquitoes to transmit the virus.

Concurrent, or nearly so, with changes occurring in the virus, there also was selection for genetic resistance within the rabbit population. Development of less-virulent strains of virus allowed survival of more infected rabbits that aided development of resistance (Kerr and Best 1998). At one site in Australia, 78% of young rabbits born the year following introduction of the virus were descendants of the few rabbits that had *evaded* infection. In following years when less virulent viruses were becoming common, almost all offspring were born to parents that had *survived* infection. These resistant rabbits survived infection with any strain of virus for longer. Ross (1982) suggested that "as resistance appears and increases, survival times in the optimal (18–27 days) range will be produced by strains which are more and more virulent to non-resistant rabbits," which may explain the increase in the average virulence of virus that occurred after about 2 decades.

In myxomatosis, there was reduction of virulence over time, but this occurred only to a degree at which rabbit numbers recovered to a density well below premyxomatosis levels. This experiment in nature has proceeded for about 50 years. How it will proceed in the future is still a subject for speculation. Fenner and Ross (1994) suggested that most changes in both the rabbit and the virus genotype that can be selected for readily have already occurred and that the disease will continue with moderate virulence and "appreciable mortality."

There still may be surprises to come. Seven of 11 virus strains isolated in Australia during the 1990s were equivalent in virulence to the original virus released (Kerr and Best 1998), and strains of virus that affected the respiratory tract and appeared to be transmitted by the respiratory route rather than by the usual arthropods have been reported in France (Joubert et al. 1982).

It is unclear how generally experience with myxomatosis can be applied to other diseases. The myxomatosis experiment was unusual in that there was no natural host for the virus in Australia or Europe, so that "the virus had to persist in the very species whose eradication was sought" (Zúñiga 2002). Ebert and Bull (2003) have cautioned against using myxomatosis as support for the trade-off model for disease virulence because the species involved was not the usual host for the virus, and virulence of the original virus "was chosen to be unusually high" so that the results might not be applicable in more natural situations.

Three other basic features complicate an understanding of virulence and of how it might evolve in a host-agent relationship. The first is that in nature, in contrast to experimental situations, an animal is never confronted with just one potential disease-causing agent at any one time. Animals are confronted by a range of agents for each of which the animal has potential cost/benefit trade-offs in relation to resistance and defense. If, for example, an animal makes a major commitment to resist intestinal worms, it will have less resources available not only for growth and reproduction but also for defense against respiratory viruses and ectoparasites, so that their virulence might increase. This diversity relates not only to different species but also to different genotypes of individual agents that may have very different virulence. Various infectious and noninfectious agents may interact in a range from totally antagonistic, through indifference and additive effects, to synergism in which the combined virulence is more than the sum of the individual components. In some situations, one agent may utilize its own pathogenicity to reduce the population density of another agent (Dobson 1985). We know very little about the interaction among disease-causing agents and particularly about their coevolution.

A second factor is that many infectious agents are capable of infecting more than one host species. There are relatively few truly single-host parasitic conditions among those diseases of greatest concern to wildlife ecologists. Almost every infectious disease that is of serious concern in wild animals is caused by a multihost agent. Single-host agents may evolve to some optimal level of virulence in that host, but the situation is much more complex for an agent that can infect many species. In a multihost system, each host species has a different relationship with the agent. Some hosts may contribute little or nothing to the agent's fitness so that there is little or no selective pressure on the agent to use those hosts prudently. (In these hosts, the parasite has the equivalent of a "free shot on goal" with little to lose from being virulent.) Multihost agents are particularly dangerous for small populations such as those of endangered species. A specialist parasite that only infected the endangered species must be somewhat prudent in order to maintain a sufficient level of transmission for its own persistence. This probably requires a certain critical host population size (see chapter 11). A multihost agent can be maintained in one or more abundant hosts (in which its virulence is under some control) but spill over into the endangered species without consequences for its own persistence. Studies of population ecology and virulence have been preoccupied with one-and two-species systems because of the "sheer difficulty" in collecting and analyzing data from a multispecies system (Begon and Bowers 1995).

A third factor is that very little is known about how changes in environmental factors (the third corner of the agent-host-environment triangle) influence virulence. Subtle alterations in some abiotic or biotic factor might alter an animal's resistance to an agent or increase the amount of exposure to the agent so that the pattern of virulence changes dramatically. Brown et al. (2003) used the term "context-dependent virulence" for situations in which seemingly benign disease agents that may occur at high prevalence in a host population can have a severe negative effect on the host only during stressful periods in the life-history of the host. Although much of the empirical evidence now available comes from parasites of insects, the phenomenon of increased virulence at times when animals are unable to compensate for increased costs of disease resistance is probably very common. Environmental factors, such as temperature, also can have a direct effect on the virulence of many contaminants affecting wild animals (Rattner and Heath 1995).

SUMMARY

- Virulence is used here as a measure of the ability of an agent to cause harm to an animal.
- Virulence is not a static feature of any disease. The ability to cause harm may change as a result of changes in the animal, the causative agent, or other environmental factors.
- Virulence may occur for a variety of reasons. Some forms are coincidental, some benefit the agent, and some are a result of coevolution of the agent and host.

- Virulence is not an inherent feature of a disease agent. The response to the same pathogen in different species, different individuals within a species, and different environmental conditions may vary from undetectable to acute lethality.

- Virulence in many infectious diseases appears to be the result of an arms race in which evolution acts on the genetic heterogeneity in the agent and host, selecting those genes that allow each to approach optimal fitness under the circumstances existing at a given time.

6
Defense, Resistance, and Repair

To pathogenic microparasites (viruses, bacteria, protozoa, or fungi), we and other mammals (living organisms at large) are little more than soft, thin-walled flasks of culture media.
—B. Levin and R. Antia

Every wild animal is exposed many times each day to potentially harmful agents and factors yet, despite these constant challenges, individuals and species persist. Levin and Antia (2001), cited above, introduced a discussion of factors that interfere with the ability of bacteria to "cause disease and lead to our rapid demise." The defense and repair mechanisms of the body have been characterized in great detail from a medical perspective but they are less well understood in an ecological sense.

A feature of defense mechanisms that is important for understanding disease in the individual and in populations is that these are active processes that require the commitment of resources both for establishment and for maintenance and operation. The concept that organisms allocate limited resources among maintenance, growth, reproduction, and defense is strongly established in plant ecological theory and is central to the idea of life history trade-offs (Bergelson and Purrington 1996). This concept has received less attention in human and veterinary medicine and is seldom mentioned in discussion of disease in wild animals, although it provides a valid foundation for discussing resistance to disease in all species (Sheldon and Verhuist 1996; Gemmill and Read 1998; Buttgereit et al. 2000; Rigby and Moret 2000; Lochmiller and Deerenberg 2000). (In this discussion, I will use resistance as an overarching term for all of the defense mechanisms used to withstand diseases.)

Each animal has limited resources and must make trade-offs in how it uses those resources. If resources are allocated to resist disease, less will be available for other activities. Conversely, if additional resources are allocated to activities such as reproduction, less will be available for defense (Deerenberg et al. 1997; Gustafsson et al. 1997). The notion of trade-offs related to disease resistance also provides a perspective for thinking about the impact of disease. An infection or damage caused by a noninfectious agent could be well controlled by an animal's defenses and never result in overt disease but still have an enormous impact on the animal's resource budget and fitness, because of the cost of resistance. Trade-offs also help to explain why animals at certain stages of their life-history or in circumstances of resource shortage are particularly susceptible to disease.

Resistance to disease seems to be a good thing, so one might expect that all individuals should be resistant to all potential disease agents. However, that is not what we see in nature. From personal experience, we know that there are differences in resistance among individuals, as in "I get colds frequently, while John never has a cold!" There are striking differences in resistance among groups, populations, and species. For instance, Spieker et al. (1996) found that all ducks of the genus *Anas* could be infected with duck plague virus but the result varied from peracute death in blue-winged teal to complete absence of any clinical effect in northern pintails. Some resistance is heritable, for example, Smith et al. (1999) demonstrated "significant heritable variation in resistance" to parasites among free-ranging Soay sheep.

If an animal is going to invest resources in defense, it makes sense to resist those conditions that are likely to be encountered and that are likely to cause severe harm. Resistance is like insurance in this regard. If there were no cost for insurance, everyone would be insured against every possible calamity. In reality, we decide if we can afford to have or not to have certain types of insurance. Life history theory would predict that for me, as a 60-something male, it would be unwise to invest resources in insuring myself against injuries associated with playing professional hockey or childbirth, conditions that I am unlikely to encounter.

Because it is costly to maintain active resistance to a disease that is unlikely to be encountered, new diseases often have a dramatic effect when first introduced into a population. Resistance to myxoma virus was rare in European rabbits in Australia prior to introduction of the virus in 1950–51, consequently 99.8% of infected rabbits died in the first year (Kerr and Best 1998). However, resistance was not totally lacking in the rabbit population, and under severe selective pressure exerted by the disease, it became widespread. In order to be able to follow the development of resistance to myxomatosis, rabbit kittens captured each year at one site were challenged with a standard dose of virus of known virulence over a period of years. Following the second annual epizootic, about 88% of kittens died, but 5 years later (after 7 years experience with the virus by the population), only 26% of kittens died after challenge. Kerr and Best (1998) concluded that "development of resistance must have required the existence of polymorphism in the population at one or more critical genetic loci as resistance is unlikely to have depended on novel mutations occurring over such a short time period."

The continuous presence of effective resistance is costly in the absence of disease but highly beneficial when disease is present (Møller 1994). Because of the trade-offs involved, resistant genotypes should perform better in terms of overall fitness than susceptible genotypes under high levels of challenge by disease agents but worse than susceptible genotypes when disease agents are uncommon or absent. The optimal level of resistance may be one that includes some risk, because complete defense against disease is probably too costly.

The defense system is complex and composed of many parts. As in a military campaign, an animal's defenses consist of strategic siting or movement to reduce contact with the enemy; a series of physical barriers analogous to walls, moats, and battlements; and defenders with various specialties and weapons. Some defenders are on constant alert, others respond when an alarm is raised, and there is the potential to recruit and mobilize other reserves if time allows. The overall cost of resistance has not been measured in any species, although the relative cost of some parts of the system has been estimated in a few situations (Kraaljeveld and Godfray 1997; Lochmiller and Deerenberg 2000; Whitaker and Fair 2002). The total bill must include the resources to produce and maintain the system together with the cost to repair the damage that the defenders cause to the body during battle. Even in a successful engagement in which the defenders are victorious, there inevitably is destruction on the tissue battlefield and there may be collateral damage to areas far removed from the site. The "friendly troops," particularly inflammation and immunity, cause much of the injury in many diseases. This is a very good reason to use these defenses only when necessary. In some circumstances, it may be to an animal's advantage to tolerate the effects of a disease rather than suffer the damage that will occur in defending against it.

Combes (2000) proposed that the relationship between hosts and parasites is controlled by two "filters" that he called "encounter" and "compatibility." An alternate name for encounter might be exposure since this filter relates to the amount of contact between disease agent and animal. Compatibility relates to all the events that happen after contact and that influence the "durability" of the relationship. The concept of these two filters is useful for thinking about resistance to all types of disease, not just those caused by parasites, because an animal's defenses are designed to either reduce exposure or to end the relationship by making the body less compatible (e.g., by killing an invading organism or by metabolizing and excreting a poison).

There are four general lines of defense: (1) behavioral avoidance, (2) physical barriers, (3) innate responses, and (4) acquired immune responses. The first two relate primarily to reducing exposure, and the third and fourth are concerned mainly with compatibility.

BEHAVIORAL AVOIDANCE

How various diseases affect the behavior of wild animals will be discussed elsewhere. Here we are concerned with the behaviors that animals use to reduce exposure to potential causes of disease. Avoidance behavior is seldom discussed as such in human medicine, but we are all advised regularly to avoid certain risky behaviors. Avoiding smoking and not drinking too much usually save rather than cost the individual resources. In animals, behavioral avoidance has a cost, and in the absence of the disease agent, avoidance behaviors are reduced or lacking (Moore 2002). Animals expend resources by moving away from areas where exposure to disease agents is likely as well as through engaging in activ-

Table 6.1 Behaviors Thought to Reduce or Avoid Exposure to Disease-Causing Agents or Substances

Behavior	Species /disease
Avoid contact	Caribou move to windswept areas or snow patches to avoid bot flies.[1]
	Brown pelicans abandon nests because of ticks.[2]
Avoid dead animals	Wild geese avoid close contact with birds dead of avian cholera.[3]
Avoid infected nests and nestborne ectoparasites	Great tits avoid nests containing fleas.[4]
Assemble in groups or herds	Ungulates in large groups receive fewer bites/individual from biting flies.[5]
Avoid fecal material	Sheep avoid grass contaminated with feces and parasite eggs.[6]
Grooming, preening	Many species respond in this manner to ectoparasites.
Nest "fumigation"	Starlings add plants containing bactericidal materials to nests.[7]
Select good mates	Female sage grouse avoid males with hemorrhages associated with lice.[8]
Avoid concentrations of ticks	Cattle avoid concentrations of tick larvae.[9]
Adjust posture	Deer adopt a "reduced silhouette" posture in response to attack by horseflies.[10]

[1] Mörschel and Klein (1997).
[2] King et al. (1977).
[3] McLandress (1983).
[4] Christe et al. (1994).
[5] Mooring and Hart (1992).
[6] Hutchings et al. (1999).
[7] Clark and Mason (1988).
[8] Spurrier et al. (1991).
[9] Sutherst et al. (1986).
[10] Hoy and Anderson (1978).

ities such as scratching, preening, running, and tail switching to discourage or remove agents. They may eat less-nutritious foods, not use part of their habitat that contains resources, restrict their choice of mates, or forgo mating to reduce the chance of exposure. Examples of avoidance behavior in wild animals are shown in table 6.1. Hart (1997) and Moore (2002) provide detailed discussion of behavioral resistance to infectious diseases.

Many examples of avoidance behavior are intriguing. Female sage grouse select against mating with males that have hemorrhages on their air sacs, typical of those found in birds with lice (Spurrier et al. 1991). This raises a question: Are the louse-infested males impaired in other ways recognized by females or are the hemorrhages a signal that females use to choose mates? This has been answered experimentally: males without lice but with artificial hemorrhages (painted on by the researchers) were discriminated against, indicating that the females recognized the hemorrhages as a signal. A larger question remains: Do female grouse discriminate to avoid becoming infected themselves (ectoparasites are often transmitted during sexual contact) or do

they perceive males with lice to be "lousy" in other regards and, hence, less fit as potential sires for offspring?

Clayton and Tompkins (1995) studied the effectiveness of grooming as a behavioral defense against lice. They placed a small "bit" on pigeons that created a 1–3 mm gap in the bird's bill. After a few weeks, the average intensity of louse infestation on birds fitted with the device quadrupled in the absence of effective grooming, clearly demonstrating the value of this behavior. Grooming and preening can be influenced by many factors that could have a dramatic effect on ectoparasitism (Day and Edman 1983; Hart 1988). As an example, waterfowl with botulism are unable to groom effectively. These birds often have large numbers of leeches in their eyes and nostrils (fig. 6.1) and suffer considerable blood loss that adds to their misery and probably increases the case fatality rate.

Hutchings et al. (1999) examined the relationships among avoidance of feces, nutrients in forage, and parasitism in sheep. They found that sheep have a strong aversion to sheep feces that outweighs the attractiveness of high nitrogen forage growing near

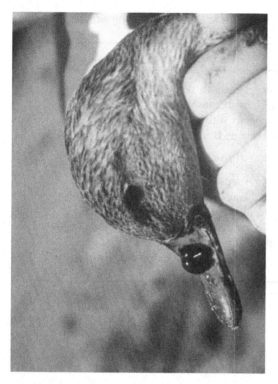

Fig. 6.1. Infestation with leeches occurs commonly in nostrils and eyes of ducks with botulism that are unable to groom.

horn sheep (Thorne et al. 1982).

Behaviors to reduce exposure to infectious agents seem to be widespread, but there is little empirical evidence that wild animals avoid exposure to many important noninfectious causes of disease. Wild ungulates probably avoid poisonous plants, but there are no data to show that wild animals avoid circumstances that result in poisoning by lead, mercury, pesticides, PCBs, endocrine disrupting compounds, or oil. It may be that exposure to this type of environmental contamination has occurred so recently that there has been inadequate time for selective processes to occur, or that the selective pressure caused by these agents has been inadequate to result in behavioral adaptation. It seems strange that waterfowl appear not to have developed avoidance of type C botulinum toxin, which is probably an ancient constituent of wetlands. Nonspecific neophobia (fear of new things) may save some wild animals from being exposed to noxious substances. It is interesting that parasite infection may decrease an animal's fear of novel situations and reduce reactivity to noxious stimuli (Webster et al. 1994; Kavaliers and Colwell 1995a), hence, the presence of one disease agent might influence behavioral avoidance and risk of other potential disease agents.

The final word in this discussion belongs to Moore (2002): "the avoidance of parasites is a nontrivial task, one that is costly, and by implication, worth the cost."

PHYSICAL BARRIERS

The epithelial surfaces between the external environment, and the internal structures of the body are the second line of defense. The skin and surface of the alimentary, respiratory, and urogenital tracts that extend into the interior of the body (fig. 6.2) are exposed constantly to agents that could cause disease, but the tissues directly below these epithelial surfaces are normally free of these agents. Skin is liberally endowed with defensive properties. The first of these is a thick, multilayered outer surface (the epidermis), the outermost layers of which are composed of dead cells that are being shed continuously taking adherent disease agents with them. Secretions from glands deeper in the skin bathe the surface with oils and organic acids that inhibit bacterial growth and prevent penetration of liquids. Epithelial cells can directly produce antimicrobial substances and emit signals that attract other defense cells (Ganz 2002). Relatively few infectious agents can penetrate intact skin directly, but many agents can enter through breaks in the skin or via bite wounds

feces. The level of aversion to feces was greater in animals with subclinical parasitism than in unparasitized animals, suggesting that avoidance of exposure to parasites may be a powerful factor in ruminant foraging strategy (Gunn and Irvine 2003). Avoidance of parasites in this manner seems to parallel behavioral avoidance of predators ("predator sensitive foraging") that also may lead to use of areas containing lower quality nutrients (Banks and Powell 2004).

Avoidance or reduction of contact with disease agents may be an important advantage for species or groups that migrate or regularly shift to new areas. Stear et al. (1998) suggested that the "ambulatory and migratory behaviour" of many herbivores may have evolved with two goals: increased access to food and reduced exposure to nematodes. Inability to move freely because of habitat loss may result in animals being confined for extended periods in areas that become progressively more contaminated. Prolonged usage of contaminated areas may be one factor in the emergence of avian cholera as an important disease of waterfowl on wintering areas (Wobeser 1992) and in lungworm infections in big-

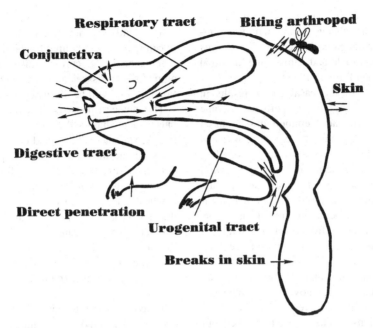

Fig. 6.2. Portals of entry through which agents may enter the body and by which agents can leave the body. Most agents enter through the digestive, respiratory, and urogenital tracts, which communicate directly with the external environment. (Note beaver are unusual among mammals in having a cloaca that is a common orifice for the digestive and urogenital tracts.) Direct penetration of intact skin is limited to a small number of actively invasive agents. The agents of some superficial infections, such as with ectoparasites and some fungi, are shed directly from the skin surface. (Adapted from *Mim's Pathogenesis of Infectious Disease*, 5th Edition, Mims et al., p. 11, 2001 with permission from Elsevier.)

by arthropods or larger animals. Penetration through the skin is an uncommon route of entry for toxins in wild animals.

The digestive, respiratory, and urogenital tracts are important portals of entry for disease agents. The external portion of these systems (the anterior nose, oral cavity and esophagus, distal urinary and genital tract) is covered by thick stratified epithelium similar to the skin. Deeper in the body these passages are lined by thin, delicate epithelium with only one layer of cells separating external from internal in the alveoli of the lung, the intestine from stomach to rectum, tubules of the kidneys and testes, and the uterus. This cell layer is replaced continuously so that damage to individual cells does not constitute a complete breach in the wall. The rate at which cells are destroyed and the rate at which they can be replaced determines the effect that many diseases have on the body. For example, coccidia are protozoal parasites that live and multiply within cells, particularly epithelial cells of the intestine. When each generation of intracellular multiplication is complete, coccidia burst from the host cell resulting in the cell's death. If the number of host cells that die is limited and the integrity of the epithelial surface can

be maintained by replacement, there is no apparent disease. However, if more host cells are killed than can be replaced, severe disease occurs. (As noted in chapter 3, the intensity of a parasitic infection often determines the outcome.) Newborn animals are particularly susceptible to many intestinal infections because the rate of replacement of their intestinal epithelium is much slower than in older animals.

The digestive tract is not sterile, but hydrochloric acid in the stomach is an important defense that kills many bacteria and viruses that have been ingested so that the upper small intestine contains very few microorganisms. Secretions into the intestine dilute noxious substances and contain antimicrobial substances. Continual movement of ingesta by peristalsis limits contact time with cells and results in expulsion of harmful material. There are progressively more microorganisms lower in the intestine, with the colon containing an amazing density and complexity of microorganisms. The community of microorganisms in the alimentary tract is very stable and protects the animal from colonization by new harmful species. Conditions that disrupt this normal intestinal microflora may allow the establishment of other damaging species. This is believed to occur in a disease called "necrotic enteritis" of wild geese in which an abrupt diet change during autumn migration allows the pathogenic bacterium *Clostridium perfringens* to proliferate and damage the intestinal lining (Wobeser and Rainnie 1987).

The architecture of the nasal cavity results in swirling of inspired air so that particles become trapped on the mucus-laden epithelium. The nasal cavity and trachea have mucus-secreting glands and cells with cilia that beat continuously, propelling mucus backward from the nasal cavity and upward from the bronchi and trachea toward the pharynx, where the material is swallowed. This moving blanket of mucus, the "mucociliary escalator," is important in preventing material from reaching the lung as well as in removing foreign material from the lung. (This escalator also is the route by which lungworm eggs and larvae leave the lungs.) Most particles and bacteria in inspired air are removed by the mucociliary system before they can reach the lungs. The mucus and secretions also neutralize inhaled chemicals and have antimicrobial actions. The principle defense within the alveoli of the lung are specialized cells called macrophages ("big eaters") that ingest and degrade particulate material. Mammals have abundant macrophages in their alveoli at all times, while birds have few resident macrophages in their lungs and depend on the influx of cells when needed (Toth 2000). Normally, the lungs are almost sterile; however, many factors including viral infections, exposure to air-borne pollutants, and chronic stress can impair the defenses of the respiratory tract and allow microorganisms to establish in the lung and cause disease.

The principle barrier in the urinary tract, which is normally sterile, is the regular flushing by urine and the desquamation of lining cells together with invading organism. The female reproductive tract is protected by acidity of the vaginal mucus, closure of the cervix, and downward flow of mucus.

INNATE DEFENSES

Although the skin and other surface membranes are effective barriers, disease agents enter the body's interior. When this occurs, other mechanisms attempt to remove both the invaders and the tissues that have been injured so that repair can occur. These defenses are of two types: innate defenses that are ancient and shared with our invertebrate ancestors, and acquired immunity that is a vertebrate feature. Hoffmann et al. (1999) estimated the age of the two systems at >1 billion years and about 450 million years, respectively. The innate system works to control agents directly after invasion and before acquired immunity can respond. No prior experience with the particular invading agent is required by the innate system, but there is the need to correctly distinguish between the animal's own tissues and foreigners. (The recognition of "self" will be discussed a little later.)

The innate response is elicited by a system of signals and mediators that is "normally in an idling state" (Spitznagel 1993) and consists of a complex array of antimicrobial peptides, proteolytic compounds, and phagocytosis (literally eating by cells) of foreign matter by cells. The major feature of the innate defense system is *inflammation*, a response that is not manifest in most tissues most of the time but that can be called up or evoked by stimuli. (In locations such as the intestine where there is constant exposure to harmful organisms and substances, some degree of inflammation is always present.) Inflammation is defined as the "reaction of vascularized living tissue to local injury" (Slauson and Cooper 2002), and it "is simultaneously the most important and most useful of our host defense mechanisms and the most common means by which tissues become injured. More animals have died of inflammatory diseases than all other causes combined, yet without an adequate inflammatory response, none of us would be living" (Slauson and Cooper 1990). Words used to describe inflammation in different tissues usually consist of a root denoting the tissue that is involved, followed by the suffix "itis," as in hepatitis for inflammation of the liver and nephritis for inflammation of the kidney. There are exceptions to this rule, for example, inflammation of the lungs usually is called pneumonia rather than pneumonitis.

The body has a limited repertoire of inflammatory responses, so that the initial reaction tends to be similar regardless of the initiating insult. Inflammation can be divided into acute and chronic stages; however, this is an arbitrary division since the actual process is a continuum of overlapping events. Acute inflammation is the immediate and early response to tissue injury and consists of three major components:

1. Changes in blood vessels so that blood flow increases to the injured area,
2. Structural changes in small blood vessels so that fluid and large molecules can leave the vessels and enter the injured tissues, and
3. Movement of white blood cells out from the vessels into the focus of injury.

When you have a sliver in your finger, the immediate area becomes reddened and warm within a few hours because of increased blood flow. The site is swollen because of extra fluid and cells in the area, and your finger is painful because of chemicals released during inflammation and because of pressure on nerves. There may be loss of function of the finger because of the swelling and pain. These features (heat, redness, swelling, pain, and loss of function) are the classical signs of acute inflammation. Although the actions seem simple, a complex array of chemical messengers or mediators and different cells is involved. Some mediators are released from damaged tissue and others are produced by the cells that respond to the injury. Because the response is very powerful and potentially damaging, there also are systems in place to control its extent and duration.

The goal of acute inflammation is to neutralize and remove injurious agents or material and damaged tissue, and to prepare the way for repair. The main white blood cell involved in acute inflammation in mammals is the neutrophil (a cell with similar function in birds is the heterophil) and its function is aided by chemical defenses including complement and lysozyme. Neutrophils are produced in bone marrow and are always present in circulating blood. They adhere to the lining of small blood vessels adjacent to sites of injury and then move through the vessel wall into the tissue. They are motile and are attracted along a concentration gradient of factors released by damaged tissues and disease agents so that they accumulate in areas of injury. Neutrophils actively engulf particulate material and pathogenic organisms. Levin and Antia (2001) likened the control of bacteria that enter the interior of the body to a predator-prey system in which bacteria are the prey and phagocytic cells are the predators. Engulfed organisms and particles are destroyed by powerful enzymes and toxic materials generated by the neutrophil. Neutrophils have a short life span in tissue (a few hours), so they need to be replaced continually. The bone marrow has a huge reserve from which large numbers of neutrophils can be released into the blood. In severe injury or infection, mediators released from the inflammatory process stimulate the bone marrow to produce and release even more neutrophils and these pour into the damaged area. As neutrophils die, their potent enzymes are released and continue breaking down and liquefying tissue.

The number of neutrophils attracted to an area of tissue injury depends upon the agent causing the damage. Certain bacteria such as *Arcanobacterium pyogenes* and *Staphylococcus aureus* produce potent attractants for neutrophils. Tissue destruction associated with the resulting massive inflow of neutrophils results in formation of semiliquid pus, consisting of liquefied tissue debris, live and dead neutrophils, and microbes, within the damaged area (fig. 3.1). A pocket filled with this liquid material (called an abscess) may form in the tissue (fig. 6.3). Other causative agents such as viral infections stimulate accumulation of fewer neutrophils and, depending on the cause, the acute inflammatory reaction may be dominated by the outpouring of fluid into the injured area (e.g., a blister), which is termed a serous reaction, or by accumulation of a coagulated protein called fibrin, in which case the lesion is described as fibrinous.

Other white blood cells also play an active role in inflammation. The most important of these are macrophages. Some macrophages are present in tissues and others come from the blood. They arrive in the injured area later than neutrophils and increase in number as time progresses. Macrophages actively engulf and remove damaged tissue and are well armed to kill invading agents such as most bacteria. Macrophages also produce many chemical substances that mediate the continuing inflammatory

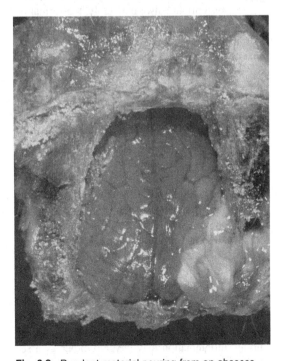

Fig. 6.3. Purulent material pouring from an abscess within the brain of a male mule deer. Brain abscesses in male deer are usually associated with skull injuries that allow penetration of bacteria.

response and assist in tissue repair. Among these are chemicals called cytokines that have very important and widespread effects. They affect blood vessels in the area, attract more neutrophils to the injured area, stimulate proliferation of fibrous tissue (as part of the repair process), and induce production of a variety of other chemical mediators. Cytokines are responsible for the systemic effects including fever, lack of appetite, and general malaise that are present in many diseases, and they are extremely important in development of acquired immunity.

The outcome of inflammation depends on the speed and completeness of the process and the regenerative ability of the tissue that is injured. If the inflammatory reaction is prompt and successful in removing the offending material, and the damaged tissue can regenerate, function will be restored with little or no residual damage. If the inflammatory response is prompt and successful in removing the agent and damaged tissue but the tissue has poor regenerative ability, the damaged tissue will be replaced by less-specialized tissue in the form of a fibrous scar. If the acute response is unsuccessful in removing the offending material and damage continues to occur, the process will proceed to a chronic stage with involvement of new players (the acquired immune system) and also, inevitably, the formation of scar tissue.

Although acute inflammation is basically the same in all tissues, the effect on the animal depends on the location and the extent of the inflammatory process. A red, swollen, painful spot on your finger in response to a sliver is an annoying inconvenience. The same basic response in the lungs may fill the airspaces with inflammatory fluid and cells that interfere with gas exchange creating a life-threatening situation. Even a small volume of extra fluid and cells within the confined space of the cranium, as a result of inflammation of the brain (encephalitis) or the meninges (meningitis), may lead to death because of compression of the nervous tissue.

If the stimulus causing inflammation persists, the processes of tissue injury, inflammation, and repair continue to occur, and this prolonged response is dominated by infiltration of macrophages, lymphocytes, and plasma cells. As the lesion becomes more chronic, there is less fluid in the affected area, and the response is dominated by white blood cells. Chronic inflammation may develop either as a sequel to acute inflammation that has not been resolved or as the initial response to certain specific stimulating agents such as the *Mycobacterium* spp. that cause tuberculosis in various animals. The

eosinophil is another cell involved in inflammation, particularly in inflammation in response to macroparasites, allergic reactions, and fungal infections. A special feature of eosinophils is that they can adhere to helminths and release proteins that are toxic to these parasites.

Differences in innate resistance to infectious disease agents have been reported among subpopulations of wild animals, including plague in northern grasshopper mice (Thomas et al. 1988), malaria in Hawaiian birds, morbillivirus infection in seals, and epizootic hemorrhagic disease in white-tailed deer (Gaydos et al. 2002a). Differences in innate resistance are likely the result of selection over time, and variation in resistance could have major implications for management programs such as translocation, if "susceptible" genotypes are moved to an area where a disease occurs regularly or new agents are introduced to areas in which the population is genetically susceptible.

It is difficult to characterize defenses against noninfectious causes of disease, such as poisons and toxins, as innate or acquired because they may have features of each type. It also is difficult to separate the direct response to the agent from the response to the tissue injury that the agent may cause. One important defense mechanism against poisonous materials is metabolism of the chemical, usually to make it more water soluble and, hence, more easily excreted. This metabolism, or biotransformation, is catalyzed by enzymes that often are most abundant in the liver. Some of the enzymes involved are nonspecific and in that sense resemble innate defenses against living organisms. The most important oxidative reactions of this type are catalyzed by an enzyme system called the cytochrome P-450 monooxygenase system that includes a collection of isoenzymes. This system is inducible, that is, exposure of an animal to a compound leads to an increase in enzyme activity and a change in the toxicity of the compound. Wild animal populations can develop genetic resistance to noninfectious causes of disease (see, for example, Webb and Horsfall 1967), but there is no evidence that this has occurred in the case of the most problematic environmental toxicants.

ACQUIRED IMMUNITY

The innate defenses are nonspecific and do not increase in intensity as a result of prior exposure to a particular agent or insult. The innate defenses may allow an animal to recover, but it remains fully susceptible should it encounter the same disease agent again. If all foreign material that entered an animal's body could be engulfed and destroyed quickly and completely by the innate system, there would be no need for the acquired immune system.

However, if foreign material persists, it acts as a stimulus for acquired immunity that has two major features not seen in the innate system: *specificity* and *memory*. Specificity relates to the ability to recognize individual invaders or foreign substances. As noted earlier, it is critical for both the innate and acquired systems to differentiate between self, that is, "the tissues, cells and molecules present as an integral part of the organism" (Ziegler 1993) and nonself (everything else, including abnormal cells such as cancer cells). The challenge in defense is to be able to recognize and deal with the massive number of nonself materials that enter the body while doing as little damage as possible to self tissues. Memory involves remembering and recognizing individual nonself entities when they are encountered again, so that the body responds more rapidly and forcefully to eliminate them on secondary exposures than occurred on the first (primary) encounter with the material.

The acquired immune system is based upon a group of blood cells called lymphocytes. A central concept in acquired immunity is that there are millions of different lymphocyte clones each of which recognizes and reacts with only one particular nonself item or "antigen epitope." An antigen is any foreign substance that can stimulate an immune response. Antigens are usually organic macromolecules and particularly proteins. An epitope is a site on the surface of the antigen that combines with a receptor on the lymphocyte. Individual antigens have multiple epitopes, and large organisms, such as helminths, have many antigens with many epitopes. In theory there will already be a few lymphocytes present that will recognize and react with any antigen that might enter the body. I visualize this part of the defense system as one in which there are a great many policemen (lymphocytes) patrolling the body. Each policeman has the photograph of only one particular potential alien that he hopes to nab.

The acquired immune system has two branches: the humoral and the cell-mediated components. Both branches are induced in all infectious diseases, but the magnitude, strength, and importance of the response by the two branches is highly variable in different diseases. Extracellular "exogenous" agents (most bacteria, many protozoa, helminths, and foreign antigens that originate outside the body and are located outside cells within the body) are dealt with primarily by the humoral immune response. Cell-mediated immunity is more important for dealing with "endogenous" antigens including organisms that live within the body's cells (viruses, intracellular bacteria, and protozoa) and cancer cells.

HUMORAL IMMUNITY

The humoral response is based on production of soluble proteins called *antibodies*, some of which circulate in serum and some of which are released in specific locations such as on mucosal surfaces. Each antibody has specific antigen-binding capacity and binds with only one epitope. Antibodies have many defensive properties including neutralizing toxins, such as those of botulinum and anthrax, preventing microorganisms from attaching to host cells; promoting phagocytosis and killing of microorganisms by macrophages; enhancing inflammatory responses; assisting in the lysis of some organisms; assisting other cells to kill host cells infected with virus; and inhibiting motility, metabolism, and growth of certain invading organisms.

The primary cell involved in the humoral response is a class of lymphocyte called the B cell. Each B cell has receptors on its surface for one specific epitope. (You and I each have B cell "policemen" looking for about 10^9 different antigen epitopes.) B cells tend to stay in the lymphoid organs (spleen, lymph nodes) and wait for antigens to come to them via the lymph. The production of antibody is complex and involves interaction of B cells with other cells that provide costimulation. The most important of these is another line of lymphocytes, the helper T cells, so named because they assist in immune processes. When B cells encounter their appropriate antigen, and are assisted by activated helper T cells, they undergo clonal proliferation, that is, they produce offspring all with the same antigen specificity. Most of these cells differentiate into plasma cells, which are protein-producing factories dedicated to production of antibody. A small proportion of the offspring become long-lived "memory cells" that are a reserve to be called upon if the animal is ever exposed again to the same antigen in the future. When an antigen is detected for the first time (the primary response), the amount of antibody produced is small and the response is slow, because there are only a few suitable B cells available (i.e., policemen with that antigen's photo). However, if the same antigen enters the body again, there are many suitable B cells available, so that antibody is produced more rapidly and in larger amounts in this secondary response.

Specificity and memory are the basis for all types

of immunization. When we vaccinate an animal, a small amount of antigen (the vaccine) is introduced into the animal and it induces a primary response. (The vaccine is often a killed agent, an agent that has been modified to reduce its virulence, or only a portion of the organism.) If the animal meets the antigen again later in life, this time in the form of an infectious agent, there will be a robust and protective secondary humoral response.

The humoral response takes place primarily in the spleen and lymph nodes, from which antibodies are exported in serum, and directly beneath the epithelium of the respiratory tract and intestine. Although small amounts of antibody are formed locally within a few days, antibody is not detectable in serum for about a week after exposure. Antibody to a particular antigen may be detected in serum for months or years after an animal is exposed to that antigen. Detection of antibody forms the basis for serological tests, and the strength of the response (the amount of antibody) is expressed in terms of the dilution of serum that still shows activity in a test. For instance, if we were interested in antibody that inhibited the growth of a virus when added to infected tissue culture, sera from the animal would be diluted sequentially, and the highest dilution that inhibited the virus would be termed the "antibody titre" for that animal.

Two additional features of humoral immunity deserve mention: *passive transfer* and *herd immunity*. Young animals are born or hatch into an environment that is filled with potential disease agents. While the young animals may be able to develop an immune response, this is a primary response so that it is relatively slow and weak. Some of their other defenses also may be less effective than those of older animals. One mechanism to protect these vulnerable newborns is through transfer of antibodies from their mother. This "passive" transfer occurs through the egg yolk in birds and through either the placenta (in primates) or the first milk (colostrum) in most other mammals. This "maternal" antibody circulates in the offspring's blood for days or weeks, gradually waning, and eventually disappearing. For example, in double-crested cormorants, antibody to Newcastle disease virus was not detectable in chicks older than 1–2 weeks of age (Kuiken 1999); the half-life of passive antibodies to canine distemper virus in raccoons was about 10 days (Paré 1997); and maternal antibody to the oribiviruses that cause epizootic hemorrhagic disease of deer and bluetongue disappear between 17 and 23 weeks of age in white-tailed deer fawns in Texas (Gaydos et al.

2002b). Passive transfer is short-term resistance only, but it provides the offspring a degree of protection against disease agents to which their mother has been exposed (and which are likely to be present in the area). Passive immunity explains why young animals may not be susceptible to some infections early in life but become susceptible as antibody acquired from their mother disappears. Passive immunity also may interfere with immunization, so that vaccination programs may have to be delayed until after passive immunity has waned. Failure of passive transfer of antibodies (usually as a result of failure of offspring to nurse) is a very important veterinary problem in neonatal domestic animals but has not been identified as such in wild animals. It could be a problem if there is inadequate suckling by the young, as occurs in deer fawns born to malnourished does (Langenau and Lerg 1976).

Herd immunity is a population concept and relates to the buildup of immunity to reinfection within a population to a point at which there are no longer adequate susceptible animals remaining to maintain transmission of the disease, and it fades out. This form of immunity relates to humoral immunity and is probably significant only in diseases caused by microparasites.

CELL-MEDIATED IMMUNITY

Cell-mediated immunity is mediated by another group of lymphocytes, the T cells, one type of which, the helper T cell, has been mentioned. As with B cells, T cells recognize individual specific antigens. However, T cells only bind to "their" antigen when it is presented to them in a specific manner by cells called antigen presenting cells (APC). (T cell policemen only recognize their felon when he has been captured, hand-cuffed, and presented to them in a specific manner by an APC. Moreover, only a specific type of handcuffs will do!) The details of this process are beyond this book, but briefly, APC are cells, including macrophages, that take in antigen, degrade it, and bind a portion of the processed antigen to specific molecules on their cell surfaces. The molecules that bind these fragments are coded for by a complex of genes present in all vertebrates called the major histocompatibility complex (MHC). The antigen fragment and MHC molecule are said to be "presented" on the surface of the APC. (The MHC molecules are the handcuffs in the policeman analogy.) Because of their specificity, the MHC genes control antigen processing and presentation and are the major genetic component of disease resistance and susceptibility (Tizard 2000).

Genes of the MHC are highly polymorphic and heterozygosity enables recognition of a wider range of antigens, but there may be an optimal level of heterozygosity (Wegner et al. 2003). Social animals in which there is a greater likelihood of frequent contact with infectious agents have greater pleomorphism in MHC genes than do solitary animals such as carnivores.

Unlike B cells, T cells go out in search of foreign antigens. There is a regular traffic of T cells from the blood stream into tissues and then back into blood via the lymphatics, providing surveillance throughout the body for nonself antigens. When a T cell encounters the correct antigen (the one it is looking for) presented on the surface of an APC, the T cell becomes activated and undergoes clonal proliferation. Different types of T cells have different actions. One type called the cytotoxic T cell recognizes nonself antigen on the surface of cells and destroys the cell. (More correctly, they induce the cell to commit suicide.) This is particularly important in killing virus-infected cells before the virus has had time to multiply. It also is important in removing abnormal cancer cells. Activated T helper cells also are involved in the cell-mediated response by assisting macrophages so that these cells can destroy intracellular organisms such as *Mycobacterium bovis* and *Toxoplasma gondii* that they have ingested, and by attracting inflammatory cells to a site of injury. Circulating T cells accumulate where antigen is located, and cell-mediated immune responses are recognizable to the pathologist because of the accumulation of lymphocytes and macrophages at the site. Cell-mediated immunity is brief and only evident when antigen is present. Memory occurs in cell-mediated immunity but is less well understood than memory in the humoral branch.

This has been only a skeletal introduction to acquired immunity, a subject that is extremely complex. There are many classes and subclasses of MHC molecules, several types of antibody, different types of helper T cells, many chemical mediators and effectors, feedback loops, redundancies, and much more interaction between the two arms of the acquired immune system and with the innate system than I have described. A single infectious organism has many antigens, and both arms of the system are activated when these antigens enter the body. The type of response that occurs varies with the type of antigen, how it is introduced into the body, and the length of time that it persists. Different portions of the immune system are of primary importance in defense against different disease agents. The acquired immune system includes exceptionally powerful and dangerous reactions for which the body has developed a series of inhibitory mechanisms.

DIAGNOSTIC TESTS AND THE DEFENSE SYSTEM

Most tests used to detect and diagnose disease in animals consist of measuring the reaction of the innate and acquired defense systems rather than detecting the actual causative organism. The number and type of white cells circulating in the blood are good general indicators of the type of causative agent involved and the probable course of the clinical disease. For example, bacterial diseases usually cause large numbers of neutrophils to be present in the circulating blood, whereas large numbers of circulating eosinophils may be indicative of parasitic or allergic disease. Detecting antibodies in blood serum (serology) is the most commonly used method to determine if animals have been exposed to an infectious disease agent. Serology is based on the specificity of the humoral immune system. The type and concentration of antibodies present in an animal's serum may reveal not only that the animal was exposed to an agent but also approximately how long ago the exposure occurred. The presence of increasing levels of antibody in samples taken a few weeks apart from an individual is good evidence of recent exposure, and sequential sampling can be used to monitor the spread of disease through a population. The cell-mediated immune response is used less commonly but is important in tests such as the tuberculin skin test. In this test, antigen is injected into the skin and the extent of resulting skin swelling, because of influx of cells, is used to judge whether an animal is diseased or not. Other tests depend on the ability of lymphocytes to react to antigens and measurement of specific mediator compounds produced by macrophages and lymphocytes.

OVERVIEW OF DEFENSES

Resistance to disease consists of a series of defenses. It appears that the costs escalate as the different methods are used sequentially, beginning with avoiding exposure and ending with use of the immune system. Discretion likely is the better part of valor, that is, it probably is better to run away to avoid contact where possible or to stop invaders at an outer wall rather than having to defeat the agent once it is within the body, because of the inevitable risk of injury from the battle. Lochmiller and Deerenberg (2000) suggest that short-lived species under intense predation pressure (such as small rodents) may depend more on the rapid protection of the innate system to allow them to survive until they can reproduce once, while long-lived species would benefit from well-developed innate and acquired immune systems that would allow them to live to reproduce several times. Hanssen et al. (2003) also indicated that immunocompetence may be particularly important for long-lived species in which infection may reduce future reproduction. A host may be selective, producing a long-lasting immune response to some agents and not to others, based on the relative costs and benefits (Boots and Bowers 2004). We usually view resistance from the vertebrate's perspective. However, in diseases caused by living organisms, the agent and host are in a coevolutionary struggle involving the interaction of two genetic lineages. Agents may be able to exploit most of the animals in a population when first introduced, as occurred with myxomatosis in Australia, but those few hosts with resistance have a selective advantage, and their genotype will become more common in the population. Individuals within the agent population that have an ability to circumvent the defenses are successful, and through selection, their offspring become abundant in the population until the host population develops a new defense, and so on in an adaptation-counteradaptation arms race described in chapter 5. Plaut (1993) has described some of the mechanisms that microorganisms have developed to subvert the host defense systems.

SUPPRESSION OF THE DEFENSE SYSTEM

Study of interference with resistance is a topical subject in all branches of medicine. This is most often described as immunosuppression, because the effects on acquired immunity have been studied most thoroughly. In humans, the effects of certain infectious agents, particularly the human immunodeficiency viruses (HIV), in causing immunosuppression are paramount at this time. It is unclear how important similar infections may be in wild animals, but we know that immunodeficiency viruses similar to HIV are widespread in wild cats and primates (Worley 2001), and there is no reason to think that similar viruses do not occur in other wild animals. However, factors other than viruses that influence resistance are likely to be of greater importance in wild animals. The following examples are intended only to illustrate the range of potential interactions that may occur among various factors and the defense system. Nutrition, infection with one agent, stress, environmental contaminants, and gender can all be factors.

Nutrition Alters Resistance

The most important single factor that affects the immune system is nutrition. Restricted energy intake if prolonged leads to suppression of the immune system and increased susceptibility to infections (Klurfeld 1993; Lochmiller and Deerenberg 2000). Protein intake is also important. For example, protein deficiency reduced the effectiveness of immunization of mice against a nematode parasite (Slater and Keymer 1988); and cell-mediated immunity was stronger in nestling barn swallows given supplemental protein-rich food; and chicks in larger broods, with assumedly lower nutrition, had lower responses (Saino et al. 1997; Naguib et al. 2004). Vitamin A affects many parts of the defense system and has been called the anti-infection vitamin. Suppression of the immune response may be adaptive during periods of intense stress and resource limitation when the cost of the response might be greater than the expected cost of an infection (Hanssen et al. 2004).

Infection with One Agent May Alter Resistance to Other Agents

Mice infected with a trematode *(Schistosoma mansoni)* had more circulating malarial parasites than did mice infected with malaria alone, and mice with malaria had reduced defense factors directed against the trematode (Helmby et al. 1998). Mice infected with *S. mansoni* also had delayed clearance of a virus (Actor et al. 1993) but had improved defenses against an intestinal nematode (Curry et al. 1995). Many viruses including influenza virus in birds (Suarez and Schultz-Cherry 2000) modify various parts of the immune response, and myxomatosis appeared to make European rabbits more susceptible to helminths (Boag 1988).

Stress Alters Resistance

When mallard ducklings were given a standardized number of nematode larvae, ducklings "stressed" by crowding retained more of the worms and the worms were larger than in ducklings that were not crowded (Ould and Welch 1980). Cold-stressed mice had depressed humoral response (Cichoń et al. 2002), which was likely related to resources being allocated to thermoregulation rather than to resistance. The reduced response occurred in mice exposed to cold long term but not in mice exposed to cold only for a short period. Stress is not always associated with reduced immune response and "the stress response suppresses particular immunological mechanisms while enhancing others" (Apanius 1998). Saino et al. (2000) reported an affect of reproduction but not of population density on humoral immunity in bank voles. Stress will be discussed more fully in chapter 7.

Environmental Contaminants Alter Resistance

Many contaminants have been shown in the laboratory to influence some part of the immune response, and some have been shown to increase susceptibility to experimental challenge with different infectious agents (Fairbrother 1994), but there are few examples from the field in which this effect is clear. As with other stressors, the effect of contaminants may be to decrease some aspects of the immune response and increase others (Grasman and Fox 2001). The suggestion that the immunosuppression seen in harbor seals fed contaminated herring (Ross et al. 1995) may have played a part in the occurrence of morbillivirus epizootics is one of the better documented examples of immune suppression at this time. Biser et al. (2004) observed, "unfortunately, threshold levels of exposure that impact immune systems in wild animals are not known."

Gender Matters

In several species of mammal, males have reduced immunocompetence and increased susceptibility to a variety of parasites (Olsen and Kovacs 1996; Poulin 1996; Schalk and Forbes 1997). Nestling male Eurasian kestrels had decreased cell-mediated immunity compared to females when raised under limited food conditions (Farrgalo et al. 2002), but testosterone did not affect antibody production in red-winged blackbirds (Hasselquist et al. 1999).

Some of the observed effects of other factors on the immune system can be explained in terms of resource trade-offs, while others may be related to effects on individual cells or mediators. Many people believe that immune suppression is important in wild animals. It is often sited as a potential effect when residues of contaminants are detected in wild animals or when it is difficult to explain a disease in other ways. However, there is a paucity of empirical data to support the allegations. Many studies to examine immune suppression have used unusual antigens such as bovine serum albumen, sheep red blood cells, or pokeweed antigen, delivered in unusual ways, to test the immune system. When an effect is demonstrated, its significance in the real world is unclear. To my knowledge, there is no example in which immune suppression has been docu-

mented to result in decreased survival or reduced fitness in a wild species. However, Møller and Saino (2004) presented evidence from meta-analysis of publications to show that production of a strong nonspecific immune response in birds is associated with improved survival. The effects of some contaminants in influencing immune function are probably "real" but extremely difficult to dissect from among all of the other factors that may influence resistance.

Hanssen et al. (2004) have described a fascinating study in which nesting female common eiders were injected with novel antigens (sheep red blood cells, diphtheria-tetanus toxoid). Because these birds do not feed during reproduction, they are under severe resource limitation. Only about 50% of the birds produced antibodies in response to immunization (as might be expected in resource-limited animals). The unexpected finding was that overwinter survival, as measured by the return rate to the colony the following year, was 27% for birds that produced antibody compared to 72% for birds that failed to mount an immune response. While this seems counterintuitive, immunosuppression may be adaptive under conditions of severe resource limitation, especially if exposure to disease is minimal at the time, such as in birds that are not feeding and that are relatively isolated on the nest. (In simple terms, this example supports the idea that insurance is costly if you don't need it!) This apparent downregulation of the immune response resembles downregulation of the acute stress response in arctic nesting birds reported by Wingfield et al. (1995). It was suggested that this occurred so that reproduction would not be delayed by response to short-term stressors such as storms.

RECOVERY AND REPAIR

Recovery of normal function depends upon either repairing injury or developing an alternate method of functioning. Some aspects of repair were mentioned in the discussion of inflammation because the two processes are inextricably linked. According to Slausen and Cooper (2002), "without effective inflammatory responses, bacterial infections are difficult to contain, wounds do not heal well, and damaged tissues do not repair." Repair of tissue injury occurs by one of two processes: *regeneration* or *scarring*. Regeneration involves regrowth of the *functional* cells or parts of an organ or tissue, that is, replacement of lost tissue by tissue of the same type. Invertebrates have an incredible ability to regenerate damaged or lost tissues, but this is one of the things we vertebrates sacrificed to become "higher" animals. Scarring involves replacement of functional tissue with less-specialized connective tissue and, consequently, carries the penalty of reduced function. (We vertebrates are good at scarring.)

There are two basic requirements for regeneration to occur: (1) the functional cells involved must be capable of renewing themselves, and (2) there must be a residual framework on which these cells can grow. Cells within the body are of three basic types: labile, stable, and permanent. Labile cells are in constant turnover and are being replaced regularly in life. Examples include cells in the bone marrow; the epithelium of the skin; and the epithelium lining the respiratory, digestive, urinary, and reproductive tracts. These cells have an excellent ability to regenerate. As long as a defect is not too large, and a tissue framework remains, regeneration is expected. The small ulcer (a cold sore) that occurs on a person's lip as a result of *Herpes hominis* infection is a good example of this process. Cold sores involve death and destruction of epithelium in a local area. The "lesion" heals rapidly by cellular proliferation from the margin of the ulcer, and function of the lip is restored. However, if a large area of skin is injured very deeply, as in a severe burn, and the germinal cells of the skin are destroyed, regeneration is delayed, fibrous tissue is laid down, and when the area eventually is covered by epithelial cells growing in from the margins, the skin will lack hair follicles and glands and be less functional.

Stable cells are cells that normally have a rather low rate of turnover but that retain the ability for cell division and replication. Examples include cells of the liver, the kidney tubules, bone, and fibrous tissue. The liver is an outstanding example of the ability of a tissue composed of stable cells to regenerate. Experimentally, 70% of the mass of the liver can be removed surgically and it will be restored. However, there must be a tissue framework, particularly basement membranes, to provide an architectural scaffolding for this regeneration. Without this framework, regeneration may occur, but it may be disorganized and not fully functional. This can be seen in diseases that occur in the kidney. Damage to epithelial cells in kidney tubules by the protozoan parasites that cause renal coccidiosis in ducks is limited to the epithelium. Although the parasite kills cells, the injury is repaired by regeneration because the basement membrane remains intact as a scaffolding for regeneration. In contrast, in some bacterial diseases of the kidney, the epithelium *and* the

underlying basement membrane are destroyed and fibrous scarring occurs.

Permanent cells are those that have little or no ability to regenerate. The best examples are nerve cells in the brain and the muscle cells of the heart. If these cells die, they are not replaced.

Scarring involves replacement of functional cells by less-specialized collagen-rich connective tissue. Scarring occurs wherever there is lack of cellular replacement or extensive damage to the connective tissue framework. It is promoted by the chronic persistence of inflammatory exudates, including pus and edema fluid, in an area.

These features allow us to predict the probability of repair and recovery in different types of injury (fig. 6.4). They also help in understanding the pattern we see in various diseases, for example why the same agent may have very different effects in different organs. To illustrate this point, consider the nematode *Baylisascaris procyonis,* a common intestinal parasite of raccoons. If an animal such as a grey squirrel ingests eggs of this parasite accidentally, the larvae that hatch migrate through many tissues of the squirrel, including the liver and brain. Functional cells are destroyed by the larvae and by the resulting inflammation in both the liver and brain. Injured liver cells are replaced rapidly, so there is little or no scarring and no diminishment of liver function. However, the squirrel may develop severe neurological disease because damaged nerve cells are not replaced and because of the effects of inflammation (fig. 6.5) within the confined space of the skull. Different agents affecting the same tissue also may have dramatically different effects. For example, both canine distemper virus and *Mycobacterium bovis* (the cause of bovine tuberculosis) infect the lung. Canine distemper has a short clinical course, and if an animal survives the initial damage caused by the virus, damaged cells are removed and replaced and there is little or no residual loss of function. In contrast, *M. bovis* persists in the tissues and within macrophages, stimulating chronic inflammation and cell-mediated immunity, leading to abundant scarring around the "tubercles" (fig. 6.6).

SUMMARY

- Resistance to disease agents and their effects consists of multiple interlocking and overlapping components.
- Resistance is costly for an animal in terms of resources and involves trade-offs with other factors such as growth and reproduction. It

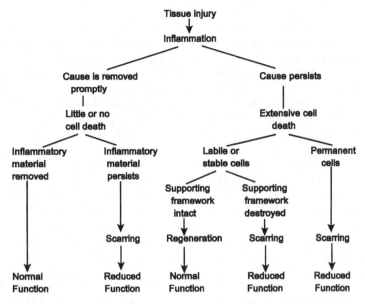

Fig. 6.4. Schematic overview of the probable outcome of various types of injury and repair. (Modified from Slauson and Cooper 2002, with permission.)

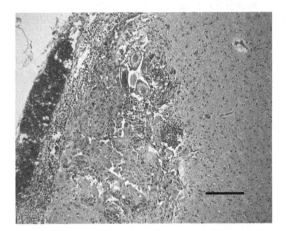

Fig. 6.5. Photomicrograph of tissue in the brain of a grey squirrel damaged by a larva of the raccoon nematode *Baylisascaris procyonis*. (Histologic slide provided by D. G. Campbell, Canadian Cooperative Wildlife Health Centre.) (Bar = 200 µm)

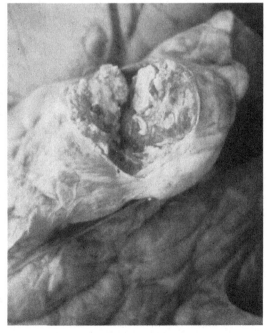

Fig. 6.6. Chronic granulomatous inflammation caused by *Mycobacterium bovis* infection within the lung of a wild wood bison. (Photograph courtesy of Dr. S. V. Tessaro, Canadian Food Inspection Agency.)

may not always be wise to invest heavily in resistance.

- Maintaining defenses is like having insurance: the costs are high in the absence of disease but justified when disease is present.
- Resistance involves either reducing exposure to the agent or limiting or ending the relationship.

- Behavioral avoidance is a common defense toward infectious agents. There are few documented examples of behavioral avoidance of noninfectious causes of disease.
- The body is well equipped with physical barriers to limit entry of disease agents.
- The innate defenses are an ancient system that acts as a nonspecific first-responder to invasion of the body. The most powerful feature is inflammation, the goal of which is to neutralize and remove injurious agents and damaged tissue to allow repair. Inflammation is a powerful double-edged weapon without which no animal can survive but which causes most of the tissue injury in disease.
- Acquired immunity is a newer system that is well developed in vertebrates. It has two arms: humoral and cell-mediated immunity. Acquired immunity has two special features: specificity and memory. Specificity means that the system recognizes individual foreign invaders, and memory means that the system recognizes and responds more vigorously to antigens that it has met previously.
- Humoral immunity involves production of specific soluble proteins called antibodies that have many functions. Humoral immunity is particularly useful for agents such as bacteria, protozoa, helminths, and foreign substances that are located outside cells.
- Cell-mediated immunity involves close interaction among certain types of lymphocytes, macrophages, and other white blood cells. It is important for dealing with intracellular organisms (viruses, some bacteria, and protozoa), fungi, and cancer cells.
- Both types of immunity are activated when foreign agents enter the body, but the relative response is highly variable.
- Many factors influence the strength and type of the immune response.
- Repair of injury involves regeneration and scarring. Regeneration requires functional cells able to regenerate and a residual framework on which regeneration can occur. If either of these is missing, scarring (replacement with less-specialized connective tissue) will occur resulting in decreased function.

7

Environmental Interactions

The natural factors that operate do so within habitats whose extent and productivity are largely influenced by human activity.
—I. Newton

Animals and disease agents do not interact in a vacuum. In chapter 2, I used the agent-host-environment triangle and the analogy of the environment as a sliding fulcrum on which agent-animal interactions are balanced to emphasize that environmental factors modulate the interaction between cause and effect (see figs. 2.6 and 2.8). Environmental factors may affect the animal or the agent, and the action may be to modify animal abundance and density, the degree and type of exposure to the agent, the degree of resistance of the host, and even the virulence of the agent. It is not possible to identify or consider all of the possible environmental factors that might modify any animal-agent relationship, so I will discuss only selected examples.

I have divided the subject into abiotic and biotic factors, but it is important at the outset to state that the effect of human population is an overarching feature involved in every disease relationship. Even climate, that most basic of abiotic factors, has been modified by humans, and the effects of humans on water, land, vegetation, and animals are obvious. No wild animal lives in a truly pristine environment unaffected by humans. An urban raccoon is more affected by humans than his country cousin, but even Arctic polar bears and Antarctic penguins carry residues of persistent contaminants in their tissues and are affected by receding ice as part of global warming. Animals deep in tropical jungles are affected by forest clearing, chemical residues, and increased interaction with domestic animals. If the human population reaches 12 billion before the close of this century, as has been predicted by some experts, one cannot guess what sort of disease "prob-

lems" will occur. I think that it is safe to speculate that things will not get better, and that disease specialists will not be short of work, because disease in all its many forms flourishes in disturbed environments and times of resource shortage.

One of the most basic features of the investigation of any disease occurrence is to set it in time and place. Determining the spatial and temporal relationships among the factors involved in a disease often provides important clues as to what is causing the disease and why the disease occurred. Where a disease occurs, the location of affected individuals and outbreaks, and its general geographic distribution are determined by the presence of factors that are suitable for the animal(s) involved, for the agent(s), and for agent and host to interact. Most diseases have a restricted geographic distribution. Pavlovsky (1966) used the term "nidality" (derived from Latin *nidus*—nest) to describe the tendency of infectious diseases to be localized. He described the study of this phenomenon as "landscape epidemiology," which involves trying to understand how features of the environment influence disease. Although the concept of landscape epidemiology was developed for infectious disease, it is equally applicable to noninfectious conditions. The distribution of many noninfectious diseases is determined directly by human activities, such as where contaminants are used or released, while the distribution of other conditions is influenced by topography, bedrock, and where wind blows and water flows.

Individual environmental factors may have a direct or an indirect impact on disease. Mouritsen and Poulin (2002) divided the anticipated effects of climatic oscillations into those that have a direct effect on parasite life cycle (especially transmission) and those in which there were more complex cascade effects on host-parasite interactions. As examples of direct effect, the number of lice on some birds is directly influenced by the relative ambient humidity (Moyer et al. 2002), and temperature and solar radiation have a direct effect on the survival of nestling birds on a beach (Overstreet and Rehak 1981).

The following are three situations in which cascade effects have been identified. Engelthaler et al. (1999) linked a dramatic increase in precipitation with increased resources for rodents, which led to a marked increase in rodent populations and, subsequently, to the occurrence of human cases of hantavirus pulmonary syndrome in the Four Corners region of the United States. Jones et al. (1998) described a "chain reaction" in which increased production of acorns by oak trees led to increased deer mouse populations and increased density of the larval and nymphal ticks involved in transmission of Lyme disease. However, the density of ticks was not related directly to that of mice. The increased tick density was a result of deer infected with adult ticks being attracted to the acorn-rich area. Adult ticks that had completed feeding on deer dropped off and laid eggs that subsequently hatched and infected mice in the area. Spalding et al. (1993), Frederick et al. (1996), and Coyner et al. (2002) have documented a link between human effects on wetlands (disturbance and nutrient pollution with sewage effluent or agricultural runoff) and infection with the nematode *Eustrongylides ignotus* in ciconiform birds in Florida. This parasite is a major mortality factor in nestling ciconiform birds. Disturbed and polluted wetlands had a higher density of oligochaetes (the first intermediate stage of the nematode), a higher density of fish (the second intermediate host), and a much greater prevalence of infection with the parasite in both intermediate host species than occurred in undisturbed wetlands. The disturbed areas are attractive feeding areas for heron-like birds because of the density of prey fish.

Environmental factors may be associated closely in time with a disease event, for example, when poisoning occurs directly after the use of a pesticide in the area or when an outbreak of a vector-borne disease follows rainfall and availability of water for mosquito breeding, or the precipitating event may be separated from the effect by a considerable time delay. For instance, Moss et al. (1993) found that rainfall early in the previous summer explained most of the variation in the number of eggs of *Trichostrongylus tenuis* passed by red grouse. In the situation involving acorns, deer mice, ticks, and Lyme disease referred to earlier, the greatest risk to humans from Lyme disease occurred 2 years after an abundant acorn crop (Jones et al. 1998) and re-

flected the June moisture index 2 years earlier (Subak 2002).

When surveying potential environmental factors that might have an effect on disease, it is necessary to consider both macroelements, such as climate, as well as events in the microenvironment, such as temperature and humidity within a burrow or under the leaf litter of a forest where larval ticks must survive until they can find their next host. Although conducted a quarter of a century ago, a study of the environmental factors involved in Colorado tick fever (Carey et al. 1980) remains a model of how such studies should be conducted. Another example of a landscape study, this time involving extensive use of models, is a study of the distribution of the heartworm *Dirofilaria immitis* in California coyotes (Sacks et al. 2004). Many of the factors that influence disease occur stochastically, and it may be very difficult to determine which factors among the environmental "noise" are important. Jonzén et al. (2002) commented, "for a given population, the relevant environmental noise to be taken into account is not a single abiotic factor, but rather the combined effect of all abiotic and biotic factors affecting birth and death rates."

STRESS AND DISTRESS

The term "stress" appears frequently in literature related to disease in all species and has become an everyday part of our vocabulary, as in the "the stress of modern life" or "nutritional stress." There are many definitions, but stress is probably best viewed as a complex process or system that includes input (stimuli), processing of this input, and output (responses). According to Levine and Ursin (1991), "this system affects many other biological processes and may function as a common alarm and drive system, whenever there is a real or apparent challenge to the self-regulating systems of organisms."

My preference is to call stimuli that elicit the system "stressors." Stressors may be anything that threatens or disturbs the homeostatic equilibrium of an animal and may differ in intensity and duration. They may be extrinsic factors such as weather, lack of food, a chemical toxicant, social interactions, presence of a predator, human disturbance, or intrinsic factors such as pain and fear. Stressors may be multiple and may interact in various ways. Information about stressors is processed and evaluated by the brain. For a response to occur, the animal must sense a stimulus to be above some threshold level that is perceived to represent a threat to homeostasis. This threshold is influenced by many factors including the animal's genotype, sex, age, prior experience, reproductive and nutritional state, and the presence of other stressors, thus, individual animals or populations may perceive a stressor differently and have different responses.

When a stressor exceeds the threshold, a cascade of reactions occurs that is under neuroendocrine control and involves a variety of hormones and mediators. The response has been subdivided into primary, secondary, and tertiary components, although these are parts of a continuum. The hormones involved in all vertebrates are catecholamines and glucocorticosteroids. In the primary response, catecholamines are released within seconds and glucocorticosteroids are released within a few minutes. These lead to the secondary response, which includes influences on the cardiac system (increased output) and mobilization of glucose by catecholamines in preparation for "fight or flight," metabolic changes that result in new glucose production at the expense of protein and fat induced by cortisol, and activation of elements of the immune response by cytokines. The tertiary response consists of whole-animal changes including changes in behavior, muscle catabolism, and organ function. The changes induced by catecholamines are very brief (minutes), while those induced by glucocorticosteroids are longer lasting. Changes also occur at the cellular level that are designed to protect against macromolecular damage and promote cellular stability (Kültz 2003).

A critical factor in evaluating the significance of the stress response is its duration. In general, a short-term stress response can be viewed as an adaptive emergency reaction that "promotes survival until the stress passes" (Wingfield et al. 1997). In the process, some other activities may be suppressed temporarily, including reproductive and territorial behavior, while energy metabolism is increased and some measures of immune function may be enhanced. When the stress subsides, glucocorticosteroid levels decline and suppressed activities resume. A robust glucocorticosteroid response to an acute stressor is regarded as indicative of a healthy individual (Wingfield and Romero 2001). In contrast, prolonged activation of the adrenocortical response as a result of a continuously or repeatedly active stressor is highly deleterious. When biological functions are disrupted as a result of prolonged response, the resulting state may be referred to as "distress" (Wendelaar Bonga 1997). Wingfield et al. (1997) listed effects of chronic stress to include inhibition of the reproductive system, suppression of

the immune system, promotion of severe protein loss, disruption of cellular messenger systems, death of neuronal cells, and suppression of growth and metamorphosis. Another result of chronic stress is believed to be damping or suppression of the ability to produce a corticosteroid response to an acute stressor so that such individuals are vulnerable because they are "less capable of responding to further stressors" (Homan et al. 2003). Some of these effects may be a result of diversion of energy, and it may be difficult to differentiate between the direct effects of some disease agents (e.g., by causing tissue damage) from their effects via the stress response.

Many environmental influences on disease occurrence may be explainable through the stress response, but little is known about how most wild species respond to different stressors, and interactions are likely to be complex and unexpected. For example, females of some bird and reptile species may be able to down-regulate their acute stress response during the breeding season to prevent minor stressors from interrupting breeding behavior (Wingfield and Romero 2001); social stress in pregnant bank voles leads to increased aggression in their male offspring (Marchlewska-Koj et al. 2003); and acute stress (from restraint) accelerated wound healing in Siberian hamsters (Kinsey et al. 2003). Lafferty and Holt (2003) suggest that stress may have different effects on host-specific (one host) diseases than on multihost diseases.

ABIOTIC FACTORS

The principal abiotic factors that I will discuss here are topography, climate and weather, water, bedrock, and soil. These are not independent, for example, topography influences local climate, soil formation, and the distribution of water on the landscape. Nor are abiotic factors independent from biotic factors, for example, soil nutrients, aeration, texture, and microclimate have a major effect on the vegetation that grows on a site and on the animals that inhabit the area.

In considering the distribution of disease events, it is important to think in three dimensions, because altitude affects where and how diseases occur (table 7.1). Topography influences distribution of contaminants and infectious agents by altering wind direction, speed, and dispersion of air-borne materials and by influencing water flow. Topographical orientation influences the degree of solar irradiation, precipitation, vegetation, and how land is used by humans. Topography may influence the distribution of

Table 7.1 Altitude and the Occurrence or Prevalence of Disease

Disease (species)	Altitudinal effect
Anthrax (livestock)	Not seen above 3000 m, perhaps because temperatures are not warm enough for significant sporulation[1]
Elaeophora schneideri (mule deer)	Prevalence of infection related to preferred altitude of the horsefly intermediate host[2]
Hantavirus pulmonary syndrome (humans)	Most exposures between 1800 and 2500 m, none >2500 m (corresponds with altitude with highest density of rodent hosts)[3]
Leucocytozoon simondi infection (ducks)	Birds elevated even a few meters above ground level seldom become infected (Foraging blackflies look for ducks on the shore, not up in trees!)[4]
Malaria (Hawaiian birds)	Highest prevalence at midelevations where vector mosquitoes are most abundant. Some native birds persist only at high altitude.[5]

[1]Hugh-Jones and de Vos (2002).
[2]Hibler and Adcock (1971).
[3]Engelthaler et al. (1999).
[4]Fallis and Bennett (1966).
[5]van Riper et al. (1986).

some infectious disease directly, for example, rabies in foxes in Switzerland spread along mountain valleys and did not spread across mountain ranges to adjacent valleys (Steck et al. 1982). In some situations, it may be difficult to untangle the interrelationships among factors, one of which might be altitude. Caley et al. (2001) found that the prevalence of tuberculous lesions in brushtail possums declined significantly with altitude and steepness of slope. However, the highest prevalence of infection also correlated with habitats capable of supporting the highest density of possums. The number of *Ixodes scapularis* ticks on deer declined with altitude and distance from the coast in Maine. This effect might have been a result of enhanced tick survival in the higher humidity near the coast and/or the dispersal of ticks along the coast by coastal migrating songbirds (Rand et al. 2003).

Climate is used here as the generally occurring weather conditions of a region averaged over many years. Climate has a major effect on the geographic distribution of animal and plant species, disease agents, and human activities. The effect of climate on distribution is most obvious in those infectious diseases that involve an invertebrate as a vector or intermediate host, because poikilothermic animals are particularly sensitive to temperature, precipitation, and humidity. These affect the rate of invertebrate development, their longevity, their activity, and the rate of development of disease agents within them. For example, "geographically variable tick population dynamics are determined principally by

climatic factors, temperature that drives development, and moisture availability that determines mortality" (Randolph et al. 2001). Because of these effects, a disease may behave in a very dissimilar manner under different climatic conditions although the host, vector, and agent involved are at least superficially the same. For instance, the oribiviruses of bluetongue and epizootic hemorrhagic disease in wild deer are transmitted by *Culicoides* spp. midges throughout the range of these diseases but the pattern of disease is very different at different latitudes. Most deer in Texas have been exposed to the viruses but there is little or no obvious disease. Deer in the northern plains states and southern Canada usually have had no prior experience with these viruses so that when hemorrhagic disease occurs sporadically, there is high mortality. Howerth et al. (2001) believes that the "differences probably reflect the combined effects of latitude and altitude on climatic variables controlling *Culicoides* populations." Because climate has a major effect on human activities, including agriculture, it also has an important indirect effect on the distribution of toxicants such as insecticides.

Prevailing wind patterns are responsible for the long distance transport of contaminants and the distribution of these in wild animals. Precipitation (rain and snow) has a major influence on the distribution of animals and disease agents. There has been considerable interest in the effect of climate change on diseases of humans and animals, and many recent reviews (Mellor and Leake 2000; Gubler et al. 2001;

Mouritsen and Poulin 2002; Harvell et al. 2002; Hunter 2003) have concentrated on infectious disease and particularly on vectorborne diseases.

Weather is the state of atmospheric conditions (temperature, wind, humidity, precipitation, sunlight) at a specific time. Weather conditions have a strong effect on the local and immediate occurrence of disease and can also be a direct cause of disease (e.g., hyperthermia, frostbite, dehydration, and starvation) in individual or groups of animals. Ambient temperature may interact with disease agents in many ways (table 7.2). Some effects of temperature may be related to energy metabolism and trade-offs. Much of the recent emphasis on temperature as a factor in disease has been on high temperature, but low temperature also may be related to disease. Cold ambient temperatures prolong the survival of many disease agents in the external environment, and disease may render affected animals more susceptible to the effects of cold weather. The most obvious of such situations are animals with impaired thermal insulation, such as coyotes with sarcoptic mange or birds with oiled plumage. In addition, animals with extra costs because of more subtle forms of disease may have fewer resources available for maintenance activities, including disease resistance, and affected animals may be the first to die during inclement weather. Howe (1992) found no effect of parasitic blowfly larvae on sage threshers in one year, but in the following year, in which there was cold wet weather, parasitized nestlings had reduced survival compared to unparasitized nestlings. Some observed effects of temperature are unexplained, for example, high environmental temperature had a sparing effect on rabbits infected with some strains of myxoma virus (Kerr and Best 1998).

Wind has obvious effects on the distribution of disease. Many airborne pollutants are distributed downwind from the source, some viruses may be carried as aerosols over long distances (Gloster et al. 1982), and arthropod vectors such as *Culicoides* spp. midges may be transported into new areas by favorable winds. The distribution of cyanobacteria and of carcasses of birds dead of botulism and avian cholera in wetlands is determined by wind direction. Even infected live birds may be displaced for long distances by strong winds. Malkinson et al. (2002) described a situation in which West Nile virus was "imported" into Israel by white storks blown from their normal migratory path by strong, hot, westerly winds.

Precipitation in all its forms may have many effects on disease. Lack of precipitation (drought) may concentrate animals about remaining water bodies or suitable habitat, enhancing contact and transmission of infectious agents. For instance, spring drought in Florida concentrates birds and vector mosquitoes together in the remaining wet areas, facilitating trans-

Table 7.2 Ambient Temperature Influence on Disease

Factor affected	General direction of change
Survival of agents in the external environment	In general but not invariably, survival of infectious agents is inversely related to temperature. Some contaminants decompose more rapidly at increased temperatures.
Biting rate by blood-feeding arthropod vector	Increases with increasing temperature up to a point and then may decline[1]
Hatchability of bird eggs	Reduced at higher temperature[2]
Proliferation of cyanobacterial blooms in water	Increased at higher temperature[3]
Survival of vector arthropods	Variable
Rate of development of agents within vector or intermediate hosts	Increased with increasing temperature
Population of blowflies on carcasses	Increased with increased temperature
Decomposition and disappearance of carcasses	Increased with increased temperature
Invertebrate reproduction	Breed at younger age and smaller size with increased temperature

[1]Otto and Jachowski (1981); Mellor and Leake (2000).
[2]Cook et al. (2003).
[3]Hunter (2003).

mission of St. Louis encephalitis virus (Shaman et al. 2002b). Snowfall and particularly snow depth influence the availability of forage for ungulates and increases the costs for locomotion (Fancy and White 1985) with a marked negative effect on resource availability for all functions including resistance to disease and reproduction (Albon et al. 2002). Rainfall, presence of standing water, and humidity have a major effect on the distribution and survival of mollusks involved in transmission of many macroparasites, the survival of agents such as worm eggs and larvae, and bacteria free in the environment, and the population density of vector arthropods. The effect of precipitation on disease may be direct or indirect. For example, the incidence of rabies in cattle in Mexico increased during the rainy season. This was a result of the timing of the breeding season of vampire bats (the reservoir for rabies) and the influx of large numbers of susceptible bats into the population, rather than a direct effect of rainfall on rabies (Lord 1992).

Water is involved in some manner in the ecology of virtually every disease (table 7.3) and must be considered during the investigation of any condition. Changes in distribution, level, temperature, chemistry, and biota all may influence disease. Unfortunately, much of the water available for use by wild animals, except in very remote areas, has been used and often abused by humans. Even in "pristine" environments water contains contaminants.

Two diseases, anthrax and selenium poisoning, are excellent examples of the many ways in which water may influence disease. Anthrax, caused by the bacterium *Bacillus anthracis,* is primarily a disease of herbivorous animals (Dragon and Rennie 1995; Hugh-Jones and de Vos 2002). The bacterium has a spore stage that is extremely resistant in the external environment. Animals become infected by ingesting or inhaling spores. Anthrax outbreaks often occur in hot, dry weather following heavy rains and may be associated with low-lying areas. One explanation is that buoyant spores in soil are carried to the low-lying areas by running water and become concentrated there as the water evaporates. Animals grazing in these areas, which often have more lush forage than the surrounding areas, are exposed to spores. Spores also may be dispersed from carcasses by water, and outbreaks in bison in northern Canada have ended with the onset of heavy rain and flooding, perhaps because of dispersal of spores concentrated about carcasses into the soil. Tabanid flies are important transport hosts for anthrax in some areas, carrying the bacteria on their mouthparts. These flies require aquatic environments for breeding, so that their distribution and abundance is dependent on surface water. During dry weather in Africa, waterholes serve to concentrate animals. Vultures that have fed on carcasses of animals dead of anthrax congregate at these waterholes where they bathe, defecate, and occasionally regurgitate in the water, contaminating the water with *B. anthracis.*

The story of selenium poisoning in wild waterbirds illustrates the effect of human manipulation of water on disease. Selenium is a naturally occurring element that is an essential trace nutrient for animals, but it is toxic at high concentrations. In the interior valleys of California, natural wetlands used by wintering waterbirds were drained to create agricultural land. Irrigation was needed for efficient crop production, so water was added back to the environment but in a different manner than had occurred naturally. Soil salinization (a common problem in irrigated

Table 7.3 Water and the Ecology of Disease in Wild Animals

Water mechanism	Examples
Fomes[1] for infectious agents	Leptospirosis, tularemia, avian cholera, toxoplasmosis
Habitat for intermediate host(s)	*Fascioloides magna* and other trematodes that use aquatic snails
Breeding habitat for vector	West Nile virus, *Leucocytozoon* spp. infections.
Breeding habitat for transport host	Tabanid flies (*Elaeophora schneideri*, anthrax)
Carrier of dissolved toxins	Selenium poisoning
Habitat for toxin-producing agents	Cyanobacteria, algae that produce domoic acid and other marine toxins
Concentrate animal populations	Anthrax
Concentrate disease agents	Anthrax
Modify local climate	Ticks on deer in coastal areas

[1]Inanimate object or substance that may be contaminated with infectious agents and become a vehicle for transmission.

areas) occurred for which a partial solution was subsurface drainage of excess irrigation water. However, this drainage water contains many chemicals, including pesticides and minerals leached from the soil. Where the soil is naturally rich in selenium, toxic levels of selenium may occur in drain water. This was first recognized at Kesterson National Wildlife Refuge in California where drain water was collected in a reservoir used by waterbirds. Selenium accumulated in plants and animals used as food by birds resulting in adult mortality as well as marked effects on reproduction, including many chicks with deformities (Ohlendorf 1996). Thus, the selenium story involved at least five separate manipulations of water: drainage of wetlands, irrigation, subsurface drainage of irrigation water, collection of drainage water into reservoirs, and finally drainage and filling of the reservoir (with loss of wetland habitat) to discourage use by birds and prevent poisoning.

The soil of an area reflects the parent bedrock and the long-term climate of the region and has a major influence on the distribution of vegetation and animals. Soil and bedrock can influence disease in many ways, and important features include its chemical, physical, and moisture content (table 7.4). As an example of the importance of soils, Guerra et al. (2002) found that the presence of *Ixodes scapularis* (the tick that transmits Lyme disease and several other diseases in North America) is positively associated with sandy or loam sand soils overlying sedimentary rock, and its absence is associated with acidic clay soils and Precambrian bedrock.

BIOTIC FACTORS

VEGETATION

Many diseases are associated with a particular type of vegetation. In some instances, this may reflect simply the distribution of the animals that are affected, or it may be related to the particular climatic or soil features of the area. In other cases, the type of vegetation may have an effect on survival of a disease agent while it is outside the host. For instance, both *Ixodes scapularis* and *I. ricinus* (the vector tick

Table 7.4 Bedrock and Soil Interaction with Disease Conditions in Wild Animals

	Disease relationship	Characteristic
Chemical composition	Deficiency of required nutrients	Calcium[1]
		Selenium[2]
		Copper[3]
		Sodium[4]
		Phosphorus[5]
	Toxic concentrations of elements	Selenium (from plants)[6]
		Lead in mine tailings[7]
		Cadmium[8]
		Fluoride[9]
	Reservoir for agents	Calcium content influences *Bacillus anthracis* persistence[10]
Physical features	Sedimentation of lead pellets beyond reach of waterfowl[11]	
Moisture and nutrient content	Reservoir for disease agents	*Histoplasma capsulatum*
Microorganisms	Conversion of toxins	Methylation of mercury in sediment

[1]Graveland and Drent (1997).
[2]Shaw and Reynolds (1985).
[3]Flynn and Franzmann (1974).
[4]Botkin et al. (1973).
[5]Hanley and McKendrick (1985).
[6]Fowler (1983).
[7]Beyer et al. (2000).
[8]Klok et al. (2000).
[9]Shupe et al. (1984).
[10]Hugh-Jones and de Vos (2002).
[11]Bellrose (1959).

for Lyme disease in North America and Europe, respectively) rarely are found in open grassland areas, probably because ticks that fall there are exposed to desiccation and die. Forested areas buffer climatic extremes and, because leaf litter is important for the survival of immature ticks, these species are more abundant in deciduous forests than in coniferous forests (Guerra et al. 2002; Lindström and Jaenson 2003).

ANIMALS

In considering the environmental effects of animals on disease, I will not deal with those organisms that have already been discussed in chapter 3 (microparasites and macroparasites). This section will deal briefly with intraspecific and interspecific relationships among larger animals.

Intraspecific Interactions

In many diseases, other members of the same species are the most important environmental influence on disease. Their abundance, distribution, density, susceptibility to disease, and current disease status may be important. Other members of the population may influence the rate of exposure to the agent and the relative resistance of individuals to the disease. (I will define population more precisely in chapter 11. Here I will use it simply as a group of animals of the same species.)

Population size and density are subjects of great interest to those working with disease, and there is a general belief that disease in wild animals is "more important" when animal populations are large and/or dense. A disease might be considered to be more important when populations are large or dense because (1) it is more apparent, (2) it occurs more commonly, (3) it involves a larger proportion of the population, or (4) the effect on individuals is proportionately greater.

To illustrate the first of these, assume that on a wetland in 1 year there are 100 ducks of which 10 die of disease X. A few years later, the duck population is much larger and more dense with 10,000 birds on the same area, of which 1000 die of disease X. In the second year, the absolute number of ducks that died was much larger (100 times that in year 1), but the mortality rate, the proportion of the population that died, is the same (10%). Because a die-off of 1000 birds is much more likely to be detected than one involving 10 birds, finding dead birds in the second year might lead to the mistaken conclusion that disease X only occurs in large/dense populations.

In some situations, disease may occur more commonly over time in a large population than in a small population. A minimum number of animals may be needed to allow the agent of some directly transmitted diseases to persist in the population. For example, the minimum population size required for measles to persist in a human population is estimated to be about 300,000 to 500,000 persons (Black 1966). If the disease is introduced into a smaller population, the disease dies out and disappears because there are not enough susceptible individuals to maintain the infection. In this type of disease, the disease agent is present all the time in large populations, while it may only be present periodically or sporadically in small populations. To return to the wetland example, disease X might be present consistently when the population is 100,000 but only occur periodically when 100 ducks are present.

Disease might be more important in dense populations if a greater proportion of the individuals that make up dense population is affected, that is, the occurrence of the disease is density-dependent. Disease transmission within a species generally is believed to be density-dependent (Kermack and McKendrick 1927), based on the assumption that the rate of contact among individuals will be greater when populations are dense. This seems intuitive but requires that mixing within the population be homogenous (i.e., that each individual has an equal opportunity of contacting every other individual). Homogenous mixing may be appropriate for some diseases but may not apply to diseases transmitted through contacts that are not density dependent, such as through mating (Caley and Ramsey 2001). Although the rate of contact among animals is a basic factor in disease transmission, and an estimate of contact rate is required for models proposed to explain the quantitative aspects of disease, very little is known about the actual contact rate among conspecifics and with other species in most diseases of wild animals. For instance, despite the importance of raccoon rabies in North America, a small observational study of interactions among 12 raccoons at a garbage dump over about a 3 month period (Tottin et al. 2002) provides the only field data concerning contact rate for this species. (Raccoons in the dump bit a conspecific about once every 3 nights while feeding.)

It is difficult to measure population density and disease prevalence in wild animals. When both have been measured, the results have not always indicated that there is more disease in dense populations. For instance, Duncan et al. (1978) compared the abundance of ticks on red grouse in populations at different densities and found that there were less ticks per capita in dense populations. One possible explanation might be that the ticks, or louping-ill virus carried by the ticks, were causing mortality of grouse, so that the more ticks that were present the more severe the effects on the grouse. Root et al. (1999) measured population density and prevalence of hantavirus infection in two populations of deer mice and found that the prevalence of infection was higher at the site with the lower population density. The two sites differed in vegetation type and density, and mice at the site with higher disease prevalence traveled longer distances, "potentially encountering more conspecifics." In other situations, disease occurrence has increased with host density. Rand et al. (2003) reported a weak positive relationship between deer density and the abundance of ticks on deer. Moss et al. (1993) found a weak positive relationship between the density of grouse and the number of *Trichostrongylus tenuis* eggs shed by grouse. A factor that may complicate such assessments is that the effects of population density on disease prevalence may not be immediate: Mills et al. (1999) found delayed density dependence in hantavirus infection of deer mice.

The generally accepted assumption that the prevalence of disease is density dependent is not a trivial one, because reducing animal density is one of the most frequently used methods to manage disease. The results of these management activities have been mixed, and the effectiveness of population reduction as a management tool has seldom been tested (see chapter 13).

A disease also might be more important if the effect on individual animals is proportionately more severe in dense populations than in sparse populations. I am not aware of a situation in which this has been documented in the field, however, other density-dependent effects, such as on the availability of resources in dense populations, might limit the ability of animals to resist disease agents. The effect of stress from crowding is sometimes inferred to be important in disease of wild animals. Ould and Welch (1980) compared the response by mallard ducklings stressed by crowding with that of uncrowded ducklings to experimental infections with *Echinuria uncinata* (a nematode that infects the proventriculus). Although all ducklings were given the same number of larval worms, more worms were retained, the individual worms were larger, and there were more severe pathologic lesions in the crowded ducklings. The crowded ducklings had enlarged ad-

renal glands and reduced size of lymphoid organs, and it was thought that the stress of crowding interfered with immune defense against the parasites. It would be very difficult to dissect this type of effect of crowding from that of greater exposure to disease agents and from relative malnutrition that might occur in crowded populations in the field.

The best test to determine if population density influences disease prevalence or severity would be to manipulate the population density and measure the effect on disease prevalence and/or effect. There have been few such studies. When the population density of coyotes in an area of Texas was reduced by about 50% for 2 years, the abundance of 5 of the 12 helminth species present decreased in coyotes from the low-density area compared to those from the high-density area (Henke et al. 2002). The abundance of *Ixodes scapularis* ticks declined in areas where the density of deer was reduced (Stafford et al. 2003). Sharing of dens by brushtail possums (a factor that might influence transmission of *Mycobacterium bovis*) declined as the density of the population of possums was reduced on one site in New Zealand (Caley et al. 1998).

The distribution of animals may have a profound effect on disease, particularly if animals are concentrated in a small area, such as by artificial feeding. In such a situation, the overall population size may not be large but the local density is high, facilitating contact and exchange of disease agents. This is thought to be a major factor in the occurrence of tuberculosis in white-tailed deer in Michigan and brucellosis in elk on western feeding grounds. Other intraspecific factors that may influence the occurrence of disease agents are the age and sex composition of the group, behavioral patterns, innate and acquired immunity (including prior experience with the agent), the presence of other coexisting diseases (particularly if they cross-react with and may protect against virulent agents) (White et al. 2001), and general resource availability.

Interspecific Interactions

Interactions with other species may influence disease in a variety of ways (table 7.5). In this discussion, I will refer to the species of primary interest as the "target species." The effects of other species are not easy to predict and may either exacerbate or ameliorate a disease condition. For instance, assume that we are interested in the effect of an intestinal nematode on mountain sheep. Nematode eggs passed with the sheep's feces develop in the external environment and infective larvae crawl up vegetation and are ingested accidentally by grazing animals. Let us further assume that wild sheep behave like domestic sheep and avoid grazing near feces as a way of reducing the likelihood of infection (Hutchings et al. 1999). The sheep share range during part of the year with deer, elk, and cattle, and there is substantial dietary overlap. Interspecific competition reduces the nutrients and the choice of forage available to the sheep. One result of interaction among the species might be that hungry sheep have less aversion to grazing near feces containing infective larvae and, thus, have increased exposure to the worms. If nutrient intake is reduced, another effect might be that sheep have fewer resources to allocate to disease resistance (including resisting and expelling the nematodes), and the sheep would be more likely to succumb to starvation because of the combined effects of parasites and malnutrition during times of food restriction. However, if the competing species consume many infective larvae along with the forage that they eat, this might reduce the level of exposure of the sheep. Alternate grazing of pasture by cattle and sheep is done intentionally to remove infective worm larvae from the pasture (Urquhart et al. 1996), the theory being that one species will "vacuum up" many larvae belonging to the other species.

Predators are thought to preferentially select prey with disease (i.e., that have some dysfunction). The effect depends upon the disease and the circum-stance. In some diseases, it is to the agent's advantage to enhance predation, and in other cases, the animal may have reduced resources for antipredator behavior because of disease. As an example of the latter, red shanks respond to energetic stress by taking additional risks related to predators (Quinn and Cresswell 2004). Disease agents that have a major energetic cost also could favor predation in a similar manner. In avian botulism outbreaks, many paralyzed birds are killed by predators. If a predator kills and eats a bird that would have survived and recovered from botulism, predation adds to the mortality related to botulism. However, if the predator kills and consumes a bird that was going to die of botulism, predation may reduce the probability of more birds dying, because it removes potential substrate within which more toxin could have formed. (Botulism is unique among poisons in that the victim becomes substrate for production of more toxin and of maggots that carry the toxin to subsequent victims.) Infections caused by macroparasites are characterized by an aggregated distribution (fig. 3.6) in which most of the parasites are concentrated in a few individuals within the population. If predators selectively remove these heavily infected individuals, the effect should be to reduce the overall level of infection in the population and to remove a major source of infection for other animals. Thus, predator removal, a common wildlife management practice, may have negative effects on populations affected

Table 7.5 Interaction of Target Species and Other Animal Species in the Occurrence of Disease

Type of interaction	Effect(s)
Competitor	Reduce availability of resources for target species, potentially reducing fecundity and resistance to disease in the target species
Predator	Remove affected individuals preferentially; increases mortality rate, may reduce prevalence of agent in population
Scavenger	Remove potentially infectious materials, e.g., scavengers remove waterfowl carcasses before type C botulinum toxin develops; may transfer disease agents to new sites
Intermediate host	Facilitates transmission
Vector	Facilitates transmission
Transport host	Facilitate transmission, e.g., mosquitoes transport avian poxvirus on mouthparts among wild turkeys
Bioaccumulator	Concentrate agent and pass to next trophic level, e.g., methyl mercury is concentrated in fish and effects piscivores
Alternative host for multihost agent	Facilitate persistence, act as reservoir of infection for target species
Modify habitat	Create habitat suitable for disease agent or vector, e.g., beaver create ponds suitable for insect vectors or aquatic snails

by some types of infectious agents (Packer et al. 2003). Even the perceived risk of predation may affect a disease. Navarro et al. (2004) found that house sparrows exposed to predators had reduced immune response and a larger load of blood parasites than birds not exposed to predators.

Many of the most important infectious agents of wild animals are generalists or multihost parasites. In considering the effect of other species in disease caused by these agents, it is critical to determine what role each species capable of infection plays in the disease. A *maintenance* host is one in which the agent can persist independently within the population without external sources of infection. A *spillover* host is one in which the disease agent can persist in the population for a time (i.e., there is some transmission) but will die out without an external source of infection. A *dead-end* host is one in which the disease is only acquired from an external source.

The various types of host also can be defined on the basis of R_0 (the basic reproductive rate) of the disease agent. (R_0 will be discussed in chapter 8, but for now R_0 must equal at least 1 for a disease to persist indefinitely in a population). In maintenance hosts, $R_0 \geq 1$, in spillover hosts, $0 < R_0 < 1$, and in dead-end hosts, $R_0 = 0$ (Caley et al. 2002). In New Zealand, many species of feral and domestic animals have been found infected with *Mycobacterium bovis*. Of these, the brushtail possum and domestic cattle are maintenance hosts; the ferret is probably a spillover host in most circumstances (Lugton et al. 1997; Caley and Hone 2004); and the rabbit, hare, feral goat, and domestic cat are dead-end hosts. Similarly, white-tailed deer are the maintenance host for *Parelaphostrongylus tenuis* and moose are a dead-end host. Under certain circumstances, a disease that is shared by two or more species may have severe consequences for one or more of the hosts in what is termed "parasite-mediated competition." The ring-necked pheasant, grey partridge, and red-legged partridge can be infected by the cecal nematode *Heterakis gallinarum*. The pheasant is a maintenance host, and the two partridge species are at best spillover hosts in which the parasite cannot persist (Tompkins et al. 2000, 2001b, 2002). The parasite does not have a severe effect on pheasants or red-legged partridge but has serious effects on grey partridge, leading to the suggestion that this parasite may have contributed to a population decline and exclusion of grey partridge from areas where pheasants occur in Britain (Tompkins et al. 2000, 2001b).

Humans have a greater overall effect on disease in wild animals than does any other single factor or species. Some examples of the many ways in which we interact with disease are shown in table 7.6. Many human-induced environmental changes occur at a much faster rate than natural disturbance, and animals may be unable to make appropriate behavioral decisions to deal with the change. Woods and Hoffmann (2000) compared the effects of natural climate change and introduction of a toxic chemical on animals. They suggested that animals often have been able to evade climate change in the past by altering their geographic distribution as new favorable habitats were created by the climate change. Toxic chemicals do not create new favorable environments suitable for colonization, so that animals may not have the option of moving and must either adapt or face extinction locally. Schlaepfer et al. (2002) used the term "evolutionary trap" for situations "where sudden anthropogenic change in the environment causes an organism to make a decision that normally would be adaptive, but now results in a maladaptive outcome." A simple example of this type might be the occurrence of a high prevalence of lead pellets in the gizzard of certain diving ducks, which suggests that the birds are preferentially selecting pellets during feeding, perhaps because they mistake the pellets for small mollusks.

I have used the example of a noninfectious disease (lead poisoning in waterfowl) (table 7.7) and a hypothetical infectious disease (table 7.8) to illustrate some of the diverse environmental factors that may have an influence on a disease.

I find it useful to think of the occurrence of a disease as consisting of a series of steps that can be arranged in a flowchart type of pattern. Each step has a probability of occurring that varies from 0 (never occurs) to 1 (always occurs). Environmental factors influence the probability of each step occurring and, hence, the overall likelihood of disease occurring (fig. 7.1).

SUMMARY

- Every disease is influenced by a range of factors that are lumped together as environmental influences. These factors are not constant, and many occur in a stochastic manner.
- Environmental factors may affect the disease agent or the animal, and the action may be to modify animal abundance or density, the type and degree of exposure to the agent, or the degree of resistance of the animal.
- It often is difficult to ascertain which factors are important among all of the environmental "noise" that surrounds a disease.

Table 7.6 Human Activities and the Occurrence of Disease in Wild Animals

Activity	Examples
Noninfectious diseases	
Release human-made biocides	Insecticides, rodenticides
Move, concentrate, and release natural toxic materials	Lead, mercury, fluoride, cadmium
Eutrophication of water stimulates growth of organisms producing toxins	Cyanobacteria, organisms producing domoic acid, red tides
Mycotoxins grow on agricultural crops used by wildlife	Mycotoxins on peanuts caused poisoning of sandhill cranes[1]
Acidification alters mineral availability	Ca deficiency in passerine birds[2]
Infectious diseases	
Translocate agents intentionally	Myxoma virus to Australia and Europe, rabbit hemorrhagic disease virus to Australia and New Zealand
Translocate agents unintentionally with wild animals	*Fascioloides magna* to Europe, *Elaphostrongylus rangiferi* to Newfoundland, raccoon rabies from Florida to Virginia
Translocate agents unintentionally with domestic animals	Bovine tuberculosis to New Zealand
Introduce new disease vectors	Mosquitoes into Hawaii, *Aedes albopictus* into North America
Introduce new intermediate or alternative hosts	Voles into Svalbard (*Echinococcus multilocularis*), brushtail possum into New Zealand (bovine tuberculosis)
Concentrate animals artificially, promoting disease transmission	Tuberculosis in deer in Michigan, brucellosis in elk in Wyoming
Introduce susceptible species into area occupied by an indigenous disease	Whooping cranes into eastern United States where eastern encephalitis virus occurs
Change water regime providing habitat for intermediate host or vector	Irrigation provides habitat for snails and mosquito vectors
Habitat change favoring "human-friendly" species	Proliferation of urban populations of raccoons and foxes
Humans as reservoir for infection in wild animals	Staphylococcal infection in eagles, tuberculosis in suricates and mongooses

[1]Windingstad et al. (1989).
[2]Graveland and Drent (1997).

Table 7.7 Lead Poisoning Among Waterfowl and the Influence of Environmental Factors

Factor	Environmental influences
Density of pellets	Hunting activity in the past, which was influenced by bird density, hunter success, and style of hunting. Compliance with current restrictions on the use of lead shot determines if any additional new shot are added.
Availability of pellets	Influenced by the physical character of the pond bottom (sinking rate of pellets), water depth (determined by weather and humans), location of pellets relative to areas used by feeding birds (determined by where shot was deposited by hunters, distribution of food stuffs and food habits of birds).
Use of pond by birds	Influenced by the availability of food (vegetation, invertebrates), water depth, presence of predators, hunters, disturbance, and alternative habitat.
Feeding habits of birds	Determined by the species of bird, bird behavior, and the food available.
Ability to resist or survive exposure to lead	Determined by the amount of lead ingested, the bird's diet, sex, nutritional condition, age, vegetative cover in which birds can hide, and number and type of predators present.

Note: This table lists some environmental factors that might influence a noninfectious disease (lead poisoning among waterfowl on a wetland where lead shot was used in the past). The probability of birds dying of lead poisoning is related to the abundance, density, and availability of lead pellets, the type of birds using the pond, and their ability to withstand or survive exposure to lead.

Table 7.8 Factors That Might Influence the Transmission of Infectious Agents

Factor	Environmental influences
Will animal A become infectious?	All of those factors, including nutrition, intercurrent disease, and other stressors that influence the ability of animal A to resist the disease and to recover without becoming infectious.
Will animal A survive to transmit the disease?	Survival may be influenced by the virulence of the agent, the resistance of animal A, the abundance and avidity of predators, and other factors such as inclement weather, intercurrent disease, and nutrition.
Will animal A contact another animal of the species?	Influenced by the abundance and distribution of animals, which is determined by habitat conditions, predation including by humans, weather, and species-specific behavior.
Will the contact be sufficiently intimate for transmission to occur?	Influenced by the sex and age of the individuals, the behavior of the species, and the circumstance in which they meet. Factors that concentrate animals such as artificial feeding increase the probability of effective contact. The ability of the agent to survive in the external environment will be influenced by temperature, moisture, and solar irradiation.
Will animal B be susceptible to infection?	All of those factors, including nutrition, intercurrent disease, and other stressors that influence the ability of animal B to resist the disease. Age, sex, and prior exposure to the agent will have a major influence.

Note: This table looks at the probability of a hypothetical infectious agent being transmitted from one member of a population (animal A) to other animals of the same species. Animal A has become infected recently and transmission requires close (nose-to-nose) contact.

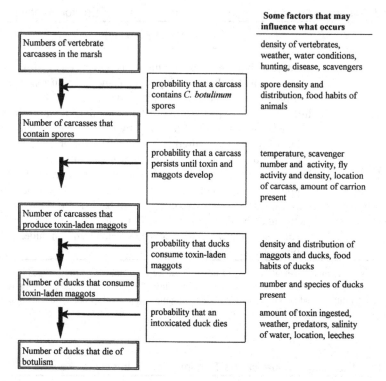

Some factors that may influence what occurs

Numbers of vertebrate carcasses in the marsh	density of vertebrates, weather, water conditions, hunting, disease, scavengers
probability that a carcass contains *C. botulinum* spores	spore density and distribution, food habits of animals
Number of carcasses that contain spores	
probability that a carcass persists until toxin and maggots develop	temperature, scavenger number and activity, fly activity and density, location of carcass, amount of carrion present
Number of carcasses that produce toxin-laden maggots	
probability that ducks consume toxin-laden maggots	density and distribution of maggots and ducks, food habits of ducks
Number of ducks that consume toxin-laden maggots	number and species of ducks present
probability that an intoxicated duck dies	amount of toxin ingested, weather, predators, salinity of water, location, leeches
Number of ducks that die of botulism	

Fig. 7.1. Type C botulism of waterfowl occurs when birds ingest preformed toxin. Spores of *Clostridium botulinum* type C are common in wetlands, although the density is variable among wetlands. The organism grows and produces toxin in warm, anaerobic, protein-rich substrates such as vertebrate carcasses. Animals living in wetlands ingest spores frequently but the spores do not "germinate" in living animals. If an animal dies while it has spores in its intestine or tissues, the bacteria may begin to grow as the carcass becomes anaerobic. Toxin that forms is ingested by maggots (saprophytic fly larvae) and birds become poisoned by eating toxin-laden maggots. This model examines some of the factors that influence the probability that animals dying in a wetland may lead to the occurrence of a botulism outbreak in which many birds are poisoned. A single factor, such as temperature or water conditions, can influence the probability of many of the steps.

- The single overarching factor that affects every disease of wild animals is the effect of human population.
- An essential component of studying any disease is to determine the spatial and temporal relationship among events and factors.
- Many environmental factors act as stressors and trigger a stress response. In general, the acute stress response is adaptive and helpful, and chronic stress is harmful.
- Abiotic factors include topography, climate, weather, bedrock and soils, and water.

- Biotic factors include vegetation, and intraspecific and interspecific interactions with other animals.
- Anthropogenic environmental changes are a particular problem because they occur at a rate faster than natural disturbance, not allowing time for appropriate behavioral or adaptive change.
- It may be useful to construct a stepwise model of how a disease is thought to operate, showing the various steps involved and listing the environmental factors that might influence the probability of each step occurring.

8
Transmission and Perpetuation of Infectious Disease

Obligate disease agents are dependent upon their host for many essentials, but in most cases the relationship between host and agent is only fruitful for the agent for a limited period of time. At some point, the host may no longer provide a hospitable environment. In a minority of instances (highly virulent infections), this is because the agent was too demanding and the host died. More often the host rebels and mounts an immune response that makes the environment unpleasant or even lethal for the agent. From an agent's perspective, each host animal is an island of suitable habitat surrounded by an inhospitable external environment. To persist as a species, some of the agent's offspring have to cross this external sea to find and colonize another suitable island. The phenomenon of passage from one animal to the next (transmission) is central to understanding any infectious disease as well as to developing methods to manage the condition.

Disease agents invest considerable resources toward increasing the chances of successful transmission. Some produce huge numbers of offspring in the hope that a few will reach a suitable new island, others produce offspring that are highly protected (e.g., by an impervious outer membrane) for the external voyage, still others produce offspring that actively seek new hosts, and many produce reproductive stages only at the time and place most appropriate for successful transmission.

Transmission consists of three steps: exit from the host, passage across the external environment to find or be found by a new host, and entry and colonization of the new host. Success of transmission is dependent upon the number of organisms that exit, their persistence in the external environment and success in finding a new host, and the number that are able to initiate an infection in that host.

EXIT FROM THE HOST

Infectious agents have to leave the body of the host for transmission to occur, except for those agents that are transmitted through predation or scavenging, in which the agent can wait in one host until consumed by the next. (Agents that "wait" in living animals may be hidden from the host's reactions or impair the host in some way so that they facilitate predation of the host.) Routes of exit used by disease agents together with examples of diseases in which each route is important are shown in table 8.1. Most agents are shed from the body's surfaces, and agents often are shed in more than one secretion or excretion. For example, canine distemper virus is shed by infected animals in respiratory, oral, and ocular secretions; urine and feces; as well as directly from the skin and through the placenta to fetuses in the uterus. However, often only one of these potential routes is important and accounts for most of the actual transmission of the disease. In canine distemper, oral and respiratory secretions are most important.

CROSSING THE EXTERNAL ENVIRONMENT AND FINDING A NEW HOST

Infectious agents have developed an amazing diversity of methods for voyaging from one host to the next. As with most attempts to categorize natural processes into a rigid set of rules, systems for classifying disease transmission are not completely successful. Those concerned with microparasites tend to classify routes of transmission differently than do those concerned with macroparasites. The system shown in figure 8.1 is a compromise, derived in part from Nokes (1992).

Table 8.1 Point of Exit from the Body of Infectious Stages of Disease in Wild Animals

Route of exit from host	Examples of disease in which this route is important
Respiratory tract secretions (aerosol)	Foot-and-mouth disease, tuberculosis, canine distemper
Saliva	Rabies, feline leukemia, feline immunodeficiency
Gastrointestinal excretions (feces)	Salmonellosis, parvoviral infections, giardiasis, many helminths, avian influenza, avian tuberculosis
Skin	Papillomavirus infections, poxvirus infections, sarcoptic mange
Blood (often by way of arthropod)	*Leucocytozoon* spp. infection, bluetongue virus, malaria
Genital secretions	*Herpesvirus simaiae* infections, pseudorabies, brucellosis
Urine	Infectious canine hepatitis, hantavirus infections, renal coccidiosis, leptospirosis
Milk	Tuberculosis, *Uncinaria lucasi* (seal hookworm) infection
Ocular discharge	Canine distemper
Via fetus or egg	Duck plague, pestivirus infections
Postmortem decomposition of carcass	Anthrax, avian botulism, *Calodium hepatica* infection
Consumption of body by predator/scavenger	*Sarcocystis* spp., many helminths, avian cholera

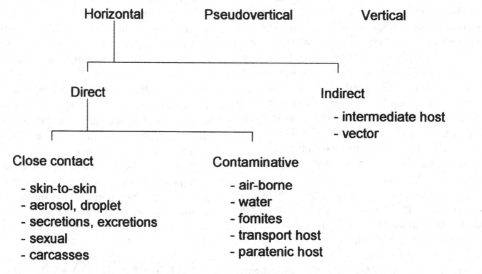

Fig. 8.1. A classification system for methods of disease transmission.

VERTICAL TRANSMISSION

Vertical transmission involves passage of an agent from parent to offspring. This may occur through passage of agents in semen, through the placenta or milk, or through the egg in egg-laying species. Toma et al. (1999a) observed that in animals, "vertical transmission occurs exceptionally in a great many diseases and is the rule in only a few." Vertical transmission occurs but is uncommon as an ecologically important method among wild animals.

Duck plague, a herpesviral disease of waterfowl, is an infection that can be transmitted vertically. Ducklings hatching from eggs laid by infected females may be infected in the egg and are likely to remain infected for an extended period (Burgess and Yuill 1981).

A disease in mammals in which vertical transmission is important is infection of bighorn sheep by the lungworm *Protostrongylus stilesi*. Adult worms produce eggs from which first-stage larvae (L_1) hatch in the sheep's lung. The L_1 are coughed up and swallowed, and exit in the sheep's feces. In the external environment, L_1 enter certain snails or slugs, where they molt twice and become infective third-stage larvae (L_3) that can infect another sheep, if it ingests the mollusk. Ingested L_3 migrate to the lungs and mature there. This pattern of using a mollusk intermediate host is typical of nematodes in the superfamily Metastongyloidea and is a form of indirect horizontal transmission to be described later. *Protostrongylus stilesi* also has an alternate method that involves vertical transmission. If L_3 are ingested with a mollusk by an adult sheep that is already infected, the larvae reach the lungs but do not develop to the adult stage, perhaps because of host immunity. These L_3 are said to be "arrested" in development and accumulate in the lungs. In pregnant ewes, the arrested L_3 leave the lungs during the last 6 weeks of pregnancy, pass in the blood to the uterus, and cross the placenta into the liver of the fetal lamb. The L_3 move from the liver to the lungs when the lamb is born and complete their development. By about 20 days of age, lambs have adult worms that are producing eggs. Unfortunately for the lamb, there is a marked inflammatory response to the eggs and the L_1 that hatch from them. If the inflamed lungs become infected secondarily with bacteria, "summer lamb pneumonia" may result, which has caused very high mortality in some bands of sheep (Hibler et al. 1977, 1982).

Another nematode *(Uncinaria lucasi)* that occurs in the intestine of northern fur seals and northern sea lions uses a different form of vertical transmission. Arrested L_3 in blubber and mammary tissue of adult females are transferred in milk to the pup shortly after birth. The worms develop rapidly in the pup's intestine and begin to pass many eggs in the pup's feces within about 2 weeks. The adult parasites feed on blood in the intestine and heavy infection may result in severe anemia because of blood loss (Lyons and Keyes 1978). L_3 that develop in eggs shed by pups remain viable in the external environment of the rookery until the following year, infect returning adults and yearlings by penetrating their skin, and then localize in blubber and mammary tissue as arrested larvae. (This form of direct contaminative transmission will be discussed later in this chapter.) This unusual life cycle is thought to be a method of circumventing the inability of adult worms to survive during the 9-month period when the seals are at sea (Anderson 1992).

Other examples of infections that may be transmitted vertically include *Bartonella* spp. in rodents (Kosoy et al. 1998) and brucellosis (*Brucella abortus* in bison and elk, *B. suis* type 4 in caribou). In brucellosis, infection of the placenta often results in severe inflammation (placentitis) causing the offspring to die in utero and be expelled or to be aborted in a weakened state.

PSEUDOVERTICAL TRANSMISSION

Pseudovertical transmission involves passage of agents to neonates shortly after birth or hatching and before they have been exposed extensively to the outside world. Transmission is often from parent to offspring, because of their close association, but parents are not the only source of infection. Pseudovertical transmission has been used to describe transfer of bovine tuberculosis to European badger kits before they emerge from the den (Anderson and Trewhella 1985). Transmission could be from any badger sharing the communal den and not just from the parents. *Oslerus osleri*, a nematode that inhabits the large airways of coyotes and dogs (fig. 8.2) also uses a method that can be considered pseudovertical transmission. L_1 produced by adult worms normally

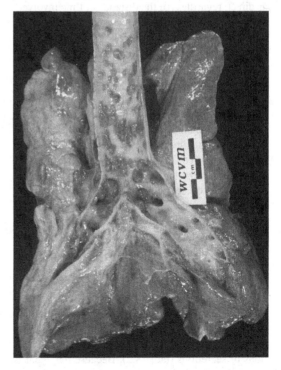

Fig. 8.2. Respiratory tract from a coyote. The trachea and bronchi have been opened to show the many nodules containing coiled adult *Oslerus osleri* nematodes, which are present just beneath the respiratory epithelium.

pass up the trachea to be swallowed and passed with the animal's feces. However, wild canids typically feed the young with regurgitated food so that larvae can be passed with food from any adult that feeds the pups.

HORIZONTAL TRANSMISSION

Horizontal transmission involves transfer of infection from one animal to other individuals in the population, independent of their parental relationship. This is by far the most common method of disease spread and takes many forms. Several methods for subdividing horizontal transmission have been described. Those dealing with microparasites tend to use the term "direct transmission" for situations in which transmission occurs by "close physical contact/proximity between individuals or by common use of an enclosed airspace." "Indirect transmission" is used when there is "intermediary involvement or action of another individual, object or substance" (Toma et al. 1999b). Scientists working with macroparasites tend to regard any transmission that occurs from one individual to another of the same species without the need for involvement of another species as direct, regardless of the distance or time involved. If two or more species are required for completion of a life cycle, the transmission is considered to be indirect. The requirement for involvement of one or more additional species as a basis for subdividing types of transmission seems to make sense. In the classification system shown in fig. 8.1, direct transmission includes any situation in which infection passes from one individual to another without the requirement for involvement of another species. Included within this definition are some forms of direct transmission that may involve other species but in which the other species is not required for transmission to occur. Indirect transmission is used for those situations in which transmission does not occur without the involvement of at least one species in addition to the target species.

Direct Transmission

The simplest forms of direct transmission are those in which intimate contact between infectious and susceptible animals allows exchange of infectious particles through skin-to-skin contact or in excretions or secretions (table 8.2). Because the agent is exposed to the external environment only briefly, agents transmitted in this manner may be rather fragile. This form of transmission is more likely to occur within a social group (e.g., a family or territorial group) than among unrelated animals of the same species or between species, because of the greater frequency and intimacy of contact.

Skin-to-Skin Contact. Although some fleas, lice, ticks, and mites have developed alternate strategies for moving among hosts, most ectoparasites are dependent upon close physical contact for transmission. For example, *Sarcoptes scabei,* the cause of sarcoptic mange in wild canids (fig. 2.1), chamois, wombats, and many other species, lives its entire life on the host animal. The mites don't hop, jump, or fly and are dependent on direct contact for transmission. Lice are somewhat more mobile, but they survive for only a very limited time away from a host and also are largely dependent upon direct contact for transmission. Ringworm (dermatophycosis), caused by the fungus *Trichophyton verrucosum,* is a common skin disease of domestic cattle that also occurs in mule deer. Most lesions in deer are on the face and legs (fig. 3.4). The fungus is likely spread primarily by direct contact with infected individuals, but, because the fungal spores are very resistant, it also may be spread by fomites (see below), such as brush or thorns along trails.

Short-Range Airborne Transmission. Transmission via aerosols or droplets is the principal method of transmission for many respiratory infections in which the agent leaves one animal on the expired air and enters another in inspired air. However, only droplets <5μm in diameter are capable of remaining suspended in air for an extended period of time. (A micron, or μm, is 1/1000th of a millimeter). Most expired droplets are in the range of 15–100μm and do not remain suspended for more than a few seconds. Thus, direct infection by this route is limited to the area immediately in front of the infected animal, that is, virtually nose-to-nose contact. This type of contact might occur between sparring male deer or bison and could be a means of spread of tuberculosis in these species. Aerosols also may be generated from secretions other than the respiratory tract, and these may be inhaled. (Long-distance airborne transmission will be discussed as a form of contaminative transmission.)

Secretions and Excretions. Secretions and excretions often contain many agents that can be transmitted through close contact. These might be inhaled in the form of aerosols generated by sniffing or, more commonly, ingested through licking and grooming, aggressive behavior, or from contamination of the immediate surroundings. It may be diffi-

Table 8.2 Form of Contact for Direct Transmission of Diseases in Wild Animals

Form of contact	Disease	Species involved
Skin-to-skin	Sarcoptic mange	Wild canids, many others
	Ringworm (*Trichophyton verrucosum* infection)	Mule deer
	Contagious ecthyma	Wild sheep, mountain goats
	Mycoplasmal conjunctivitis	House finches
Respiratory aerosol or droplets	Canine distemper	Canids, mustelids
	Foot-and-mouth disease	Ungulates
	Tuberculosis (*Mycobacterium bovis* infection)	Ungulates, European badger, brushtail possum
Secretions, excreta		
Saliva, licking	Rabies	Kudu
Saliva, bite wounds	Rabies	Many species
	Bovine tuberculosis	Wild ferret[1]
Feces	Classical swine fever	Wild boar
	Salmonellosis	Many species
Urine	Infectious canine hepatitis	Canids
Genital discharges	Brucellosis	Bison, elk, caribou
Discharge from lesions	Tuberculosis	Brushtail possums to cattle
Sexual	Brucellosis	Bison, elk, caribou
	Rabbit syphilis (*Treponema cuniculi*)	European rabbit
	Chlamydiosis	Koalas[2]
Contact with carcass of infected animal	Tuberculosis	Ferret from possum[1]
	Brucella abortus infection	Wolf from bison

[1]Lugton et al. 1997).
[2]Whittington (2001).

cult to determine the actual route of transmission involved among animals in close contact. For example, rinderpest, a disease that has had devastating effects on cattle in Africa and can infect many African wild ungulates, is caused by a very fragile morbillivirus that usually can survive for a few hours at most outside the host. It is shed in all secretions and excretions of infected animals, and transmission occurs during close contact. The actual route is unclear and airborne spread is thought to be unlikely in the wild.

Some agents are shed specifically in saliva, and transmission via saliva is important in a small number of diseases. The best known example of salivary transmission is rabies in which the normal route of transmission is via bite wounds. Animals infected with rabies virus usually die from the infection, and secretion of virus in saliva only occurs during the final stages of the disease. The abnormal and often aggressive behavior caused by inflammation of the brain in rabid animals facilitates transmission by

this route. Rabies in kudu may be transmitted by a variation of salivary transmission. Kudu sick with rabies and drooling saliva profusely were licked and groomed by other kudu that subsequently developed the disease. Saliva from the sick animals caused rabies when placed experimentally on the oral mucosa of healthy animals (Rupprecht et al. 2001). Bite wounds are one method by which tuberculosis (*Mycobacterium bovis* infection) is transmitted among wild ferrets in New Zealand (Lugton et al. 1997), and hantavirus is spread in rodents (Escutinaire et al. 2002).

A great many infectious agents are shed in droppings, and vast numbers of infectious particles may be present per gram of feces. However, in most conditions direct transfer from fresh feces is unlikely except in situations where animals are abnormally crowded and fecal contamination of skin or food supplies occurs. This may apply in *Salmonella* infections of passerine birds concentrated at bird feeders. Thing and Clausen (1980) associated intensive use of areas with short-cropped vegetation ("lawns"), heavily seeded with bacteria, with increased risk of *Escherichia coli* infection of caribou calves in Greenland. In some herbivores, there is active avoidance of fecal material. This aversion is thought to reduce exposure to helminths, and subclinical parasitism increased the level of aversion to feces (Hutchings et al. 1999). Spatial separation of feeding and fecal deposition documented in several wild ruminants may serve the same purpose (Gunn and Irvine 2003). In most situations in which fecal-oral transmission occurs, it is through contaminative transfer and involves resistant organisms that can survive in the external environment for long periods.

The primary habitat for some disease agents (e.g., bacteria of the genus *Leptospira*,, the protozoan *Encephalitozoon cuniculi*, and renal coccidia) is within the kidney tubules. These agents exit the body primarily via urine. In other diseases, such as infectious canine hepatitis in canids and type B tularemia in voles, the infection may be more generalized, but shedding of organisms in urine may occur for months and is a major source of infection for other animals. Agents are shed in urine in many other diseases. Transmission of leptospirosis may involve direct contact with urine (Bolin 2000), but, as with feces, direct contact with freshly voided urine is probably not a common method of disease transmission among wild animals. However, many of the agents shed in urine, including leptospires, *Francisella tularensis,* and the adenovirus causing infectious canine hepatitis, are durable and can persist and be transmitted via contaminated water or fomites.

Genital Discharges. Transmission of bacteria of the genus *Brucella* among terrestrial mammals is primarily through contact with fetal fluids, vaginal exudates, and aborted fetuses. This takes the form of licking an infected fetus, placenta, or the genital region of an animal after abortion or parturition. Rhyan (2000) related the frequent occurrence of brucellosis among male bison to the intense interest shown by young bulls in materials associated with the birth process: "the most interested animals are the 2-year-old bulls. Following parturition, cows with attached placentas are often followed by young bulls who continue to sniff and lick the placentas and fluids." Leptospirosis and pseudorabies also may be transmitted through contact with placental fluids.

Discharge from Lesions. Massive numbers of organisms may exit the body through open, draining lesions such as abscessed lymph nodes that have ruptured to a skin surface. This is probably an infrequent route of transmission, but occurs in European badgers and brushtail possums with tuberculosis.

Sexual (Venereal) Transmission. Transmission through sexual contact is a specialized form of direct transmission adopted by some infectious agents including such highly successful human diseases as syphilis, gonorrhea, chlamydiosis, genital herpes, and HIV. Venereal transmission has been documented in a variety of diseases of wild animals, such as brucellosis, but in general this appears to be a minor route of transmission except in a few diseases. These diseases include rabbit syphilis, caused by the bacterium *Treponema cuniculi* in European rabbits and hares (Small and Newman 1972; Lumeij 1996); *Mycoplasma* infection in geese (Stipkovits et al. 1986); and one form of chlamydiosis in koalas (Whittington 2001). Many other diseases may be transmitted at the time of breeding, although the actual route is not venereal. This may be very important in solitary species in which breeding is one of the few times that conspecifics have contact (Altizer et al. 2003).

Contact with Carcasses. The carcass of an animal that died of infectious disease may contain massive numbers of infectious agents. Direct contact with carcasses is probably not a common route of *intraspecific* disease transmission. McLandress (1983) suggested that wild geese avoided contact with dead conspecifics thereby reducing the likelihood of direct transmission of avian cholera, but whether aversion to carcasses is widespread in other species is unknown. Contact with aborted fetuses is an important route of transmission of *Brucella* spp. Cook et al. (2004) placed bovine fetuses in the field to mimic abortions caused by *Brucella abortus* in bison and elk. They observed frequent sniffing, licking, and chewing of the fetuses by elk. More than 100 elk had contact with one fetus and >150 elk had contact with a another fetus. Cannibalism (intraspecific scavenging and predation) is probably infrequent as a method of disease spread, but it is important in the transmission of *Calodium (Capillaria) hepatica*, a nematode that occurs in rodents and less commonly in other species. The adults of this worm live and deposit eggs within the liver of the host, and the eggs remain in the liver until released by predation, decomposition, scavenging, or cannibalism. Cannibalism is a major method of transmission of this parasite among deer mice (Herman 1981). *Interspecific* spread of disease through scavenging is a more common occurrence. For instance, we have seen avian cholera in common crows, gulls, and bald eagles that had scavenged waterfowl dead of the disease. Scavenging is also important in the transmission of *Echinococcus granulosus* between sheep and foxes (Gemmell 1959) and between moose and coyotes (Samuel et al. 1976).

Many diseases are transmitted between prey and predators as a form of indirect disease transmission, which will be discussed later. Occasionally, disease agents are transmitted directly in this manner: wolves become infected with *Mycobacterium bovis* from feeding on infected bison, and raptors may acquire *Trichomonas gallinae* (a protozoan parasite) from eating infected pigeons and doves. Mustelids appear not to have specific fleas of their own but carry ectoparasites picked up from their rodent prey. King (1976) suggested that most fleas on British weasels were acquired from nests and runways of prey rather than directly from the rodents, so perhaps this should be considered a form of contaminative direct transmission.

Direct transmission from predator to prey also may occur occasionally. Many carnivores carry the bacterium *Pasteurella multocida* in their mouths, and Mims et al. (2001) suggested that "bites from tigers and cougars can lead to *P. multocida* infection as well as bad dreams" in humans. This method of transmission occurred in a caribou population in Newfoundland that was in severe decline as a result of poor calf survival. Many calves were found dead on the breeding ground with abscesses on their necks and with generalized infection (septicemia) caused by *P. multocida*. Through skillful detective work this was linked conclusively to attacks by lynx (Bergerud 1971). Removal of lynx from the caribou breeding grounds resulted in caribou calf survival to 6 months of age increasing from 27 to 63%. (The proportion of calf deaths due to direct predation versus bacterial infection from thwarted predator attacks is not known.) I have seen bite wounds compatible with attack by a lynx (fig. 8.3) on mountain caribou calves from British Columbia that died from *P. multocida* septicemia.

Contaminative Transmission. The term "contaminative transmission" is used here for forms of direct transmission in which there is separation in time and/or space between the infectious individual and susceptible animals. For this to occur, the agent must be sufficiently robust to survive in the external environment. In many situations, some intermediary

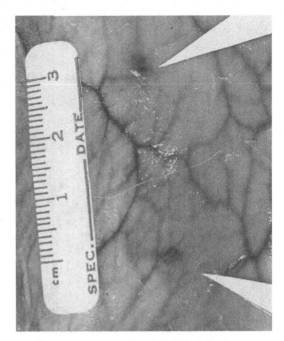

Fig. 8.3. Bite wounds compatible with attack by a lynx in skin from the neck of a caribou calf that died of *Pasteurella multocida* infection. Lynx have *P. multocida* in their oral cavity, and it is assumed that the bacteria were injected through the bite wound. This is a rare example of direct spread of an infectious disease caused by a microparasite from a predator to a prey animal.

or "vehicle" is involved. This might be water, air, inanimate objects, or a living organism of another species. In the latter case, participation by the other species is not required for transmission. Avian pox in wild birds (fig. 8.4) illustrates contaminative transmission. The causative virus can be transmitted through direct skin-to-skin contact among birds. Because the virus is extremely hardy, birds also can be infected by contact with virus surviving on perches used by an infected bird. The mouthparts of biting insects, such as mosquitoes, may be contaminated with poxvirus when the insect feeds on affected skin of a bird. Virus on the mouthparts can then be introduced into the skin of the next bird fed on by the mosquito. Both the perch and the mosquito's mouthparts are contaminated with virus; the mosquito is not infected by the virus. Neither the perch nor the mosquito is essential for transmission, but they increase the dispersion of the virus in space and time and, hence, enhance the probability of transmission.

The term "fomites" is used for inanimate objects, such as the perch, that convey infectious agents.

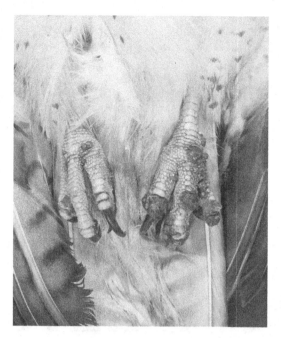

Fig. 8.4. Proliferative and destructive lesions on the feet of a red-tailed hawk caused by infection with avian poxvirus. Avian poxviruses can be spread by direct contact, inanimate fomites, or biting insects acting as a transport host.

Many terms have been used to describe animals, such as the mosquito, that are contaminated with an infectious agent that does not multiply or replicate in the animal. These include "mechanical carrier," "mechanical transmitter," "passive carrier," "flying pin," "flying needle" (the latter to suggest that the insect is equivalent to a contaminated hypodermic needle), "transport host," and "mechanical vector." On balance, I prefer transport host, with the implication that the agent is simply being transported. Mechanical carrier may be appropriate, but the term "carrier" is used to describe animals with persistent infections that shed organisms without having obvious disease. (The most notorious carrier was Typhoid Mary Mallon, a cook who while healthy herself infected many people with *Salmonella typhi.*) I prefer to reserve the term "vector" for those other species in which the infectious agent undergoes either some required part of its life cycle or multiplication, neither of which is true of the mosquito in the case of avian pox. Examples of contaminative direct transmission are shown in table 8.3.

Long-Distance Airborne Transmission. Most droplets originating from the oral or nasal cavities are only infectious within a short distance from their origin. However, particles <5 μm may remain in suspension for extended periods and may be carried long distances. This might occur through evaporation of water from droplets, resulting in "desiccated droplet nuclei" of an appropriate size to remain suspended indefinitely (Thrusfield 1986). It is believed that long-distance aerial spread of foot-and-mouth disease virus has occurred to livestock on several occasions including from France to the Channel Islands in 1974, from Denmark to Sweden (~100 km) in 1960, and from France to the Isle of Wight (~250 km) in 1981 (Donaldson et al. 1982; Gloster et al. 1982). The conditions under which this type of transport can occur have been well characterized (Gloster et al. 1982), and it is thought that airborne transmission is much more likely to occur over the sea than over land. However, humans up to 1700 m downwind from a contaminated cooling tower became infected with *Legionella pneumophila*, the bacterium that causes Legionnaire's disease (Mims et al. 2001). These examples demonstrate the potential for long-distance aerial transmission, but, to my knowledge, no instance of extreme long-distance transmission of disease by this route has been documented among wild animals. Examples of shorter distance airborne transmission include rabies virus in bat caves where extremely high humidity may stabilize the virus, hantavirus transmission to humans in the form of fine-particle aerosols from rodent excreta (Tsai 1987), and aerosolized anthrax spores in dust clouds created by rutting bison (Dragon and Rennie 1995). Opportunistic fungi that live in the external environment (e.g., *Aspergillus fumigatus*) are inhaled as spores.

Water. Many diseases are transmitted through contaminated water, and disease agents that are not normally thought of as being aquatic often survive longer in water than in the terrestrial environment. Agents may enter water from secretions, excretions, draining tracts from lesions, and from dead animals. For some diseases including avian influenza in waterbirds, type B tularemia (caused by *Francisella tularensis palearctica*) among aquatic rodents, leptospirosis in many species, and *Giardia* infection in beaver and muskrats, water is the major route of transmission. Waterborne transmission may be responsible for sudden, massive outbreaks of avian cholera and duck plague. In avian cholera, *Pasteurella multocida* is shed in large numbers in the secretions of dying birds and is released from carcasses into water when dead birds are scavenged.

Table 8.3 Method of Transfer for Contaminative Direct Transmission of Diseases in Wild Animals

Method of transfer	Disease	Species involved
Airborne (medium to long distance)	Foot-and-mouth disease	Potentially many
	Hantaviruses	Rodent excreta to humans
	Newcastle disease, chlamydia	Many birds (aerosols and dust particles)
	Anthrax	Bison (on dust particles)
Waterborne	Avian influenza	Wild waterfowl
	Leptospirosis	Many mammals
	Type B tularemia	Aquatic and semiaquatic rodents
	Avian cholera	Waterfowl
Food or pasture contamination	Many protozoa and helminths	All species
	Yersiniosis	Many species
Other fomites	Avian pox (perch)	Many species
	Contagious ecthyma (salt lick)	Mountain sheep
Transport hosts		
blowflies	Anthrax	Kudu[1]
carnivores carrying rodent fleas	Plague	Prairie dogs[2]
cockroaches	*Sarcocystis falcatula* infection	Opossum to bird[3]
flies	Infectious keratoconjunctivitis	Chamois[4]
mosquitoes, fleas	Myxomatosis	Rabbits
vultures, gulls	Anthrax	African animals[5] , bison[6]
Paratenic hosts	*Baylisascaris procyonis*	Many species to raccoons
	Dioctophyme renale	Fish, frogs to mink

[1]Braack and deVos (1990).
[2]Barnes (1982).
[3]Clubb and Frenkel (1992).
[4]Giacometti et al. (2002).
[5]Ebedes (1976).
[6]Dragon and Rennie (1995).

The bacteria survive in water for days to weeks and accumulate near the surface of the water column (Friend and Franson 1999). Healthy birds may be exposed while drinking and feeding, or by inhalation of bacteria-laden aerosols generated by bird activity.

Water also may influence transmission of disease in other ways. Runoff water plays an important role in anthrax transmission through collection and concentration of the extremely resistant spores in low-lying depressions (Dragon and Rennie 1995). Freshwater runoff into a marine environment was considered a likely route by which *Toxoplasma gondii* (a protozoan parasite whose only known final host are felids, primarily the domestic cat) reached sea otters (Miller et al. 2004a) and marine dolphins (Bowater et al. 2003).

Contamination of Food, Vegetation, Soil, and Other Abiotic Elements. Consumption of contaminated

food and exposure to vegetation and soil contaminated by organisms, particularly those shed in feces, are common routes of transmission for many important diseases of wild animals, including diseases caused by viruses, bacteria, protozoa, and helminths. The usual route of entry into the new host is via ingestion, although some organisms may enter via inhalation, through skin wounds, or by direct penetration of skin or mucous membranes. An example is the transmission of bovine tuberculosis among deer through contact with contaminated feed (Palmer et al. 2004). Survival of most organisms in the external environment is prolonged under cool, moist conditions and abbreviated under hot, dry conditions, particularly if there is high exposure to sunlight. This may have effects on the distribution of disease: Hansen et al. (2004) proposed that the spatial aggregation of larval *Echinococcus multilocularis* in voles occurs because tapeworm eggs shed by foxes fail to survive in areas with high temperature and dry conditions so that infection occurs in voles in humid areas with lower temperature. (These areas were suggested to also be areas with greater risk for human infection.)

Many organisms that utilize this form of transmission produce extremely resistant forms. Among the champions in the "sit and wait" category are embryonated eggs of nematodes of the subfamily Ascaridinae, including those of *Baylisascaris procyonis* of raccoons that can remain infectious in the environment for years (Kazacos 2001) and spores of *Bacillus anthracis*, the cause of anthrax, that may remain infective for centuries (Gates et al. 2001). It is not known how long the prions that are thought to cause transmissible spongiform encephalopathies can persist in the external environment, but mule deer became affected after exposure to pens that had not contained deer with chronic wasting disease for at least 2.2 years (Miller et al. 2004b). Some agents that spread by contaminative transmission actively increase their chances of finding another host. Infective L_3 of the seal hookworm (*Uncinaria lucasi*) remain viable on seal rookeries over winter, and then actively penetrate the skin of adult seals when they return the next year. Larvae of some nematodes that infect the alimentary tract of herbivores (e.g., *Trichostrongylus tenuis* that infects red grouse) crawl up vegetation and wait where they are likely to be ingested by browsing or grazing hosts. Larvae and nymphs of some ticks climb vegetation to a height appropriate for their desired host and wait in hopes of contacting a passing animal.

Transmission by Other Species. There are two forms of direct transmission that involve species other than the usual host for the disease. The first of these is exemplified by the carriage of avian poxvirus on the mouthparts of mosquitoes described earlier. Other examples of diseases transmitted by a transport host include mechanical transmission of the causative agents of myxomatosis, tularemia, and anthrax on the mouthparts of biting flies. Organisms also can be carried on pelage or plumage of scavengers and on the exterior of other parts of invertebrates. Some agents survive passage through the intestinal tract of animals that have fed on carcasses, secretions, or excreta. Anthrax spores may be passed in the feces of scavengers (Pienaar 1967), and cockroaches that had fed on opossum feces transmitted the protozoan *Sarcocystis falcatula* when they were eaten by birds (Clubb and Frenkel 1992). Tapeworm eggs can survive passage through the digestive tract of flies, and flies are thought to be a major means of

spread of *Echinococcus granulosus* from dog feces to other species, including humans (Lawson and Gemmell 1983, 1985). Filter-feeding invertebrates might be a route by which *Toxoplasma gondii* oocysts that are washed into the sea reach sea otters (Miller et al. 2004a).

The second form of animal transport is through "paratenic hosts." These are hosts that become infected with the organism but in which reproduction of the organism does not occur. Paratenic hosts are not required, but they may enhance the probability of transmission. Paratenic hosts usually are only recognized for macroparasites. Adults of *Dioctophyme renale*, the giant kidney worm of wild mink, live within and destroy one (usually the right) kidney of mink, and eggs pass with urine into water. The usual life cycle is indirect with larval stages developing in an aquatic oligochaete and mink becoming infected by eating the oligochaete. However, if an infected oligochaete is eaten by a fish or frog (common prey of mink), these animals become infected. The larvae persist in the tissues of the frog or fish hosts but do not develop or grow. If the frog or fish is eaten by a mink, the larvae then grow to maturity in the mink. The fish and frog are not required for transmission of *D. renale* but serve to increase the probability of its occurring.

Indirect Transmission

Indirect transmission requires the involvement of more than one species. The "other" species may be a vertebrate or an invertebrate, and more than two species may be required in some diseases. When two or more species are involved in the life cycle of a disease agent, the nomenclature used to designate the status of the different hosts is a bit problematic. By convention, parasitologists working with macroparasites call the host in which the agent reaches sexual maturity the "definitive" or "final" host (although transmission doesn't end there). "Intermediate host" is used for the animal(s) in which there is development and, perhaps, replication, but in which the parasite does not reach sexual maturity. This system works well for disease agents in which sexual maturity can be pinpointed (table 8.4).

In diseases such as malaria and *Leucocytozoon* infection, the definitive host is an arthropod and the intermediate host is a vertebrate. From the examples in table 8.4, it should be apparent that a species can be an intermediate host for some infectious agents and a definitive host for others.

Indirect transmission is very common among macroparasites, and their life cycles often are complex

Table 8.4 Indirectly Transmitted Diseases

Disease agent	Definitive host	Intermediate host
Fascioloides magna (trematode)	Elk, white-tailed deer	Snail
Parelaphostrongylus tenuis (nematode)	White-tailed deer	Snail or slug
Echinococcus granulosus (cestode)	Wolf	Moose, deer, elk, caribou
Sarcocystis rileyi (protozoan)	Striped skunk	Duck
Sarcocystis rauschorum (protozoan)	Snowy owl	Collared lemming
Plasmodium relictum (protozoan)	Mosquito	Bird
Leucocytozoon simondi (protozoan)	Blackfly	Duck
Dioctophyme renale (nematode)	Mink	Aquatic oligochaete
Sarconema eurycerca (nematode)	Swans, geese	Biting louse
Elaeophora schneideri (nematode)	Mule deer	Horseflies (*Tabanus* spp., *Hybomitra* spp.)

Note: The definitive host is the host in which sexual replication of the disease agent occurs.

and devilishly "clever." Many such life cycles are based on a predator-prey relationship in which one host must die for the parasite to be transmitted. As noted in the discussion of virulence (chapter 5), the term "parasite increased trophic transmission" (PITT) (Lafferty 1999) is used to describe life cycles in which infection alters the intermediate host in a manner that increases the chance that it will be eaten by a suitable final host. This may involve changing the intermediate host's behavior or appearance so that it is more easily detected by the predator, or impairing its ability to escape when detected. Most well-documented examples of PITT involve invertebrate intermediate hosts, but the phenomenon likely also operates in larger animals.

In a few situations, one animal may act as both definitive and intermediate host for a single agent. *Trichinella* spp. are nematodes whose adults live in the intestine of mammals. The females produce larvae that, rather than exiting the body, penetrate the gut wall and encyst in the animal's skeletal muscle where they remain viable for a very long time until eaten by a predator or scavenger. *Trichinella* spp. cause the disease trichinosis in humans that is often associated in North America with eating inadequately cooked bear meat. Larvae in the meat develop to the adult stage in the human alimentary tract. The adults produce larvae that localize in the person's musculature, and both the intestinal and intramuscular stages of infection cause illness. Heavy infections may be fatal.

It is more difficult to find suitable names for the hosts involved in indirectly transmitted diseases caused by viruses, bacteria, and some protozoa, because sexual replication is not a distinguishing feature. The species that is of greatest concern to humans (almost always the most highly valued vertebrate) is often called the "primary" host, and the other animal(s) involved are called alternate hosts or, in the case of invertebrates, vector species (table 8.5).

Table 8.5 Vectorborne Indirectly Transmitted Diseases

Disease (agent)	Wildlife host of concern	Vector
Bluetongue, epizootic hemorrhagic disease of deer (oriboviruses)	Deer, other ungulates	*Culicoides* spp. (biting midges)
Lyme disease (*Borrelia burgdorferi*)	White-footed mouse, other rodents, birds	*Ixodes scapularis, I. ricinus* (ticks)
West Nile virus	Wild birds	Mosquitoes, primarily of the genus *Culex*
Louping ill (flavivirus)	Red grouse, mountain hare	*Ixodes ricinus* (tick)
Plague (*Yersinia pestis*)	Prairie dog and other rodents	Rodent fleas
Type A tularemia	Lagomorphs	*Haemophysalis leporis-palustris* and other ticks
Ehrlichiosis (*Ehrlichia* spp.)	Deer	Ixodid ticks

The word "vector" has been used in many ways. It is used in a general sense for "anything that allows the transport and/or transmission of a pathogen" or in a more restricted ecological sense as "a living creature which, because of its ecological relationship to others, acquires a pathogen from one living host and transmits it to another" (Toma et al. 1999b). Vector will be used here in a very restricted sense for a heterogenous group of blood-feeding arthropods that are involved in the indirect transmission of disease. These arthropods are infected with the agents, rather than simply having their external surfaces contaminated, and the disease agent develops or multiplies within the arthropod.

Vector-transmitted diseases are relatively common and many are highly virulent. Ewald (1983) reviewed a large number of human diseases and concluded that, in general, diseases transmitted by biting arthropods are more severe than those transmitted directly. He speculated that because mobility of the human host was not required for transmission in these diseases, debilitation was not harmful to transmission and might even facilitate transmission if it made the human less able to avoid feeding arthropods.

There are important differences among different types of blood-feeding arthropod vectors, particularly between ticks and blood-feeding insects, that influence the pattern of disease transmission (Randolph et al. 2001). Most insects fly and are mobile, while ticks are relatively sedentary. Consequently, the geographical distribution of tickborne diseases tends to change slowly while that of insectborne diseases can change rapidly. This is exemplified by the rather stable distribution of Lyme disease (tick transmitted) compared to the explosive spread of mosquito-borne West Nile virus across North America. As an extreme example of the mobility of insects, it is suspected that *Culicoides* spp. midges infected with various orbiviruses have been carried by wind for many kilometers across national boundaries (Sellers 1980; Sellers and Pedgley 1985; Gibbs 1991). Only the adult of most insects feeds on blood, while ticks feed on blood at all stages of their development and may feed on different animal species at the larval, nymphal, and adult stages. Thus, ticks can efficiently carry a disease agent along a chain of different species. Insects tend to feed frequently, while ticks take few but large blood meals. For example, female *Culicoides* midges feed about every fourth day during their 70-day life span, while many ticks feed only once during each life cycle stage. A single insect can potentially infect many

more animals than can a tick. Transovarial (through the egg) and transtadial (from one life cycle stage to the next) transmission are less common in insects than in ticks. Ticks are long-lived and may provide a long-lasting source of infection in an area, while most insects are short-lived. (Some viruses may overwinter in infected mosquitoes that spread the disease to susceptible vertebrates the following season.) Insect transmission is rapid and requires a large transmission rate for persistence. Tick transmission may be interrupted by long delays (months) during which molt occurs from one stage to the next and persistence may occur with lower transmission rates (Hudson and Dobson 1995).

Diseases transmitted by indirect routes using poikilothermic crustaceans, mollusks, and arthropods are particularly sensitive to climatic variables such as temperature and humidity. The spatial distribution and seasonal incidence of these diseases may be sharply defined by factors such as the number of days above a certain minimum temperature each summer, the relative humidity, or the amount of rainfall. For example, outbreaks of hemorrhagic disease caused by orbiviruses transmitted by *Culicoides* spp. end shortly after the first killing frost of autumn.

MULTIPLE ROUTES OF TRANSMISSION

Many infectious diseases have more than one route of transmission. The route that is most important may vary in different situations. This is obviously of great importance in understanding how a disease is maintained. As an example, the nematode *Baylisascaris procyonis* is transmitted by different routes to juvenile and adult raccoons. Adult worms live in the intestine and eggs are passed in the raccoon's feces. After a period of development in the external environment, the eggs are directly infectious if ingested by another raccoon. This is the route by which most *young* raccoons become infected. If eggs are ingested by animals of other species (usually a rodent or small bird), the eggs hatch and the larvae migrate vigorously through the animal's tissue (a process called "visceral larva migrans") and some reach the brain. The larvae do not complete development in these paratenic hosts, but the resulting debilitation and/or death of the animal facilitates its being found and consumed by a raccoon. This is the route by which most transmission to *adult* raccoons is thought to occur (Kazacos 2001).

ENTRY INTO THE NEW HOST

The third step in transmission is invasion and colonization of a new host. Much of what we consider to be inside the body is in fact directly connected with the outside (fig. 6.2). The most important points of entry for agents are via ingestion and inhalation. Less commonly, organisms enter through the mucous membranes of the conjunctiva, the urogenital system, and the skin. Some agents never penetrate through the epithelium lining the body's surfaces. Some of these live on epithelial surfaces (e.g., *Giardia* spp. in the intestine), and others such as coccidia enter epithelial cells but do not penetrate more deeply into the body.

Mims et al. (2001) listed four general mechanisms by which agents enter the body.

1. *Agents may have special mechanisms for attaching to and penetrating the body surfaces.* These allow them to adhere to specific molecules, called receptors, in specific host cell membranes. (Receptors were not designed for disease-agent attachment, they serve other functions in the cell.) Some organisms can bind to more than one cell type.
2. *Agents may be introduced through the skin by a biting arthropod or may penetrate directly as is done by some macroparasites such as the hookworms of seals and canids.*
3. *Agents may be unable to penetrate the body surfaces and depend upon some damage to a surface to allow them to enter.* The damage may be a mechanical break in the skin or a mucous membrane, or a bite wound as used by the rabies virus.
4. *Agents may enter when there is a local or generalized defect in the body's defenses.*

Not all disease agents that reach a new host are successful in establishing an infection. The number of agents arriving at a new host usually is quite small and may be inadequate to overcome local defenses. In diseases caused by microparasites, a threshold number of organisms, the "minimum infectious dose," is required to result in infection. Little is known about the minimum infectious dose required for transmission of most diseases of wild animals, but the approximate infectious dose of some agents for humans is known, illustrating the degree of diversity. For example, *Salmonella typhi* = $\leq 10^5$ bacteria, *Shigella dysenteriae* = 10 bacteria, *Giardia lamblia* = 10 cysts, and *Mycobacterium tuberculosis* = 1–10 bacteria (Mims et al. 2001). Limited information about diseases in wild animals indicates similar diversity. About 10^7 *Brucella suis* biovar 4 were required to routinely infect reindeer even when the bacteria were instilled directly on the

animals' conjunctiva (Dieterich et al. 1991), while about 15,000 plague bacilli (*Yersinia pestis*), the number that can be transmitted in a single fleabite, were "more than sufficient" for transmission of that disease (Burroughs 1947, cited in Gaspar and Watson 2001).

The actual dose required to result in infection varies with the species, age, sex, genotype, and general condition of the animal, the particular strain of agent, the route of infection, and many other factors. The effect of any one of these factors can be startling, for example, the dose of foot-and-mouth disease virus required to infect cattle is about 10,000 times greater by the oral than by the respiratory route (Thomson et al. 2001). The need for a minimum or threshold infectious dose has a major impact on disease transmission. For myxoma virus to be transmitted by mosquitoes, infected rabbits must have at least 10^7 viable virus particles per gram of skin. If less virus is present in the skin, mosquitoes' mouthparts are not sufficiently contaminated with virus to transmit the diseases (Kerr and Best 1998). In infections caused by macroparasites, the minimum infectious dose is usually not determined, but only a portion of the infective stages that reach a host are successful in establishing an infection. For instance, <1% of *Echinococcus granulosus* eggs given orally to sheep develop to the larval stage, and <5% of larval protoscolices of *E. granulosus* from sheep result in infection when fed to dogs (Gemmell et al. 1986).

In general, the more agents that infect a host the greater the effect on the host. This is most evident in infections caused by macroparasites in which there is no replication in the host (i.e., one egg or larva only results in a single worm). In infections caused by microparasites, even a single virus particle or bacterium that becomes established can potentially result in a huge number of offspring. Less attention has been paid to the initial number of infecting microparasites, because this was thought to have little effect on the ultimate number of offspring that infect the host. It was believed that the organisms reached a certain density or "carrying capacity" regardless of the infecting dose. However, larger infecting doses are associated with a shorter clinical course and with more severe pathologic effects in many diseases, perhaps because the carrying capacity is reached more rapidly. In an experimental system where dose and effects could be measured precisely, larger infective doses of a bacterium and a fungus reduced fecundity and survival of the host *Daphnia magna* and also reduced the production of transmission stages by the agents (Ebert et al. 2000b). At very high infective doses of the fungus, the hosts died before any transmission stages were produced.

Much of what is known about the pathogenesis of disease has been obtained through experimental infections. Many such infections were transmitted by unusual means, entered the animal by unnatural routes, and involved doses that likely had little relation to natural infections. Caution must be used in extrapolating from such data to nature as the results may be very different from those resulting from natural transmission.

ESTABLISHMENT AND PERPETUATION OF DISEASE

The pattern that disease takes within a population depends upon the course of infection in the individual animal, the mode of transmission, and characteristics of the host population (demography and social structure) (Nokes 1992). I have discussed qualitative aspects of transmission to this point. Now we will make a limited foray into quantitative features that affect whether or not disease will become established in a population and if it will persist. I will use the analogy of a forest fire, because of similarities in behavior of fire and infectious disease in some circumstances.

Establishment and persistence of both disease and fire depend on the reproductive success of the agent. In disease this is expressed as R_0, the basic reproductive rate (also called the basic reproductive number or ratio), a term equivalent to the intrinsic rate of increase (r) in population models. R_0 is not a constant for a particular disease agent. It is determined by features of both the agent and the host population, and is defined differently for microparasites than for macroparasites. The basic requirement for establishment and persistence of any infectious disease in a population is that infected individuals must *on average* pass the infection on to at least one susceptible individual (i.e., R_0 must ≥1). If R_0 is <1, each succeeding generation of transmission will involve fewer individuals and the infection will fade out to extinction. Conversely, *"if each infected individual on average causes more than one new infection, a chain reaction will ensue"* (Heesterbeek and Roberts 1995), and the disease will become more prevalent.

For microparasites, R_0 is defined as the average number of secondary infections that arise from introduction of one infected individual into a totally susceptible population. This is analogous to the number of trees to which fire spreads from a single

tree ignited by lightning. Many mathematical formulae have been proposed to describe R_0 in different situations, including that

$$R_0 = ßX /(a + b + σ)$$

where ß = probability of transmission between susceptible and infectious host animals, X = host density, a = disease-induced mortality rate, b = mortality rate of uninfected hosts , and σ = rate of recovery from infection (Anderson and May 1986; Anderson 1991). In this and other models, the rate of transmission is influenced by the frequency of contact between infectious and susceptible individuals, the proportion of contacts that result in infection, host density and population size, and the rate at which animals recover (or die). For detailed discussion of modeling of disease transmission, see Grenfell and Dobson (1995) and Hudson et al. (2001).

Imagine two pine forests: forest A has few, widely dispersed trees; forest B has densely packed trees. Each tree in A or B could potentially burn (all are susceptible). But if lightning were to strike a single tree in each forest, we would expect that the rate of spread (equivalent to R_0) would be different, although the agent (fire) and the species affected (pine) are the same in each forest. The difference in rate is related to fuel-load (density of susceptibles) and the likelihood of transfer from a burning tree to a susceptible one ("transmission"). In forest A, the fire might burn locally and then die out, while in forest B it might become a raging wildfire. Similarly, we know that when disease is introduced, it may sputter and go out or it may become an epizootic. (While outbreaks may be recognized, we have no way of knowing how frequently diseases that are introduced into wild populations fail to establish.)

Because population size/density seems to be important, most models of disease assume that a population threshold exists below which R_0 is <1 and the disease will eventually disappear. However, as noted by Begon et al. (2003), "empirical evidence for thresholds of any sort has been rare." The subject is complex, and it is not clear if the same threshold applies for invasion of a disease as for its persistence and whether it is host density or total population size that is the critical feature. The nature of the relationship between host population size/density and the frequency with which contacts occur is unknown for most diseases in wild animals. Swinton et al. (2001) suggested that increased host population size or density will increase *per capita* contact rates under two circumstances:

1. *When individuals contact conspecifics within a given "socio-spatial arena" and crowding increases the number of individuals in that arena.* This might apply to transmission of avian cholera among waterfowl crowded onto refuge areas by habitat loss and to transmission of brucellosis among elk and tuberculosis among deer concentrated by artificial feeding.
2. *If social structure allows contact with most of the population during the lifetime of the disease.* Swinton et al. (2001) suggested that this might apply to morbillivirus infection among seal populations that regroup daily on haulout areas.

Threshold population density is unknown for most diseases in wild animals although it has been estimated in a few situations. About 1 fox/km^2 was thought to be required for rabies to become established in some areas of Europe (Anderson et al. 1981), and about 6.5 mountain hares/km^2 were thought to be required to maintain louping-ill virus in Scottish Highland areas (Gilbert et al. 2001). Packer et al. (1999) estimated that about 75 to 200 lions in the Serengeti area were sufficient to allow calicivirus and parvovirus infections to occur. It is important to realize that R_0 and threshold population size/density are likely to be highly site and situation specific, so that values such as these are not transferable (i.e., more or less than 1 fox/km^2 may be required to maintain rabies in areas other than those parts of Europe modeled by Anderson et al. (1981).

In diseases caused by microparasites, the host population is composed of susceptible, infected, and recovered individuals. The latter are usually immune to reinfection. The course of disease within an individual animal is a progression through these states:

Susceptible → Infected → Recovered and resistant

with an alternate outcome, death, if the disease is highly virulent. The infected stage can be subdivided into an initial period in which the animal is not capable of transmitting the disease agent and an infectious period during which transmission can occur. Duration of the infected and recovered stages is highly variable among diseases. For example, in canine distemper, the animal may be infected for 1–2 weeks and infectious for only a few days. If it survives, it is resistant to reinfection for the remainder of its life. By contrast, a tuberculous deer may be infected for months or years, infectious for some part of that period, and likely never recovers.

When fire sweeps through a forest, the available fuel is consumed, the fire "burns itself out," and we do not expect another fire until new fuel accumulates. Similarly, when disease occurs in a population, the susceptible individuals are "used up" (by death if the agent is highly virulent or by recovery and development of immunity).

Figure 8.5 illustrates the course of a disease, caused by an agent that spreads rapidly and in which the infectious period is brief, in a naive population. Initially, almost every contact by the few infectious individuals is with a susceptible animal, R_0 is maximal, and the number of infected individuals rises rapidly. As the susceptibles are used up, progressively fewer of the contacts by infectious animals are with susceptible animals, and both the reproductive rate of the disease and the number of infected individuals decline. Eventually, there are insufficient susceptibles left to maintain transmission, and the disease fades out in the same manner that a fire burns itself out without adequate fuel. The resulting epizootic curve (fig. 8.5) of the number of infected animals is typical of diseases maintained by transmission from host to host at short intervals ("short cycle," Matumoto 1969).

Diseases caused by microparasites, in which hosts are infectious for only a short period of time and then develop lifelong immunity, tend to have cyclic behavior (Dobson and Hudson 1995). Good examples are morbillivirus infections, including phocine morbillivirus among seals (Kennedy 2001) and canine distemper in dogs in isolated communities in northern Canada (Leighton et al. 1988), raccoons in New Jersey (Roscoe 1993), lions in the Serengeti (Packer et al. 1999), and a mixed carnivore community on the prairies of western North America (Williams 2001). In epizootics of these diseases, the entire course occurs over a period of weeks, and there is no time for replacement of susceptibles through recruitment or immigration. The pattern of disease is sporadic (i.e., the causative virus is introduced periodically), sweeps through the population, fades out, and does not return for a period of years until a new susceptible population has developed. Many other diseases caused by microparasites do not follow this dramatic boom or bust pattern for reasons that will be discussed later.

R_0 for macroparasites is defined as the average number of female offspring that live to reproduce produced by a single female introduced into a completely susceptible population, or "the number of 'next generation' adult parasites that would arise from one adult parasite in a totally susceptible population" (Roberts et al. 1995). Unfortunately, neither the simple SIR model that illustrates the course of

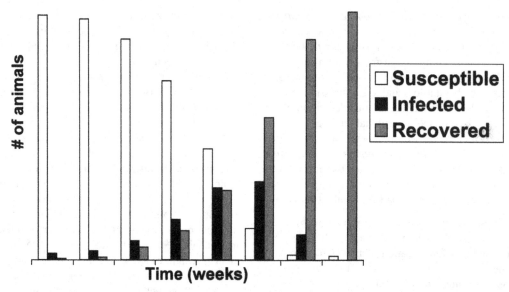

Fig. 8.5. Graphical representation of the course of a hypothetical disease outbreak in which an infectious agent was introduced into a totally susceptible population of two hundred animals. The agent was highly transmissible but of low virulence. For this model, R_0 was 2.5 in the fully susceptible population and the effective reproductive number (R_e) declined as the proportion of susceptible animals in the population decreased. Each infected animal recovered after 2 weeks and became resistant to reinfection. Contact was assumed to occur randomly among all members of the population. The number of infected individuals each week represents the "epizootic curve" for the disease.

microparasite infection nor the forest fire analogy are appropriate for describing disease caused by macroparasites. In infections by macroparasites, some individuals may be infected more than once and accumulate parasites during their lifetime (i.e., they are both susceptible and infected); recovered individuals may recycle to the susceptible pool; and resistance is relative, often transient, and may be dependent upon the presence of a current infection (i.e., an individual may be both infected and resistant). An important feature of infections caused by macroparasites is that infected individuals cannot be treated as a homogenous group because a small proportion of the infected individuals carry most of the parasites (fig. 3.6) and are responsible for most of the transmission. Many aspects of transmission are related to the intensity of infection, including the immune response by the host and the fecundity and survival of individual parasites. For these and other reasons, such as the common involvement of extra hosts and features such as arrested development of larvae, modeling of macroparasitic transmission is very complex. In comparison with microparasites, macroparasites have "more sluggish dynamics, but are less susceptible to fade-out (local extinction). This may be a consequence of the many adaptations

that allow helminth and arthropod larval stages to live for long periods of time in a dormant state; or, it may be a consequence of the complex multi-host life cycles that have evolved to allow parasites to use different host species at different times of year, or in different parts of their hosts' habitat" (Hudson and Dobson 1995).

Most infectious diseases do not fade to extinction. This raises the question as to how diseases such as canine and phocine morbillivirus infections that are self-limiting in local areas avoid disappearing completely. Detailed studies of measles (also caused by a morbillivirus) in humans indicate that two factors are involved in persistence of this type of disease (Bolker and Grenfell 1995; Finkenstädt and Grenfell 1998; Finkenstädt et al. 1998):

1. In very large populations, the disease may persist through the "epidemic trough" that follows outbreaks, because sufficient susceptible individuals remain to maintain the disease at a low level. The minimum size of a closed population within which a pathogen can persist indefinitely is estimated to be ~300,000 to 500,000 humans for measles (Black 1966). Bartlett (1960) calls this the "critical community size (CCS)."

2. The entire host population is not affected simultaneously. Although the disease may fade out in a local area, it can be reintroduced later from other portions of the metapopulation. [A metapopulation is "a set of spatially disjunct populations, among which there is some immigration" (Wells and Richmond 1995)]. This has been described in yellow fever among wild primates as "wandering epidemics moving through the population over a large area" (Yuill and Seymour 2001). (Bryant et al. [2003] found that yellow fever in an area of the Peruvian Andes appeared to be locally maintained and circulated continuously.)

Both factors may apply to canine distemper. The virus infects many species so that the combined number of susceptible canids (dogs, wolves, coyotes, foxes), mustelids (skunks, badgers, weasels, mink, otter, marten, fisher), and raccoons in western Canada where I live may form a sufficiently large community to support the disease, and the disease may occur asynchronously in different species. Tompkins et al. (2001a) suggested that the CCS required to allow phocine morbillivirus to persist in North Sea harbor seals was "several orders of magnitude greater than the known world population size" and used this as evidence that the disease was likely introduced from some other species to cause an outbreak in 1988. Swinton et al. (2001) suggested that if there is a CCS for phocine morbillivirus, it will be >50,000 individuals. Epizootic phocine morbillivirus infection reoccurred in northern Europe in 2002 after an absence of at least 10 years and at a time when almost the entire seal population was again susceptible (Jensen et al. 2002; Müller et al. 2004).

The size of population required for persistence of most diseases in wild animals is unknown, but we may be able to make some predictions (derived in part from Matumoto 1969):

* *Diseases with a short length of time from infection to the cessation of infectiousness require frequent transmission to the next host and a large CCS.* For instance, the CCS for persistence of measles is about 500 times that required for varicella (a chronic infection), which can be maintained in ~1000 humans (Black 1966). On this basis, we can predict that rabies (long latent period) and tuberculosis (extended infectious period) will require a smaller CCS for persistence than canine distemper.

* *A smaller CCS will be required for persistence of diseases in species with a rapid population turnover because of more rapid replacement of susceptible individuals.* (Thus, a smaller population size might be required to allow a disease to persist in rodents than in elephants.) However, this may not apply in diseases maintained in chronically infected animals. For example, Sin Nombre virus occurred much less frequently in a population of deer mice with a very rapid turnover than in a stable population (Calisher et al. 2001).

* *A smaller CCS will be required for persistence of diseases that have resistant stages that can survive in the external environment or in some alternate host for extended periods.* This is exemplified by tapeworm species that persist in carnivore populations composed of small numbers of widely dispersed individuals with infrequent contact. Parasites such as *Echinococcus granulosus* can persist in small, dispersed populations of wolves because much of the lifespan of the parasite is spent in the long-lived larval form in a caribou or moose. *Bacillus anthracis* can persist in areas with low animal populations (and without infecting any animals for years) because its spores are highly resistant.

Reduction of population size and/or density has been a common method suggested for management of many diseases of wild animals, with mixed results. Assumptions that "killing half the wildlife population will halve the risk of infection" are simplistic and fail to take into account many features that affect disease transmission (Swinton et al. 2001). For instance, reducing the overall size of a population may not reduce average group size or social interactions (McCarty and Miller 1998), and social perturbations as a result of culling may promote transmission (Swinton et al. 1997; Donnelly et al. 2003).

A number of mechanisms have been identified by which infectious diseases may persist, even though few susceptibles are present in the population (table 8.6). Many of these involve persistence of the agent outside the host population in a "reservoir." If more than one species are involved in a disease, one host is often designated the reservoir, and the other is the susceptible or, perhaps appropriately, the target species. Haydon et al. (2002) stressed the need for strict definition of the term "reservoir" and proposed that it be used for "one or more epidemiologically connected populations or environments in which the pathogen can be permanently maintained and from which infection is transmitted to the defined target population." This definition includes abiotic elements of the environment as reservoirs. Haydon et al. (2002) described methods that can be used to confirm the existence and identity of a reservoir, and Laurenson et al. (2003) used these to identify the mountain hare as a reservoir of louping-ill virus. The most important reservoirs for infectious disease are animal species other than the target species.

The majority of important diseases of wild animals has multiple hosts, and >81% of the animal diseases of greatest importance internationally infect multiple hosts (Cleaveland et al. 2001). Population dynamics of multihost conditions are complex, and only two features will be discussed here.

1. Host-specific diseases (diseases with only one host) are likely to fade out in very small populations because of the lack of sufficient susceptibles as fuel for maintenance. This has practical significance in conservation biology because one-host diseases are unlikely to drive a host species to extinction—the disease will probably fade out before the host species. In contrast, a multihost disease can have a severe effect on a small population if the disease is maintained in some other more numerous species. The best-known example of this phenomenon is the very close brush with extinction by the black-footed ferret as a result of canine distemper virus circulating in other more numerous hosts (Williams et al. 1988).
2. A host-specific agent should not be too virulent if this jeopardizes its own transmission and persistence. Multihost agents are not limited by this constraint in all hosts. The effect of high virulence in one species may be unimportant to perpetuation of the disease agent. This is probably the case in many situations of coincidental virulence discussed in chapter 5, such as *Parelaphostrongylus tenuis* infection in ungulates other than white-tailed deer. This nematode is dependent upon white-tailed deer, in which it is essentially avirulent, for its persistence. The coincidental death of the occasional moose or caribou has no significant effect on the parasite because these hosts represent a dead end. The intestinal nematode *Heterakis gallinae* is maintained in pheasants and cannot be maintained in grey partridge, but it is believed to be one cause of the decline of the grey partridge in the United Kingdom (Tompkins et al. 2000).

In trying to understand the dynamics of multihost diseases, it is necessary to differentiate between interspecific transmission and intraspecific transmission. Caley and Hone (2004) used a combination of modeling and experimental population manipulation to dissect the transmission of *Mycobacterium bovis* in brushtail possums and feral ferrets in New Zealand and showed that controlling possum populations was the first step in managing tuberculosis in ferrets. I will end this section with words of wisdom from Caughley and Sinclair (1994): "Transpecifics are the parasites and pathogens to watch out for."

SUMMARY

- Host animals are like islands of habitat. To persist as a species, disease agents have to cross a generally inhospitable external environment and colonize other islands.
- Most disease agents exit the host in secretions and excretions from a body surface.

Table 8.6 Mechanisms That Allow for Prolonged Persistence of Disease Agents

Mechanism for persistence	Diseases in which mechanism is operative
Very extended infectious period (months to years)	Tuberculosis, paratuberculosis, feline immunodeficiency virus, many macroparasites
Existence of a "carrier" state in which recovered individuals continue to shed infectious material	Duck plague
Extended latent period	Rabies (average 1–3 months between infection and clinical disease)
Long-lived, resistant stages that persist in the external environment	Anthrax, canine hepatitis virus, avian botulism, many macroparasites
Existence in alternate hosts in which the agent may be long-lived	*Echinococcus* spp., many other helminths

- Vertical transmission (from parent to offspring) may occur in many diseases but is uncommon as an ecologically important method of transmission in wild animals.
- Pseudovertical transmission (passage of agents to neonates shortly after birth or hatching) is an uncommon route of transmission.
- Horizontal transmission (transfer of infection from one animal to other individuals, independent of their parental relationship) is the most common form of transmission and takes many forms.
- Direct transmission includes any situation in which infection passes from one individual to another without the requirement for involvement of another species.
- Indirect transmission includes those situations in which transmission requires the involvement of at least two species.
- Not all agents that reach a new host are successful in establishing an infection. In general, the more agents that reach the host the greater the likelihood of becoming established and the greater the effect on the host. The minimum infective dose required for infection is not known for most diseases of wild animals.
- Much of what is known about the effects of some diseases is based on experimental infections that involved unusual routes of transmission and large infective doses.
- For an infectious disease to persist, infected individuals must on average pass the infection to at least one other individual in the population.
- Host population size and density are very important in disease transmission and persistence, but the precise relationship is undefined for most diseases and likely to be highly site and situation specific.
- Many diseases are able to persist in small populations with few susceptible animals through involvement of reservoirs (abiotic and other animal species).

9
Noninfectious Disease: Nutrients and Toxicants

"Noninfectious disease" is a catchall term for a wide variety of dysfunctions caused by agents or factors other than living organisms that live in or on the animals that are affected. The range of conditions that fall into this category was introduced briefly in chapter 3. Two particular subjects, nutritional diseases and disease caused by poisonous substances, deserve further attention because of their importance in wild animals.

Nutrition is important because it may be a direct limiting factor for wild populations and because what animals are eating may interact in many different ways with other disease agents. Surprisingly, nutrition has received relatively little attention in the discussion of disease in wild animals. Toxicants are important because they are widespread in the environment and because wild animals frequently carry residues in their tissues that may or may not be harmful. I noted earlier that those who study disease in wild animals usually specialize in either infectious diseases or toxicology (the study of poisonous substances), and often there is little interchange or exchange of ideas between the two groups. This does not reflect the real-life situation in which wild animals are exposed to both types of disease simultaneously. For example, while I was writing the first draft of this chapter, we were investigating a die-off among wintering crows. Early in the investigation we had to consider viral and bacterial infections, for which there was some evidence, as well as poisoning by cholinesterase-inhibiting insecticides and road salt. We also had to consider the nutritional state of the crows and how it might influence their exposure and susceptibility to both infectious and noninfectious agents.

NUTRITIONAL INTERACTIONS

At various places in this book, I have stressed the importance of nutrition in disease. I believe that it is one of the most important environmental variables that influence the course and outcome of disease in wild animals. In considering nutrition here, I will begin by identifying the components that make up nutrition and then discuss general food availability and deficiencies of particular substances.

At a basic level, nutrients include energy, proteins, water, and certain essential substances such as vitamins, minerals, and fatty acids. Each species has its own specific requirements. For example, ruminants can produce B vitamins in their digestive tracts, but animals with a simple stomach such as carnivores cannot and are dependent upon obtaining these vitamins from their diet. Relatively little is known about the requirement of most wild species for either macroelements such as calcium, phosphorus, sodium, magnesium, chloride, and sulfur or trace elements including zinc, manganese, copper, iodine, and selenium. Robbins (1993) is the most complete source available on nutrition in wild animals.

Malnutrition is a complex subject because it may involve an overall shortage of food, a deficiency of one or more specific elements, or an inappropriate balance among nutrients. Much of the information available related to nutrition of wild animals is concerned with energy. Deficiency of energy is often coupled with a shortage of protein. In humans the term "protein-energy malnutrition" (PEM) is used, and it also is likely appropriate in many situations in wild animals. PEM may result from either inadequate quantity or inadequate quality of food.

Most wild species experience some point in the year when nutrient intake is marginal or less than required for maintenance. This seasonal nature of deficiency increases the difficulty in interpreting the role of nutrition, because nutrition may be adequate or more than adequate except during these critical periods. When malnutrition occurs during the year is variable in different ecosystems. In temperate areas,

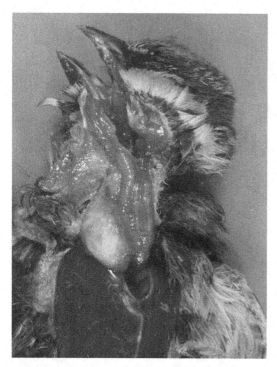

Fig. 9.1. House sparrow that died of salmonellosis *(Salmonella typhimurium* infection). Outbreaks of this disease occur in winter about backyard bird feeders and affected birds often have extensive necrosis of the crop wall as seen in this bird.

winter survival is a major fitness factor for many wild species, and in arid areas nutritional limitation may occur during the dry season. Species deal with periodic food shortage in a variety of ways that are at least partially determined by the ability to store reserves. For example, some small passerine birds must feed and store fat each day to be able to survive through the next winter night. At the opposite extreme are species such as lesser snow geese that accumulate sufficient fat during spring migration so that they may not need to feed during nest establishment, egg-laying, and incubation. The ability to withstand periodic food shortage can have a direct effect on the outcome of other diseases. Because small passerine birds such as common redpolls or house sparrows cannot survive for more than a day or two without feeding, any infection such as with *Salmonella typhimurium* (fig. 9.1), which debilitates them even temporarily so that they do not feed, may be a death sentence in winter (even without counting the increased energetic cost of fever and defenses mobilized against the infectious agent).

Fat storage represents a trade-off situation be-

cause the energy could have been used for other purposes and because storing fat has costs. The costs of storing fat in birds include increased risk of predation while feeding, reduced agility, and increased costs of flight. These are balanced against improved ability to withstand periods of resource shortage. Bird species with predictable food availability tend to store less reserves than species with unpredictable food sources (Rogers and Smith 1993).

Food availability may interact with other disease and mortality factors in several ways. For example, as food becomes less available, animals may increase feeding effort to avoid starvation at the expense of increased mortality from predation (Rogers and Smith 1993). Animals "with a high level of feeding motivation" may risk acquiring more parasites by reduced parasite avoidance behavior (Hutchings et al. 1999). Figure 9.2 illustrates some interactions that occur among malnutrition, host defenses, and infection as proposed by Keusch (1993). I have modified the diagram to show how these factors are linked to some other components of disease. In the diagram, malnutrition is used in the most general sense as faulty or inadequate nutrition. This might represent a lack of some particular nutrient or an overall lack of nutrients required to meet the demands of the animal (including those related to one or more disease agents). This depiction of the effect of malnutrition is concerned only with resistance to disease, and it does not capture the effect that malnutrition may have on exposure to disease (e.g., Hutchings et al. 1999) or the effect that malnutrition may have on reproductive success, both of which may be substantial.

Ezenwa (2003) studied the interactions among nutritional status and gastrointestinal nematode infection in African wild bovids under drought and nondrought conditions. During a drought year, six of the nine host species studied had increased fecal output of parasite eggs. The species that had the greatest increase in parasite egg output were those with the lowest quality diet (in terms of protein content). It was suggested that "as food resources declined from the drought it is probable that nutrient/protein deficient animals, mostly the low quality feeders, experienced a breakdown in immune function" and that synergy between the effects of malnutrition and parasitism might be important in population regulation in some African bovids. The relationship between infectious agents and host nutrition may be complex. In an experimental system in which mosquitoes were the host and protozoa were the parasite, Bedhomme et al. (2004) found

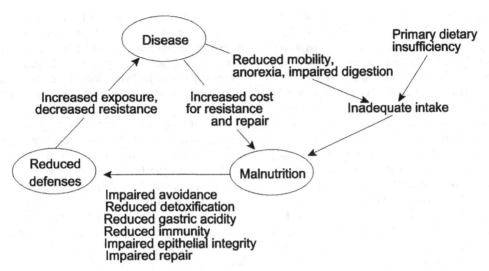

Fig. 9.2. Interactions among disease, malnutrition, and host defenses. Malnutrition may be primary, as a result of habitat conditions, or it may be secondary to the effects of disease, but the result is impairment of host defenses, with the likelihood of further disease. (Adapted from Keusch 1993)

that the virulence of the parasite was strongly related to the nutritional state of the host. At very low levels of nutrition, the parasite had no ability to express virulence (because the host animals could not develop), and at high levels of nutrition, the parasite had no effect (because of complete compensation). Virulence was only evident at intermediate levels of nutrition in this experimental system.

The ultimate state of malnutrition is one that results in death of the animal. Starvation as a result of food shortage occurs relatively commonly in some wild animals, but starvation represents only the extreme of a continuum in which lesser degrees of malnutrition reduce growth, reproduction, and general fitness. These sublethal effects are easily overlooked.

Diseases caused by deficiency of specific macroelements or micronutrients are well documented in humans and domestic animals but rarely are described in wild animals (Robbins 1993). One explanation for this might be that wild animals do not suffer such deficiencies. Fielder (1986) expressed the view that native species should have adapted to the local availability of nutrients such as minerals and so should not suffer deficiency. An alternate explanation for the lack of reports of specific nutritional deficiencies in wild animals might be that deficiencies occur but go undetected. Identification of a specific nutritional deficiency is difficult, even in domestic animals in which the exact diet is known and animals can be observed closely, because the clini-

cal features of deficiency often are subtle. Identification of a deficiency state in wild animals is even more complicated because the diet is known only in general terms, the animals are difficult to observe and follow through time, deficiencies tend to involve individual animals rather than groups, and the conditions tend to be chronic so that debilitated animals are likely to be removed by predators.

I will cite four examples of deficiency leading to disease in wild animals to demonstrate that deficiency states do occur and that these often relate to recent, human-induced habitat changes.

Example 1: Deficiency of calcium (discussed in chapter 3) appears to be affecting reproduction of some passerine birds, particularly in parts of Europe. This seems to be a result of environmental acidification reducing snail populations and, hence, the availability of calcium-rich materials for birds.

Example 2: Nutritional bone disease that resembled rickets occurred in African vulture chicks (Mundy and Ledger 1976). The underlying problem was that the large carnivores (lions, hyenas) that broke bones into portions small enough to be ingested by the vultures had been removed from the ecosystem so that the vultures did not have access to small bone chips as a source of calcium.

Example 3: Vitamin deficiency occurs in wild ducks in Saskatchewan. We have recognized vitamin A deficiency in mallards overwintering on open water below a hydroelectric dam. The birds were far to the north of their normal winter range and had fed exclusively for several months on cereal grains that contained almost no ß-carotene (Honour et al. 1995). Vitamin A deficiency has been associated with "increased susceptibility, severity and duration of infection" in a variety of species (Sijtsma et al. 1990). Some of the ducks with lesions of vitamin A deficiency died with generalized staphylococcal infection (Wobeser and Kost 1992), a disease that we have not seen elsewhere in wild ducks.

Example 4: Selenium deficiency occurred in wild black-tailed deer in an area of California. Flueck (1994) suspected that subclinical selenium deficiency might be affecting reproduction, and many deer that were sampled had less selenium in their blood than would be considered marginal for domestic sheep. Deficiency was confirmed by supplementation of does with selenium with remarkable effects on reproduction. Preweaning survival of fawns increased from 0.32 fawns/doe prior to supplementation to 0.83 fawns/doe after supplementation. Flueck (1994) proposed that selenium deficiency was limiting reproduction in the population and that selenium cycling and bioavailability had been altered by human activities.

These examples suggest that although Fielder (1986) may have been correct in the assertion that wild animals should have adapted to the level of nutrients available in their natural environment, wild animals may experience various types of deficiency when that environment is altered. Altered habitat also may be associated with other types of nutritional problems, including excessive availability of nutrients. We have diagnosed a condition called rumen overload or carbohydrate engorgement in deer, pronghorns, and moose in Saskatchewan that is related to use of unnatural foods. Affected animals had ingested a large amount of readily fermented carbohydrate in the form of cereal grain. The resulting rapid fermentation in the rumen produced a large amount of lactic acid that resulted in fatal systemic acidosis and dehydration (Wobeser and Runge 1975).

ASSESSING NUTRITIONAL CONDITION

Assessing the nutritional condition of individual animals is usually based on the amount of fat present, although lean body protein mass is also important.

In dead animals, the amount of fat in the bone marrow often is used as a measure of nutrient reserves. Because bone marrow fat is one of the last reserves to be utilized, lack of marrow fat indicates severe nutritional stress. In living animals, relative nutritional condition often is assessed using some type of condition index (i.e., the ratio of mass to some measure of body size, such as total length or wing length). Judging whether an animal's body condition is "normal" or "adequate" requires a good understanding of the biology of the species and of what is appropriate for the specific time and place where the animal is examined. This is particularly true for many species of wild birds that experience large physiologic fluctuations in body condition over a short period of time. For example, migrating bar-tailed godwits make a 1 month refueling stop in the Wadden Sea while migrating north. When they arrive in this area, fat makes up 5–10% of the body mass, and when they leave, fat makes up 25–30% of the body mass (Landys-Ciannelli et al. 2003). Both of these values are normal for the species (at different times of year), but simply measuring the condition without understanding the birds' schedule could lead to an inappropriate conclusion. Eared grebes make even more dramatic changes in body condition, doubling their mass on staging lakes by adding huge amounts of fat while their flight muscles atrophy (Rattner and Jehl 1997).

Assessing the nutritional condition of a population of animals may be difficult. Caughley and Sinclair (1994) suggested that samples of live animals taken from the population may be poor indicators of the nutritional state of the population, because the sample is likely to be biased toward healthy individuals. Those in poor condition are less likely to be sampled, and the segment of the population most susceptible to density-dependent restrictions in food supply is probably relatively small. In this regard, malnutrition may have population features similar to macroparasite infection, in which a small proportion of the population carries most of the parasites and suffers most of the harm. In human populations, severe malnutrition and parasitism tend to occur in the same individuals (Bundy and Golden 1987). This also may be true in wild animals, although I am not aware of a study that has examined the overall distribution of body condition and parasitism in a population.

Death as a result of starvation may not be a good indicator of the overall effect of malnutrition on the population. In some species, some animals will die of starvation (loss of body condition to a point at which the body cannot recover) during critical times of the year. Mass starvation is uncommon except in situations where a food supply disappears, such as in catastrophic die-offs of seabirds, or becomes unavailable for an extended period, such as under deep snow. Often there are complex interactions among factors so that the proximate cause of death of malnourished animals is predation, accident, or infection, and the effects of malnutrition on survival and/or reproduction are obscured. Baker et al. (2004) described a situation in which a population of red knots has declined dramatically in association with food shortage during a refueling stop because of overfishing of horseshoe crabs, on whose eggs the knots depend. The birds were unable to accumulate sufficient resources for migration and breeding. Although recruitment of young birds declined by 47% and survival of adults decreased by 37%, there was no mass starvation, and the dramatic population effect would not have been evident without a long-term monitoring program.

The effects of malnutrition are not distributed evenly throughout a population. Access to nutrients may be limited by intraspecific competition or territoriality, and certain sex and age groups are affected most severely. Reid et al. (2003) suggested that individuals may have to make different life history allocations because of differing ability to acquire and utilize resources. During a study of winter mortality of white-tailed deer, we found that death as a result of starvation was limited almost entirely to young-of-the-year (fawns) and older males. Fawns are vulnerable because their small body size results in increased difficulty moving in snow and proportionately higher heat loss compared to larger animals, and because they enter the winter with limited fat stores and are inexperienced in finding food. Older males are vulnerable because they enter the winter in poor body condition because of the rut.

FASTING AND DISEASE

An area that has received little attention is the interaction between disease agents and nutrition in those species that undergo prolonged fasting, either because food is not available (e.g., Antarctic penguins, polar bears, and some nesting Arctic birds) or because of voluntary fasting while food is available (e.g., rutting male deer). The physiologic events during fasting are well known (Le Maho 1983), including the occurrence of three phases in protein utilization (phase I: reduced; phase II: maintained at low level; phase III: increased—protein no longer spared), but interactions with disease resistance are largely unknown. An intriguing study by Hanssen et al. (2004) suggested that immunosuppression may be adaptive in severely malnourished animals, particularly if exposure to disease is infrequent at the time, as might occur in animals that are not taking in agents with food and are relatively isolated, such as a hibernating bear or a bird sitting on its nest.

The most convincing evidence that a nutritional deficiency is occurring in a wild population comes from demonstrating a positive response by the population to supplementation, as has been done for selenium deficiency by Flueck (1994) and calcium deficiency by Graveland and Drent (1997).

POISONOUS AND TOXIC COMPOUNDS

Discussion of poisonous compounds follows naturally from that of nutrition because many elements that are harmless or even required nutrients at low concentrations, including common salt, selenium, phosphorus, copper, zinc, and vitamins A and D, are poisonous at higher concentrations. The study of poisonous substances has its own vocabulary, and the word usage is somewhat confusing. The basic term is "poison." A poison is a substance that impairs or destroys cellular function, sometimes to the point of causing death. *Toxicity* is the state of being poisonous, and *toxic* is synonymous with poisonous (i.e., a toxic substance impairs or destroys cellular function). An animal that is showing evidence of poisoning can be said to be *intoxicated*. Substances that are poisonous (i.e., that produce cellular dysfunction) also are referred to as "toxicants," and that is the general term that I will use here. Purists refer to poisonous substances produced by living organisms (plants, fungi, algae, bacteria, and some animals) as *toxins*, and differentiate these from naturally occurring poisonous substances such as lead, mercury, and cadmium, and from artificially produced poisonous chemicals such as pesticides and rodenticides. The word "xenobiotic" (from Greek *xenos*, stranger, and *bios*, life) is used in some toxicological literature, and refers to foreign substances that are not naturally produced within an organism.

GENERAL FEATURES OF TOXICOLOGY

The first step in the interaction between a toxicant and an animal is exposure, as in infectious disease. Although a few toxicants may be inhaled or absorbed through the skin (e.g., when birds are sprayed with insecticide in forest or croplands), the majority of toxicants that affect wild animals are ingested with food or water and enter the body

Table 9.1 Routes by Which Toxicants Reach Wild Animals

Route	Examples
Inhalation	May occur in animals in areas sprayed with insecticides
Absorbed through skin	Some organophosphorus insecticides
In water	Selenium, salt, cyanobacterial and algal toxins
Direct ingestion of particulate toxicant	Lead poisoning of waterfowl, ingestion of pesticide granules, ingestion of road salt granules, ingestion of white phosphorus
Ingestion of vegetation	
Incorporated in plant	Mycotoxins in grain or seeds, selenium, cyanide
Surface contamination	Diazenon in grazing waterfowl, fluoride on plants near smelter
Ingestion of soil or sediment	Lead in mine tailings
Ingestion of invertebrate prey	Type C botulinum toxin in blowfly larvae, domoic acid in shellfish, DDT in earthworms
Ingestion of vertebrate prey	Mercury in fish, organochlorine poisoning of raptors
Through scavenging	Diclofenac in vultures, barbiturates in eagles, lead in condors and eagles, carbamates in raptors scavenging poisoned animals

through the digestive tract. Routes by which toxicants commonly reach wild animals are summarized in table 9.1.

The degree of exposure to any toxicant is determined by the distribution of the toxicant and the animals, the amount of toxicant present, and the proportion of that toxicant that is available to the animals. The distribution of a toxicant may be either localized or diffuse. Localized distribution of a toxicant is sometimes referred to as coming from a "point-source," such as the effluent from an industry. Toxicants may spread from a point-source by wind or water, and the distribution often is an important feature in identifying the source. Diffuse distribution reflects general availability of the toxicant either because of widespread use or dispersion.

The absolute total amount of elemental poisons such as lead, mercury, and cadmium in the world does not change since they are neither created nor destroyed, but the distribution and the abundance of these elements in a location can be altered dramatically, particularly through human activities. For instance, cadmium is ubiquitous in bedrock and soils at a very low concentration, but it may occur at a much higher concentration downwind from a smelter through deposition of airborne material released during smelting. The amount of natural toxins such as botulinum toxin produced by *Clostridium botulinum* and toxins produced by cyanobacteria and marine dinoflagellates is subject to vast differences in abundance. These toxins are not long-lived in the environment, but their production may be affected by weather and by anthropogenic factors

including nutrient pollution and euthrophication of water, and their distribution is influenced by wind and tides. The amount and distribution of anthropogenic toxicants such as pesticides reflect human usage and transport mechanisms (e.g., wind and water) that move the compounds around the world.

The amount of any toxicant present also is affected by its persistence in the environment. Heavy metals such as lead and mercury are neither created nor destroyed, but their chemical form and availability to animals may change. Most other toxicants break down or decompose and become inactive. The rate at which this occurs under different environmental conditions has a major influence on the likelihood of poisoning occurring. A prominent feature of organochlorine insecticides, such as DDT, is their prolonged environmental persistence. This was a desirable quality for the purpose of having a long residual effect on insect pests, but it had a very undesirable effect on other aspects of the environment. The persistent nature of organochlorine insecticides was a major reason why they were replaced by organophosphate and carbamate insecticides. Many of these alternate pesticides have greater acute toxicity but they break down more rapidly in the environment.

The availability of a toxicant to wild animals involves several features including where it is located, its concentration, and its chemical form. As a simple example, the distribution of lead shotgun pellets in a wetland is determined by where hunters were located and where they pointed their shotguns. If areas of concentrated shot deposition coincide with where birds feed, the shot will be available to birds, but if most of the shot passed across the pond and fell on the opposite shore, few ducks would be exposed. The availability of shot also is determined by the nature of the pond bottom. If the bottom is soft and if there is a high rate of sediment deposition, shot sink into the mud, are covered by new sediment, and become unavailable. Water depth also may limit availability of shot. Many years ago I saw a situation in which lead poisoning occurred in dabbling ducks on a wetland. When the water depth increased, dabbling ducks were seldom affected because they could no longer reach pellets by tipping-up. Pellets could be reached in the deeper water by tundra swans and poisoning of swans continued.

Important features of some toxicants are bioaccumulation and biomagnification. *Bioaccumulation* is a feature of the individual animal and is the result of the rate of intake of the compound exceeding the rate of elimination so that the compound accumulates over time in the animal's body. Cadmium has a long retention time and bioaccumulates in mammals because it is excreted very slowly. In humans, the concentration of cadmium in the kidneys continues to increase to about age 50 (Cooke and Johnson 1996), at which time the rate of elimination and intake are approximately equal and the concentration in the body remains relatively stable. *Biomagnification* (also called bioamplification) refers to an increase in the concentration of a toxicant at each trophic level within a food chain as a result of bioaccumulation in animals at the different levels. The classic example of this phenomenon was the accumulation of successively higher concentrations of pesticides from water → plankton → fish → fish-eating birds reported by Hunt and Bischoff (1960). With toxicants that are biomagnified in this manner, there may be no evidence of toxic effect in animals at lower trophic levels, while top predators such as birds of prey accumulate large concentrations and may be affected severely.

A study of cadmium and copper in badgers in the Netherlands (Klok et al. 2000) provides a good example of bioaccumulation and biomagnification. It also demonstrates the effect of abiotic environmental conditions on the likelihood of poisoning and that a toxicant can have an indirect effect on wild animals. Most soils in the Netherlands contain <1 mg/kg of cadmium, but earthworms can contain 10–200 times as much cadmium as the soil in which they live. The bioaccumulation of cadmium by earthworms is greatly affected by soil pH and is enhanced in acid soils. Earthworms form a substantial portion of the diet of badgers. If even a small proportion of the cadmium in earthworms is absorbed, badgers can potentially accumulate harmful concentrations of cadmium in their kidneys over time. (Cadmium in badgers accumulates because of both bioaccumulation and biomagnification.) Kidney function in mammals is considered to be compromised when the concentration of cadmium in kidney tissue reaches about 200 mg/kg dry weight. Klok et al. (2000) estimated that badgers living in areas with acid soils are at risk of developing kidney lesions within 2–4 years of life, while badgers that live in areas with alkaline soils are unlikely to develop toxic levels of cadmium in their kidneys within their expected life span. (Most badgers in the Netherlands have a life span of <6 years.) Copper acts in a different manner and has an indirect effect on badgers. It is not bioaccumulated by earthworms, but high concentrations of copper, such as occur where copper is added to orchard soils, are toxic for earthworms. There is no biomagnification, and copper toxicity has not been recognized in badgers. However, addition of copper to the soil may have an indirect effect on badgers by limiting the availability of an important food, thereby increasing foraging effort and the probability of being killed in traffic (Klok et al. 2000).

Factors that determine the availability and biomagnification of toxicants may be very localized, and individuals within a species may be exposed to much different toxicant levels, depending on their lifestyle. Bustnes et al. (2000) compared the concentration of five organochlorine compounds in the tissues of glaucous gulls breeding in two colonies on an island in the Barents Sea. One gull colony was located on cliffs at the edge of a seabird (guillemot) colony, the other was 1–2 km from the seabird colony and closer to sea level. The diet of gulls near the guillemot breeding colony contained a much higher proportion of seabird eggs, and these gulls had significantly higher concentrations of all five contaminants in their blood than did gulls from the other colony that fed largely on fish. The conclusion was that gulls in the two colonies occupied different trophic levels and, hence, were subject to different levels of biomagnication. Nygård and Gjerhaug (2001) reported a similar situation in golden eagles in Norway. Eagles from coastal locations had higher residues of organochlorine compounds and lower annual reproductive success than eagles from inland. The coastal birds fed substantially on seabirds, while the inland birds ate grouse, hares, and deer.

Absorption

⇓

Distribution ⇄ Storage

⇓

Biotransformation

⇓

Elimination

Fig. 9.3. The five basic processes by which toxicants interact with living organisms.

With the exception of toxicants that cause local damage at the site of contact, a toxicant only causes injury after it has been absorbed by the organism. Toxicants interact with living organisms through a series of five processes: absorption, distribution, storage, biotransformation, and elimination (fig. 9.3).

Absorption

Absorption involves crossing an epithelial cell barrier in the skin, lung, or digestive tract. This usually is only the first of several cell membranes that a toxicant and its metabolites must cross before the compound finally is eliminated from the body. Cell membranes consist of a biomolecular layer of lipid molecules with proteins scattered throughout the membrane. A toxicant may pass across a cell membrane by one of four mechanisms: passive diffusion, filtration through membrane pores, carrier-mediated transport, or being engulfed by the cell. (The latter two processes are active.) Passive diffusion is the most important route, and most toxicants enter by this method. The rate of passage by diffusion is determined by the concentration gradient and the lipid solubility of the compound. In general, nonpolar, lipid-soluble molecules of low molecular weight diffuse across cell membranes much more readily than do large, polar, water-soluble molecules. The absorption of toxicants is highly variable and is influenced by many variables. For example, only about 5% of ingested cadmium usually is absorbed, but if the animal's diet is low in calcium, protein,

zinc, copper, or iron, a larger proportion may be absorbed (Cooke and Johnson 1996).

Distribution

Once a toxicant is absorbed, it is distributed by the blood or lymph to other tissues. To reach the extracellular fluid and then the interior of cells, the compound must pass through at least two more cell membranes (the blood vessel wall and the target cell wall). The distribution among various tissues is influenced by many factors including the blood flow to the organ, the variation in pore size in the capillary walls (large in the liver, very small in the brain), presence of transport systems in particular cells, and special features that promote storage of compounds in individual cells. So-called barriers may limit the distribution of some toxicants. Water-soluble compounds usually do not pass across the blood-brain barrier or the blood-placenta barrier. Thus, for example, lipid-soluble methyl mercury can cross into the brain and fetus producing severe effects at both sites, but inorganic mercury does not cross either barrier. Because the small intestine is the major site of absorption of most toxicants and all blood flow from the intestine passes through the liver, the liver receives large amounts of toxicants and is frequently injured. Fortunately, the liver has a remarkable ability to repair and regenerate damaged cells.

Storage

Toxicants may be stored, which implies accumulation with no adverse effect. Some toxicants are stored by binding to plasma proteins so that they are held in an inactive form in the blood. Others, such as lead and fluorine, accumulate in the mineral portion of bone where they remain for a very long time.

Examination of lead concentration in bones is a good method for monitoring long-term exposure of animals to lead. Surveys of the lead concentration in wing bones of hunter-killed waterfowl have been used to identify geographic areas with high exposure to lead (Stendall et al. 1979). Lipid soluble compounds such as polychlorinated biphenyls (PCBs) and organochlorine insecticides accumulate in body fat. Storage has several effects. It is protective in that it reduces the amount of active compound available to cause damage, but it also reduces the rate of detoxification and excretion of the compound from the body. Stored material may be released from storage by some physiologic change, as when PCB and insecticides are released from fat in animals suffering food deprivation or starvation, so that the animals can be exposed to high levels of active compound at times when they also are under nutritional stress. Normal annual cycles in organ mass and body composition may complicate the assessment of residues in wild animals: liver mass in eared grebes may vary up to six-fold as a physiologic event (Rattner and Jehl 1997).

Biotransformation

Biotransformation or metabolism of toxicants affects their distribution, excretion, and toxicity. Biotransformation is usually considered to have two phases. Phase I involves degradation of the parent compound through some form of cleavage (oxidation, reduction, hydrolysis). The product that is produced may be less or more toxic than the parent compound. A feature of some toxicants is that they do not cause damage until they have been biotransformed, and it is the metabolic product(s) of biotransformation that cause injury. For example, parathion (an organophosphorus insecticide) is metabolized in the liver to a compound that is a much more potent choline esterase inhibitor than the parent compound. Consideration of the toxicity of DDT (an organochlorine insecticide) for wild animals has to include measurement of the metabolites DDD and DDE that also are toxic (Blus et al. 1996). Because a great deal of biotransformation occurs in the liver, this is a frequent site of injury by metabolic products.

Phase II involves synthesis in which the material (usually a product of phase I metabolism) is added to or conjugated with some endogenous molecule. The product is made more water soluble and, hence, more easily excreted and generally less toxic. Biotransformation involves many different enzymes in many tissues. For example, the cytochrome P-450 enzymes are an important family of enzymes that are involved in the metabolism of lipid-soluble compounds. Their action is to decrease lipid solubility and to increase urinary excretion. Some enzymes have low specificity and may metabolize a variety of compounds. Some enzyme systems have a remarkable ability to increase when required. Measurement of the activity of certain enzymes may be used to detect exposure to certain types of toxicant, for example, the activity of hepatic mixed-function oxidases is often measured as a nonspecific biomarker for exposure to toxicants.

Elimination

The rate of excretion of toxicants is extremely important in determining their effect. Some compounds may be readily metabolized and excreted and never reach toxic concentrations in the body.

Others such as cadmium are excreted so slowly that they accumulate in the body over time until a toxic concentration may be reached. The most important route for excretion of toxicants is via the urine. Metabolism and excretion of toxicants require active and functional organs. Injury to the liver or kidney either by the toxicant or by some other disease process may reduce metabolism and excretion, extending the half-life of toxicants in the body so that they may accumulate to toxic levels. The interaction between organ damage and impaired excretion of toxicants has not been studied extensively in wild animals, but one would expect that injury caused by one toxicant or by an infectious agent could potentially reduce excretion of other toxicants and exacerbate their toxic effect. Thus, for example, one would expect that an animal with considerable liver or kidney injury caused by a parasite might be unusually susceptible to a variety of toxicants.

Harmful Effects of Toxicant

Harmful effects of a toxicant result from biochemical interactions between the toxicant and certain structures of the organism. As with all other forms of disease, the process begins at the cellular or subcellular level and the effect is to impair cellular function or survival. If sufficient cells are affected, then a physiologic function is disrupted creating detectable disease. A few such actions may be nonspecific, and any structure coming in contact with the material may be injured, as occurs with caustic chemicals. This is probably the case for certain mycotoxins (metabolic by-products produced by fungi growing on food stuffs) that cause damage to the lining of the esophagus. We have seen injury to the lining of the esophagus of wild geese that were consuming mycotoxin-laden grain, which resembles injury in mallards experimentally exposed to T-2 mycotoxin (Hayes and Wobeser 1983).

More often the effects are specific and involve interaction with some particular subcellular component or components. These component(s) may be present at many sites in the body or at only one site. Some toxicants interact with a specific chemical grouping such as sulfhydryl or amino groups that are common to many subcellular locations so that the toxicant may interact with a wide variety of cellular components at different sites. Lead inhibits a great variety of enzymes throughout the body and has effects on the function of the nervous system, red blood cell production, liver, and kidneys, among others. When a toxicant interacts at the same subcellular site in different organs, often one particular organ is the first to show evidence of dysfunction and that organ is termed the critical organ. The highest concentration of a toxicant is not necessarily found in the critical organ. For example, methyl mercury has its major effect on the nervous system (the critical organ), but the concentration of mercury in poisoned animals is higher in the kidney and liver than in the brain.

It is beyond the scope of this book to discuss in detail the mechanisms by which various toxicants cause cellular malfunction and disease. Haschek et al. (2002) provide a wealth of information on pathology produced by toxicants. Many toxicants act by interfering with the interaction between enzymes and substrates. The effect may be to cause the enzyme-substrate response to occur (in which case the toxicant is an agonist) or to prevent the effect (the toxicant is an antagonist). Domoic acid, a toxin produced by marine diatoms and concentrated by bivalves and planktivorous fish, is similar structurally to a neuroexcitatory substance and is an agonist. It binds to receptors on neurons causing continuous stimulation and neurological disease in birds such as brown pelicans and in California sea lions (Scholin et al. 2000). A toxicant may form stable substrate-enzyme complexes that inhibit the normal action. Organophosphorus insecticides form a very stable complex with the enzyme acetylcholine esterase, which normally removes acetylcholine from the nerve synapse. Because the enzyme is inhibited, acetylcholine accumulates to toxic levels producing clinical signs resembling excessive stimulation of nerves. Carbamate insecticides also inhibit choline esterase, but the complex is less stable and is reversible.

A toxicant may replace the normal substrate so that an abnormal product is formed. Sodium fluoroacetate (1080), a potent poison that has been used for vertebrate pest control, acts by producing an abnormal product within the citric acid cycle, resulting in a generalized failure of energy metabolism, which is seen first in the nervous system and heart. (These tissues have little or no capacity for anaerobic metabolism so they are more sensitive to lack of oxygen than other tissues.) Some toxicants bind to and destroy enzymes. Injury also may occur as a result of damage to cell membranes, inhibition of coenzymes, and binding to nucleic acids. Various organochlorine insecticides act on nerve fibers by different mechanisms including effects on the sodium channels and disturbing transport of calcium.

Injury from toxicants can result in direct mortality, debilitation that indirectly leads to mortality from other proximate causes, impaired reproduction, occurrence of neoplasia (carcinogenesis), induction of genetic mutations (mutagenesis), or production of anomalies in developing unborn or unhatched animals (teratogenesis).

Unfortunately, there is no comprehensive text that deals with all the toxicants that have been associated with disease in wild animals. I have selected what I consider to be important types of toxicants and will discuss a few examples of each briefly.

TOXINS PRODUCED BY LIVING ORGANISMS

A number of organisms that live in fresh, brackish, and marine water produce toxins associated with disease in wild animals (Solter and Beasley 2002). In most of these, toxicity appears to be coincidental because causing disease in animals does not benefit the organism producing the toxin. For example, toxins produced by cyanobacteria may be of use in competing with other aquatic microorganisms, but killing cows or ducks that happen to drink water containing the toxin is probably of little benefit. Some toxins are harmful on direct exposure, others are ingested with water, and some such as domoic acid may be concentrated by shellfish or fish (Scholin et al. 2000). Botulism is unusual among diseases caused by toxins in that the carcass of victims provides ideal substrate for the growth of the *Clostridium botulinum* and production of further toxin, so that killing animals may be of advantage to the bacterium. Much of the interest in mycotoxins (metabolic by-products produced by various species of fungi) as they relate to wild animals has centered on animals consuming contaminated crops, such as contaminated peanuts (Robinson et al. 1982; Windingstad et al. 1989), but wild foods also may contain these compounds (Oberheu and Dabbert 2001). Some mycotoxins are associated with carcinogenesis (cancer causation) and several may be immunotoxic.

HEAVY METALS

Historically, the metals of most concern have been lead, mercury, cadmium, and selenium. Cadmium and selenium have been discussed elsewhere (cadmium, see above; selenium, see chapter 7). Lead is a systemic poison that affects many enzyme systems, particularly those associated with hemoglobin production. Poisoning is most common in waterbirds that have ingested lead shotgun pellets or fishing weights and in raptors that ingest lead from pellets or bullets in the tissues of animals or birds that they prey on or scavenge (Saito et al. 2000). Lead poisoning may occur from ingestion of sediment containing lead (Beyer et al. 2000) or from paint peeling from buildings (Sileo and Fefer 1987). Lead poisoning usually is a chronic disease. It was estimated that lead poisoning killed 2–3% of the North American waterfowl population each year (Bellrose 1959). Dmowski et al. (2000) analyze the effect of local heavy metal pollution (primarily lead) on populations of small mammals. Populations in polluted areas were small compared to unpolluted areas, the populations contained few young animals because of high juvenile mortality, and the populations often went extinct over winter. The polluted areas were considered to be "sink habitats" unable to sustain stable populations without recolonization from outside.

Mercury enters the environment from both natural (e.g., volcanic eruptions) and anthropogenic sources (coal combustion, chemical processes, incineration, and industrial and domestic waste disposal). It occurs in many chemical forms, but the most significant are organomercurials, particularly methyl mercury compounds. Methyl mercury compounds caused direct poisoning of seed-eating birds and secondary poisoning of raptors in Sweden when the compounds were used as seed-dressing agents. The problem disappeared when the use of the compounds ceased (Wanntorp et al. 1967). Natural methylation of mercury occurs in water resulting in bioaccumulation in aquatic organisms and biomagnification in food chains. This does not result in conspicuous die-offs of animals, but piscivorous wild animals in many areas of the world have elevated residues of mercury in their tissues, and poisoned animals are found periodically (Wobeser and Swift 1976).

Pesticides

"Pesticides are the only toxic chemicals deliberately released into the environment in large amounts," say Galloway and Handy (2003). Two groups of pesticides, insecticides and rodenticides, are particularly important in causing disease in wild animals.

Insecticides

The organochlorine insecticides include a group of compounds that have low solubility in water and high solubility in lipids so that they are stored in fats and tend to bioaccumulate. Included are chemicals such as DDT, aldrin, heptachlor, and dieldrin. Some cause neurological disease and mortality, but they are best known for their effects on reproduction in birds including failure to breed, eggshell thinning, reduced hatching, and reduced survival of young. There are marked differences in susceptibility to these effects among birds, ranging from little or no effect in chickens to profound effects in brown pelicans and some raptors (Blus 1982). These chemicals caused severe population declines in some piscivorous and bird-eating raptors. Newton (1998) suggested that in North America, this was largely an effect of DDT metabolites on reproduction, while in western Europe, mortality from aldrin and dieldrin were more important. Suspension of use of many of these compounds in some countries resulted in improved reproduction of affected species (Newton 1998), but substantial residues still occur in some birds (Nygård and Gjershaug 2001; Gill and Elliot 2003).

Organophosphorus and carbamate insecticides have replaced many organochlorine chemicals. These compounds disappear more rapidly from the environment, but many are much more directly toxic to wild animals than most organochlorine insecticides. Carbofuran, a carbamate, is particularly toxic to birds, and it has been estimated to kill at least two million birds per year in the United States (Mineau 1993). Some of these agents also are used illegally to poison "pest" species such as coyotes in western North America, and we have diagnosed many cases of secondary poisoning of eagles as a result (Wobeser et al. 2004). Walker (2003) reviewed the effects of neurotoxic pesticides on bird behavior.

Rodenticides

Several toxicants have been used to control commensal rodents (rats and mice). The most widely used are anticoagulants, the first of which was warfarin, that interfere with blood clotting. Because of development of resistance to warfarin, new second-generation anticoagulants were introduced. Compounds such as brodifacoum have greater toxicity for rodents and other species, but they are very persistent so that secondary poisoning of raptors and mustelids may occur from eating dead rodents or rodents that survived sublethal poisoning. Eason et al. (2002) provide a useful review of brodifacoum in relation to the risk to nontarget species.

Pharmaceuticals

It may seem unusual to consider drugs used for therapy in other species as a cause of concern in wild animals but recent events suggest that this is appropriate. The most dramatic event of this type is a massive decline (>95%) in the population of the oriental white-backed vulture in Pakistan, which has been linked to kidney damage caused by a nonsteroidal anti-inflammatory drug, diclofenac, used widely to treat livestock (Oaks et al. 2004). Vultures became poisoned by scavenging dead livestock. Other less-dramatic examples are poisoning of raptors that feed on improperly disposed of carcasses of livestock euthanized with barbiturates (Langelier 1993) and death of black-billed magpies exposed to organophosphorus insecticides used to treat parasites of cattle (Henny et al. 1985). The potential effect of pharmaceuticals, particularly reproductive hormones, that enter water via domestic sewage will be mentioned below.

PETROLEUM AND SALTS

Millions of metric tons of crude oil and petroleum products enter the aquatic environment annually. While major oil spills attract attention, smaller discharges account for most of this total (Jessup and Leighton 1996). Aquatic birds, particularly marine species, are most at risk. The effects include surface contamination (oiling), reproductive effects through soiling of eggs causing embryo mortality, and direct toxicity.

Increased concentration of salts in water is of concern in dryer parts of the world. Salts leached from soil accumulate in terminal wetlands that have no outflow. Because these basins are not useful for agriculture, they are not drained. They form a significant proportion of the wetlands available for wild birds in some areas. Several disease conditions have been identified including external encrustation with salt (Wobeser and Howard 1987), salt poisoning (Windingstad et al. 1987), ocular damage (Meteyer et al. 1997), and mortality of juveniles (Stolley et al. 1999).

ENDOCRINE-DISRUPTING COMPOUNDS

Wild animals are exposed to an astonishing array of human-made chemicals known collectively as "endocrine disruptors," which interfere with the reproductive, endocrine, immune, and nervous systems by interfering with hormonal and other cell-messaging systems (Colburn and Clement 1992). A variety of definitions has been proposed for these substances (Phillips and Harrison 1999). The range of such chemicals is very broad and includes substances such as estrogenic hormones from contraceptives that find their way into sewage, mycotoxins, and some insecticides. Most interest has centered on persistent, lipophilic polyhalogenated aromatic hydrocarbons (including PCBs, polychlorinated di-benzo-p-dioxins, and dibenzofurans) and

on polynuclear aromatic hydrocarbons (Rolland 2000). Because of their stability and lipophilic nature, these chemicals are found commonly as residues in wild animals, sometimes at concentrations associated with endocrine dysfunction in experimental animals. It has proven extremely difficult to establish direct causal relationships between these chemicals and effects under field conditions. Hester and Harrison (1999) and Cooke et al. (2002) provide an overview of the subject.

ASSESSING THE EFFECT OF TOXICANTS ON WILD ANIMALS

A central theme in toxicology is that there is a relationship between the dose of the toxicant and the physiological response, with the premise that for any compound there is a dose that has no observable effect and another dose that causes a maximal effect. Much of toxicology relates to determining this dose:response relationship and defining values such as the LD_{50} (the dose that is lethal for 50% of the test population) and the NOEL (the no observed effect level) for compounds. There are huge gaps between the ability to detect toxicant residues in animal tissue (often at the parts per billion level) and the ability to relate these residues clearly to harmful effects on wild animals. This applies at both the individual animal and the population level. Even the diagnosis of intoxication in a single animal is quite different from diagnosis of an infectious disease, particularly those caused by bacteria or a virus. If we isolate a pathogenic virus or bacterium from a sick or dead animal, it is not usually necessary (or possible) to quantify the organisms present in order to decide if the agent is causing disease. Many apparently healthy animals have residues of toxicants in their tissues, so the dilemma lies in knowing what concentration of the compounds is sufficient to account for the injury that has been detected. Beyer et al. (1996) provide a good discussion of the difficulties and give guidelines for interpreting tissue residues of many toxicants.

It is even more difficult to establish a cause:effect relationship at the population level. It is clear that certain organochlorine insecticides had a severe negative effect on populations of some raptorial and fish-eating birds. This effect was detectable because there were long-term data on population abundance and reproductive success, and the effect was confirmed by the recovery of the populations when the use of the chemicals ceased and contamination declined. Toxicants such as lead, mercury, and carbofuran are sufficient in and of themselves to cause the death of wild animals. Although animals may die of many other toxicants, and still other toxicants are known to affect reproduction, it is much less clear what the effect is at the population level. Many toxicants are associated with various physiologic effects, but a clear cause:effect relationship has not been confirmed. For example, Rolland (2000) reviewed 22 published field studies of the effects of toxicants on thyroid and vitamin A status and concluded that "any association between thyroid and retinoid alterations and the adverse health effects reported in these field studies is only circumstantial."

Because of the difficulty in conducting long-term studies to link contaminants to effects such as reduced survival, measurement of biomarkers in wild animals has become common. Biomarkers are changes in cellular and biochemical activity that result from exposure to toxicants. Some, such as the inhibition of the enzymes delta aminolevulinic acid by lead and inhibition of blood or brain choline esterases by organophosphorus and carbamate insecticides, are specific and very useful, both for diagnosis and for determining exposure to these toxicants among living animals as part of a surveillance program. Many other biomarkers, such as the activity of hepatic mixed-function-oxidases and the presence of various porphyrins, are less specific and may be induced by many conditions, hence, they are less useful. In general, biomarkers are easier to measure than to interpret or to link to a specific health problem in wild animals. The relationship between exposure to specific levels of specific toxicants and biomarkers has seldom been validated in wild species.

Information for assessing the effect of toxicants on wild animals comes from two main sources: (1) examination of animals from heavily contaminated environments for effects and then inferring the individual effects from the population data, and (2) experimental exposure of animals to the toxicant and then inferring population consequences from the response of individuals

The first source is useful for identifying the type(s) of effect associated with a particular toxicant, but the levels of exposure in a severely contaminated location may be much greater than that experienced by most of the population. The assumption that it is valid to extrapolate linearly from high doses to predict effects at lower doses may be invalid because different levels of exposure may elicit totally different responses (Welshons et al. 2003). There also may be difficulty in separating the influence of other factors from those of the toxicant. For example, Sagerup et al. (2000) reported a relationship be-

tween parasites and chlorinated hydrocarbon residues in glaucous gulls. One interpretation would be that the contaminants interfered with resistance to nematode parasites (i.e., a cause:effect relationship). However, the data are difficult to interpret because both the parasites and the contaminants reach the birds through their food. Birds eating a certain type of food may be exposed to both more parasites and more toxicants, confounding interpretation.

The general difficulties in extrapolating from experimental to field situations are well known, such as the inability to replicate the environmental features that occur in the field. Diet is known to have a marked effect on the toxicity of lead for birds. Experimental ducks given five lead pellets and fed only corn all died within <9 days, whereas ducks given the same number of pellets and fed commercial duck food all lived for more than 21 days (Sanderson 2002). The question that arises from these data is, which, if either, of these dose:response relationships represents the situation in wild ducks? In experimental situations, animals typically are exposed to constant concentrations of the toxicant for the period of exposure, but in the field exposure is often sporadic and to differing concentrations of toxicant. Most experimental studies are short-term while toxicants may exert an effect over the lifetime of the animal or even into succeeding generations. The length of time that a compound should be studied to understand its population consequences may be related to its environmental persistence: Laskowski (2000) suggested that a study of the effects of methyl mercury or DDT might require 50 years. There have been few studies of the effect of toxicants on long-lived species because of the difficulty in following individuals of these species through time. Most studies involve a single toxicant, whereas animals in the field are exposed to many chemicals simultaneously and toxicants in combination may behave differently than toxicants alone. Walter et al. (2002) found that a mixture of compounds was more toxic than expected although each of the chemicals was at the "no observed effect concentration."

Baker et al. (2001) demonstrate the difficulties in obtaining "statistically significant resolution when comparing populations living in contaminated to those inhabiting relatively uncontaminated sites." They studied a population of bank voles at Chernobyl that had the highest body burdens of radioactive cesium documented in any mammal. They identified increased genetic diversity at the contaminated sites but could not tell if this resulted from elevated mutation rate because of radiation injury or increased variation through immigration. Their conclusion was that variability in ecological factors such as habitat quality and community structure obscured contaminant effects without long-term studies that included massive data sets. A study of the effects of contaminants, parasitism, and predation on turtle reproductive success (De Solla et al. 2003) is one of very few studies that has tried to measure the relative effects of toxicants and other potential factors on a population parameter.

Problems in assessing the significance of a toxicant are similar to those that occur in using a statistical test. Inability to detect an effect may lead to a conclusion that a toxicant has no effect when in fact it does (equivalent to a type II error). This probably occurred for many years with DDT. Because the evidence for direct toxicity was limited, it was assumed that the compound was safe until there was overwhelming evidence of a reproductive effect in birds. The converse is that a toxicant may be considered to be important when in fact its effects are not significant (a type I error).

SUMMARY

- The occurrence and severity of almost every disease of wild animals is influenced by nutrition.
- Malnutrition may result from inadequate quantity, quality, or balance of nutrients.
- Although wild animals die directly as a result of starvation, the effects of malnutrition are more often subtle and chronic through reduced growth and reproduction, and increased susceptibility to predation and infection.
- Deficiency of specific nutrients is often associated with anthropogenic changes in habitat.
- Assessment of nutritional condition in an individual animal or population is not easy and requires a thorough understanding of the biology of the species to recognize what is appropriate at a specific time and place.
- Intervention, for example through supplementation, is the best method for establishing cause: effect relationships between putative nutritional problems and disease.
- The toxicity of compounds is dose related. Some elements are required as nutrients at one level and poisonous at higher levels.
- The dose that an animal receives is influenced by the amount of toxicant available and by the rate at which it is absorbed, distributed, stored, biotransformed, and eliminated from the body.
- Toxicants may accumulate within individual animals (bioaccumulation), and concentrations may be amplified at successive trophic levels (biomagnification). Because of these two processes, animals at lower trophic levels may be unaffected by a substance while top predators are affected severely.
- Toxic injury involves interaction of the toxicant with specific cellular components. Some toxicants react with chemical groupings that are present in many sites but usually one organ is the first to show evidence of injury.
- The ability to detect residues of chemicals in animal tissues far exceeds the ability to measure the effect of these residues for the individual animal and particularly for populations.
- Although some toxicants cause mortality or decreased reproduction directly, indirect effects that are subtle and chronic and act through reduced growth, reproduction, altered behavior, and increased interactions with nutrition and infection are probably more important.

10
Effects of Disease on the Individual Animal

The pattern of the effect is not simple, and is likely to be the result of subtle and changing interactions with other processes—a conclusion that is, we believe, almost certain to apply more generally.
—S. Telfer and Colleagues

The effects of disease on wild animals occur at many different levels, beginning at the molecule and proceeding through subcellular, cellular, organ, individual animal, and population, finally ending with the effects on communities of organisms. Each of these would be a valid focus for scientific study. What is most important for the purpose of this book is understanding how changes at one level affect subsequent levels. In this chapter and chapter 11, I will weave the various levels together. First I will deal with how various factors injure individual animals and result in the dysfunctions that we define as disease (without getting too involved in pathology). In chapter 11, I will consider the effects of disease on groups of animals.

FEATURES COMMON TO ALL TYPES OF DISEASE

At meetings dealing with disease in wild animals, there often is a separation between those interested in infections and those interested in noninfectious disease. The inference is that infectious and noninfectious diseases are inherently different and share no common ground. However, when one is actually examining sick or dead wild animals, it is obvious that they often are affected simultaneously by potentially harmful agents of both types. Various insults don't wait patiently in line for their turn to affect an animal. When a snow goose has avian cholera, it does not stop being affected by lice among its feathers, worms and protozoa in its gut, various contaminants in its fat and liver, or the effects of wear and

tear on its feathers and joints. All of these factors continue to have an impact on the bird. When we study disease, the tendency is to look at each factor in isolation and to emphasize differences rather than similarities and interactions among disease agents. Many features are common to all types of disease, and this helps in understanding why different diseases may look alike and how various conditions may interact. Six features common to all types of disease are that:

1. All disease is the result of injury to cells.
2. The location and rate of cell injury, and the capacity for repair determine the effect.
3. Reaction by the body to injury is often more damaging than the injury itself.
4. The body has only a limited number of ways to respond to injury.
5. Injury in one location often leads to injury elsewhere.
6. All disease is intimately connected with energy.

CELLULAR INJURY

Disease, regardless of cause, is the result of injury to individual cells. Injury to cells leads to the changes in the structure and function of organs such as the lung that we recognize as disease. Individual cells maintain a very narrow range of internal physical and chemical conditions within which they function. If these internal conditions are perturbed, cell function is disrupted. Conditions within a cell are very different from those outside the cell in the extracellular fluid, for example, the concentration of sodium is much greater outside than inside cells, and the gradient of potassium is in the reverse direction. The chemical gradients and the internal milieu are maintained by the cell's membranes and by active processes that require energy. Injured cells are unable to maintain the processes that regulate their internal environment. Depending on the type of cell involved, its metabolic state, and the severity of the injury, an injured cell may survive and recover, or it may die. Even in sublethal injury, functioning of the cell, such as protein synthesis or metabolism of toxins, may be reduced or absent.

An example of loss of function occurs in a condition called hepatic lipidosis in which there is accumulation of abnormal amounts of lipid (fat) within liver cells. This is a nonspecific reaction that occurs in many conditions. It occurs if excessive amounts of free fatty acids are delivered to the liver such as when body fats are mobilized rapidly. Rutting bull elk that forget to eat and live off their body fat while they are preoccupied with sex have a "fatty liver" that can be recognized grossly because it is enlarged and pale yellow. Hepatic lipidosis occurs in the early stages of starvation in all species when the animal still has fat that is being mobilized. It also occurs in many types of cell injury that reduce synthesis of protein, because protein is needed by liver cells to export lipid. Hepatic lipidosis is a reversible condition from which cells can generally recover. It resolves in bull elk as they start to feed again after the rut. But while the condition is present, liver cell functions, such as in detoxification, are impaired, and in severe cases this may result in detectable disease.

There are two basic causes of cell injury: (1) interference with the cell's energy supply and (2) direct damage to the cell's membranes. One or both of these is/are involved in all cell injury. Deficiency of oxygen (hypoxia) that interferes with energy supply to the cell is a very common cause of cell injury. Hypoxia may result from many different processes. It occurs if the blood supply to a tissue is impaired resulting in ischemia. A striking example is the death of tissues that occurs when arteries are plugged by the inflammatory reaction to the nematode *Elaeophora schneideri* in an elk (Hibler and Adcock 1971). It may result from lack of oxygen carrying capacity of the blood as occurs in anemia caused by oil or lead intoxication, malaria, or blood loss, or from inability of cellular metabolism to utilize oxygen (as occurs in cyanide poisoning). In cells deprived of oxygen, metabolism tends to shift to anaerobic glycolysis to provide energy, the internal pH falls, and mechanisms that maintain the chemical gradient across the cell membrane fail. Direct injury to the cell membranes, regardless of whether caused by a bacterial toxin, a virus, inflammation, or a contaminant, has the same basic effect. It allows the chemical gradient between cell contents and the extracellular fluid to disappear.

The fact that all disease starts with cell injury and that cells are injured by only a few basic mechanisms provides a foundation for understanding how various factors may interact. For example, cells that are under stress because of oxygen deficiency from one cause are particularly susceptible to any other factor that also reduces oxygen availability or that damages their membranes. Similarly, animals that are deficient in factors that protect cell membranes from injury are particularly susceptible to any other disease agent that injures cell membranes and to hypoxia.

Different cell types and different organs vary in their susceptibility to injury. Some cells withstand hypoxia better than others. Nerve cells in the brain and spinal cord undergo irreversible injury if deprived of oxygen for even a few minutes, whereas fibrous connective tissue cells are very resistant to oxygen deficiency. Some tissues are particularly vulnerable to injury because of the manner in which the blood supply reaches them. Tissues located at the "end" of an arterial blood supply (such as kidney tubules, the brain, and heart muscle) are particularly susceptible to any obstruction in blood supply, because they have no alternate or backup blood delivery system. In contrast, skeletal muscle, lung, and liver have many interconnecting vessels that form a collateral circulation by which oxygen-rich blood can reach them. For this reason, localized tissue death because of interrupted blood supply (infarction) occurs commonly in heart muscle but rarely in skeletal muscle.

As discussed in chapter 6, the rate at which cells are injured and the rate at which they can be replaced have a major influence on the effect that any injury will have on organ function. Some tissues are much better at repair than others. Nerve cells in the central nervous system and muscle cells in the heart are unable to replicate so that there is no replacement if these cells die. In contrast, epithelial cells in the skin or mucous membranes are replaced continuously and rapidly. But even in these tissues, the number and rate at which cells die determine the effect. If relatively few cells are destroyed by an agent, such as a coccidial organism or a virus, the integrity of the surface membrane can be maintained through replacement, and there is no clinical disease. However, if so many cells are destroyed that replacement cannot keep up, the affected organ's function is disrupted. If this type of injury occurs in the intestine, fluid is not absorbed properly and protein, inflammatory fluid, and inflammatory cells pour into the lumen resulting in diarrhea and fluid loss that may be fatal.

Injury to cells elicits inflammation and immunity. Inflammation is a defense mechanism. It is similar to a military force in that it is necessary for survival in a hostile world, but its deployment always results in damage to host tissue and, paradoxically, may cause far more serious injury than the original insult. Sarcoptic mange illustrates this point. The direct injury by the mites is trivial compared to the damage caused by the intense inflammatory and cell-mediated immune response. Affected animals scratch and chew their skin resulting in hair loss, they abandon normal behavior, and they may cease feeding completely. The inflammation results in loss of large amounts of valuable protein-rich fluid and cells on the skin surface, and infected animals usually die in an emaciated state. Although the microscopic mites cause little direct injury, sarcoptic mange was considered to be the main cause of extinction of foxes on an island in Denmark (Henriksen et al. 1993) and of a population of Spanish ibex (León-Viscaíno et al. 1999).

Other examples of this same phenomenon are infection by the liver fluke *Fascioloides magna* and tuberculosis caused by *Mycobacterium bovis*. *Fascioloides magna* are large but appear to cause relatively little direct injury to the liver (and the liver has a tremendous capacity to regenerate damaged cells). However, infected moose have such an exaggerated inflammatory response that large portions of liver are replaced with scar tissue (fig. 5.1). *Mycobacterium bovis* does not produce toxins or injure cells directly. However, the bacterium is resistant to intracellular destruction by macrophages, and its presence stimulates intense cell-mediated immunity. The tissue lesions in reaction to the bacterium eventually consist of a central area of dead tissue containing live and dead bacteria surrounded by macrophages, lymphocytes, and fibrous tissue that is called a tubercle (fig. 6.6). Chemical mediators released by the reacting inflammatory cells cause the severe generalized wasting (cachexia) that occurs in chronic tuberculosis.

The body has only a limited number of ways in which it can respond to injury, thus, different causes may produce a similar response. For example, severe damage to the lung, whether from inhaled chemicals, circulating bacterial toxins, or direct viral injury, results in increased permeability of small blood vessels and flooding of the air spaces with fluid. Pathologists sometimes use the term "end-stage" to describe chronic injury to tissues, such as the liver and kidney, because the end result of many different types of insult to these organs is the same. (This is the pathologist's equivalent of "all roads lead to Rome.")

Injury to one tissue usually leads to effects in other tissues. For instance, chronic injury to the liver, regardless of cause, affects the liver's many functions, which include production of proteins involved in blood clotting and maintenance of blood osmotic pressure, detoxification of harmful substances, and production of bile that aids in absorption of lipids including fat-soluble vitamins from the intestine. Animals with severe liver injury, caused by a variety of agents, may have secondary changes including hemorrhage at sites far removed from the liver (because of impaired clotting), collection of fluid in tissues and body cavities (because of reduced plasma osmotic pressure), diarrhea (because of reduced intestinal absorption), and brain injury (because of failure to remove toxic substances from the blood). Similarly, chronic kidney injury, regardless of cause, may lead to secondary injury to the heart and blood vessels, anemia, and resorption of minerals from bone.

INJURY AND ENERGY

Energy is essential for life. "If one were asked to pick out a single common denominator of life on earth, that is, something that is absolutely essential and involved in every action large or small, the answer would have to be energy," observes Odum (1993). We can use energy to understand the effects of individual diseases on an animal and for considering how various factors may interact. Each of the steps in energy metabolism (intake, assimilation, and use; fig. 2.3) can be affected by disease. The relationship between energy and disease is governed by two basic rules:

1. An animal cannot expend more energy than it can take in, unless it has stored energy to utilize.
2. Increased use of energy for one purpose decreases the amount available for other purposes.

Energy is a limited resource, and wild animals have limited ability to vary their intake. ("All-you-can-eat" restaurants are rare in nature.)

Disease may reduce energy intake in several ways:

1. Many diseases are characterized by lethargy, resulting in less energy being expended in foraging. This may be helpful in the short term (analogous to bed rest) but is a serious problem in chronic disease because of reduced energy intake.

2. Inappetence is a feature of many diseases: it occurs in reindeer with gastrointestinal helminths (Arneberg et al. 1996), mercury poisoning in raptors (Borg et al. 1970), and oil exposure in sea otter (Wiliams et al. 1990).
3. Animals may avoid highly nutritious foods if these carry the risk of exposure to disease agents (Hutchings et al. 1999).
4. Animals may devote more time to activities related to disease and less time feeding, for example, shorebirds exposed to oil preen more and feed less (Burger 1997).
5. Physical impairments such as degenerative joint disease in old animals (fig. 3.10) may limit mobility and ability to reach nutritious foods.

Of the energy that is taken in, the proportion that is assimilated is related to the quality of the food and to the ability of the animal to extract nutrients from the food, each of which may be modified by disease. Sheep choose to eat less-nutritious herbage in order to avoid grazing near feces (Hutchings et al. 1999). Parasites within the gastrointestinal tract compete directly with the host for nutrients from the ingesta, thereby reducing the proportion available to the host. Intestinal injury of many types, as well as injury to the liver and pancreas that provide digestive enzymes, reduce digestive efficiency leading to malabsorption. Even tapeworms that are considered "benign" reduce the digestibility of food (Munger and Karasov 1989). There may be a significant loss of nutrients, particularly of proteins, in diseases that involve inflammation of the intestine.

Assimilated energy is apportioned among maintenance (keeping the body functioning and repaired), production (growth, reproduction, and defense), and storage as fat. Animals make trade-offs in energy allocation to maximize their lifelong fitness. Disease agents may have a major effect on energy trade-offs by increasing the cost for maintenance and defense. Any condition that interferes with the insulating efficiency of the plumage or pelage increases the cost of thermoregulation, for example, oiling of waterbirds and marine mammals or hair loss in moose infested with the tick (*Dermacentor albipictis*) (Glines and Samuel 1984). There also is increased energy consumption for disease resistance, including avoiding exposure, inflammation and immune responses, and repair of damaged tissue.

The total costs of resistance are unknown (Lochmiller and Deerenberg 2000) but each component of the defense system requires energy for maintenance as well as for specific activity. For instance, stimula-

tion of a lymphocyte by an antigen results in an almost instantaneous and prolonged 35% increase in oxygen consumption by the cell (Buttgereit et al. 2000). Fever is part of the response to many disease agents. Energy consuming reactions speed up by 13% for every degree rise in body temperature, so that an animal with a fever may have a resting metabolic rate >40% above normal. When fever is coupled with impaired energy intake, an animal rapidly "burns" its fat stores and catabolizes muscle to meet energy demands. The energy costs for production of detoxification proteins and replacement of toxicant-damaged tissues also can be very high (Sibly and Calow 1989). Even the immune response to an innocuous antigen can be costly and can produce measurable effects on growth (Spurlock et al. 1997; Fair et al. 1999). Responding to an antigen resulted in asymmetry in the wings of mountain chickadees (Whitaker and Fair 2002) and delayed molt in male pied flycatchers (Sanz et al. 2004). Lochmiller and Deerenberg (2000) observed that the cost of upregulation of defenses may "push the animal beyond the minimal levels of body reserves to survive."

Trade-offs for energy can work in the opposite direction as well. Reduced availability of energy, because of extra commitments to other activities, especially reproduction, and/or because of inadequate intake can have a severe impact on disease resistance. Prolonged reduction in the intake of energy is associated with increased susceptibility to infections, especially those caused by opportunistic agents (Klurfeld 1993). Reduced intake of energy is usually accompanied by reduction in intake of protein resulting in protein-energy malnutrition (PEM). The effect of PEM is to limit not only the energy required for defense but also the amino acids required for constructing reactive proteins including acute phase proteins and antibodies, and for repair of damaged tissues. Increased commitment of resources to reproduction may lead to decreased resistance to disease agents (Deerenberg et al. 1997). Coop and Kyriazakas (1999) proposed that maintenance, including repair, replacement, and reaction to damaged tissue, will have first priority for resources and that growth and reproduction will have the second highest priority. Disease resistance, except for the early stages of immune recognition, will have lower priority. However, it is unlikely that the "rules" for trade-offs are rigid. The relative fitness value of growth, reproduction, and disease resistance is probably stochastic (Lochmiller and Deerenberg 2000) and disease may have a more or less severe effect depending on nutrition and the presence of factors that act synergistically with disease (Murray et al. 1997; Albon et al. 2002). There also are clearly defined sex-specific differences in the way that resources are allocated that may explain some differences in relative susceptibility to disease between males and females (Tschirren et al. 2003). The relationships among nutrition, disease resistance in its broadest sense, and the occurrence of clinical disease (fig. 9.2) should be considered in assessing the effect of any disease. Conclusions about the effects of a disease agent based on trials in which animals are given unlimited access to high-quality food and are free of other stressors are probably of questionable value.

TYPES OF INJURY

Traditionally, disease has been detected in wild animals through observation of sick or dead animals. This has low sensitivity as a surveillance technique because of the covert behavior of sick animals and rapid removal of affected animals from the population by predators and scavengers. This method does not detect animals with subclinical disease.

A disease is important to a wild animal when impaired function decreases its chances of survival or lowers its reproduction (Gulland 1995). When assessing the effects of a disease, we need to consider the entire lifetime of the animal because "fitness does not only depend on reproductive success, but on longevity as well" (Lochmiller and Deerenberg 2000). By extension to chapter 11, a disease becomes important to a population when it "causes sufficient reproductive failure or mortality to reduce

breeding numbers below what would otherwise occur" (Newton 1998).

Thus, "significant" diseases fall into one or both of two categories: (1) those that cause reduced survival and (2) those that cause decreased reproduction. This rather stark approach to disease is quite different from the way disease is viewed in humans (and pet animals) in developed countries where many "important" diseases affect the "quality" of life for individuals who are long past reproduction and where the average length of survival is increasing. Most wild animals don't enjoy golden years of postreproductive senescence in which they have to worry about the quality of their postretirement life. The approach to disease in wild animals also is different from the way disease is considered in domestic livestock, where important diseases interfere with production rather than with survival or total reproductive output. Most domestic animals reach the end of their lives prior to reproduction, and few survive to complete their potential lifetime reproductive output.

DISEASES CAUSING REDUCED SURVIVAL

Direct Mortality

A small minority of diseases results directly in mortality (i.e., is solely responsible for an animal's death), on a regular basis, although these are the conditions that come to mind when the public thinks of disease in wild animals. Diseases that occur in explosive outbreaks in which the accumulated dead overwhelm the normal scavenging and sanitation systems (table 10.1) are the most visible forms of

Table 10.1 Diseases That Result in Extensive Direct Mortality of Individual Animals in the Form of Conspicuous Die-offs

Disease (cause)	Species affected
Phocine distemper (phocine morbillivirus)	Harbor seals, grey seals
Plague (*Yersinia pestis*)	Prairie dogs
Avian cholera (*Pasteurella multocida*)	Wild waterfowl
Avian botulism (*Clostridium botulinum* types C and E)	Waterfowl, piscivorous birds
Oil spills	Marine birds and mammals
Hemorrhagic disease (orbiviruses)	Deer, pronghorns
Pesticide poisoning (e.g., Diazenon)	Grazing geese
Myxomatosis (Myxoma virus)	European rabbit
Rabbit hemorrhagic disease (Rabbit hemorrhagic disease virus)	European rabbit
Pneumonia (*Pasteurella trehalosi*, *Mannheimia haemolytica*)	Mountain sheep
Traumatic injury (hailstorms)	Waterfowl
Newcastle disease (Avian paramyxovirus 1)	Double-crested cormorants

Note: Conspicuous die-offs = mortality that is concentrated in time and space.

Table 10.2 Diseases That Cause Direct Mortality Dispersed in Time and Place (Carcasses Not Evident)

Disease (cause)	Species affected
Lead poisoning	Waterfowl
Rabies	Fox, skunk, raccoon, bats
Canine distemper (canine distemper virus)	Canids, mustelids
West Nile virus	Wild birds
Trichostrongylosis (*Trichostrongylus tenuis*)	Red grouse
Avian malaria (*Plasmodium relictum*)	Native Hawaiian birds
Visceral larva migrans *(Baylisascaris procyonis)*	Ground hogs, other rodents, birds
Myiasis (*Wohlfahrtia* spp.)	Voles, wild ducklings
Sarcoptic mange	Canids, chamois, wombats

disease and attract attention. Other diseases that also are directly lethal (table 10.2) attract much less attention because the victims are dispersed, removed efficiently by scavengers, and less obvious.

Infectious disease agents are unlikely to cause extensive mortality of their hosts, because of the risk of their own extinction, except under special circumstances (Yuill 1987). These include situations such as the following.

- *Serious illness or death of the host assists in transmission of the disease.* In rabies the severe terminal abnormal behavior leads to bite wounds and transmission of the virus. The persistence of anthrax depends upon killing its host, releasing persistent spores that remain in the environment (Hugh-Jones and de Vos 2002).
- *Death of the host does not hinder transmission.* For example, development of flesh flies that cause the disease myiasis (fig. 10.1) is not hampered by death of the host, because development of the fly larvae continues after the host dies.
- *The agent does not depend on that host species for its survival.* Many multihost parasites are maintained in one host in which damage is limited but cause fatal injury in other hosts. For example, plague that causes die-offs in prairie dogs is maintained in small rodents (Anderson and Williams 1997).
- *A disease newly introduced into a naive population in which very few individuals have resistance.* One example is myxomatosis in Australian rabbits.
- *A disease that moves through a population over a wide geographical area over a long period of*

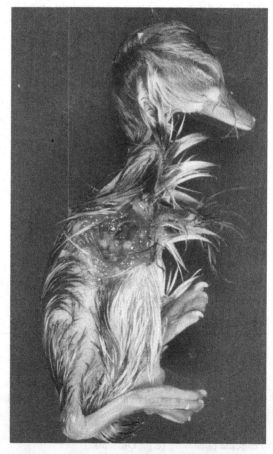

Fig. 10.1. Nestling blue-winged teal infected by the flesh fly *Wohlfahrtia opaca*. This form of infection by fly larvae in a living animal is termed "myiasis." It is somewhat unusual in that death of the host does not prevent the larvae from completing development to the pupal stage.

time so that the entire host population is not threatened. This may occur in canine distemper in some situations.

Noninfectious agents such as poisons and trauma are not constrained by the same limitations because they do not depend upon the continuation of a host for their persistence and are free to cause mortality. In type C botulism, lethality provides substrate for multiplication of the bacterium.

With diseases of the type shown in tables 10.1 and 10.2, in which the agents are known to be able to kill animals directly, the probability of an individual's dying of the disease is a function of the likelihood and degree of exposure to the disease, and the ability to resist or recover from the exposure, both of which are affected by many other factors.

Indirect Mortality

Many diseases reduce survival indirectly. This is difficult to quantify, particularly if we are dependent upon looking at the end result and trying to guess at the process that led to an animal's demise. A large proportion of the dead wild animals that I examine are in poor body condition or are emaciated. In those relatively uncommon situations in which I am confronted with a dead wild animal in good body condition, my first thought is that some acutely lethal agent such as an insecticide or a highly virulent virus is probably involved. Emaciated animals always present a diagnostic challenge. We receive emaciated hatch-year great blue herons for necropsy each autumn. Usually no single cause of death is evident but the birds have intestinal trematodes, nematodes, and cestodes, small amounts of contaminants such as mercury and various hydrocarbons in their tissues, and even mild bacterial infections or fungal infections. None of these seems severe enough in itself to kill the bird, and one is left trying to assess how the individual factors, together with malnutrition as a result of inexperience in feeding, contributed to the bird's demise.

Indirect effects leading to reduced survival may take different forms, many of which are mediated through energetic interrelationships (fig. 9.2). It is inappropriate to consider these factors as independent or the effects as simply additive. Indirect effects on survival that have been identified include:

- Increased susceptibility to predation
- Increased susceptibility to other diseases
- Increased vulnerability to accidents
- Depression of growth and maturation
- Increased susceptibility to starvation

Sublethal disease of many different types has been suggested to increase the susceptibility of animals to predators, and predators may take a disproportionate number of parasitized prey (Holmes and Bethel 1972; Temple 1987). Parasite-increased trophic transmission (PITT) (also called parasite-induced vulnerability to predation) is a feature of many parasitic infections that have a complex life cycle dependent on predation. Increased vulnerability may result from alteration in the behavior or appearance of infected intermediate or paratenic hosts, which increases the likelihood that the prey animal will be eaten by a suitable predator. For instance, rats infected with *Toxoplasma gondii* have reduced fear of cats (Webster et al. 1994), rodents infected with larval *Baylisascaris procyonis* have abnormal behavior that may make them vulnerable to raccoons, and snowshoe hares infected with larval tapeworms have delayed color change that makes them conspicuous to predators that are the final host of these worms (Leiby and Dyer 1971). Some behavioral changes that make animals susceptible to predation are unrelated to PITT and result from a general reduction in reactivity to noxious stimuli or mental acuity because of the disease. As an example, mice infected with *Eimeria vermiformis* have reduced aversion to the odor of cats, although cats are not involved in the transmission of this parasite (Kavaliers and Colwell 1995a). This type of nonspecific effect on behavior is likely a widespread phenomenon. Consider that there is an association between the intensity of infection with the intestinal roundworm *Ascaris lumbricoides* and aspects of cognitive behavior in children (Levav et al. 1995), and mice infected with a nematode have reduced spatial learning ability (Kavaliers and Colwell 1995b).

Disease may affect susceptibility to predation in other ways. Injuries may reduce the ability to escape when pursued (Harwood et al. 1996) or the ability to detect predators. Exudate in the ears of mountain sheep infected with ear mites is thought to increase their susceptibility to cougars (Norrix et al. 1995). Diseases may interact with food supply to increase vulnerability to predators. Hungry animals are more vulnerable than well-fed ones to predation for a variety of reasons but particularly because they are more active (Newton 1998) and because they may have less energy to devote to antipredator behavior. Diseased animals may need to feed to compensate for energy demands associated with disease. This was thought to be the mechanism that resulted in disproportionate predation of snowshoe hares infected with the stomach worm *Obeliscoides cuniculi* (Murray et al. 1997). Some forms of increased susceptibility to predators may be coincidental, for example, female red grouse heavily infected with the cecal worm *Trichostrongylus tenuis* are thought to emit more odor than lightly infected birds and, hence, be more vulnerable to mammalian predators (Hudson et al. 1992a). Increased susceptibility to predators extends to vulnerability to human hunters. Moose infected heavily with larval *Echinococcus granulosus* (Rau and Caron 1979) and ducks that ingested lead shot (Bellrose 1959) are more vulnerable to hunters.

Presence of one disease may make animals susceptible to other disease agents in a number of ways. The most simple of such situations occurs when injury from one agent provides a portal of entry for others, for example, openings in the skin caused by bot fly larvae allow bacteria and other species of fly larvae to enter the body (Boonstra 1977; Warren 1994). Respiratory viruses predispose to bacterial infections of the lung by interfering with the mucociliary system of the upper respiratory tract and with the activity of macrophages in the alveoli. Lethargy as a result of one disease may make animals more susceptible to biting insects that transmit other agents. Many infectious agents and toxicants, such as mycotoxins, lead, and polychlorinated biphenyls, cause immune suppression under laboratory conditions and are suspected to have a similar effect in the wild. Some forms of immune suppression are mediated through competing demands for energy, while others are the result of specific damage to organs, such as the thymus or bone marrow, or interference with chemical mediators.

Animals with impaired function because of disease are susceptible to accidents and misfortunes. For example, many coyotes with sarcoptic mange wander into farmyards and are killed by farmers or their dogs, and mountain animals with keratoconjunctivitis (inflammation of the cornea of the eye) fall from cliffs (Meagher et al. 1992; Loison et al. 1996; Cransac et al. 1997). My experience has been that a disproportionate number of animals killed by collisions with automobiles have preexisting diseases.

Growth depression is cited frequently as a sublethal effect of many infectious and noninfectious diseases. In wild animals, body size may be a factor: "body size influences social status, fecundity and survival," according to Cooch (2002), so that this effect may in fact be more than sublethal. The developmental limits of an individual are determined by

its genotype, but the ability to develop to the optimal phenotype is determined by environmental conditions, including the effects of various diseases. Conditions that occur during growth and development may have consequences throughout the lifetime of an individual (Cam et al. 2003). For instance, nutritional stress early in life was associated with increased joint disease in senescence among moose on Isle Royale (Peterson 1988). Developmental features other than size at maturity, such as asymmetry in normally bilaterally symmetrical structures, also may have significant effects on fitness (Whitaker and Fair 2002). Effects on growth and development of offspring may result from disease in the parents or because of disease in the growing animal. Parental effects may result in suboptimal time of birth, small fetal size, poor nutrition of the offspring, or inadequate maternal care. It is obvious that diseases that cause direct tissue injury to growing animals, such as leeches on ducklings (Davies and Wilkialis 1981) and mange on calves (Rehbein et al. 2003), could depress growth and development. However, it is perhaps surprising that the immune reaction to an innocuous antigen can result in significant growth reduction (Fair et al. 1999) and delay feather molt (an annual repair mechanism; Sanz et al. 2004), as can stimulation of lymphocyte response (Soler et al. 2002). "In general, stimulation of a host's immune system equates to proportional declines in growth as endogenous strategies of resource allocation shift toward survival and away from nonessential processes such as growth" (Lochmiller and Deerenberg 2000).

Growing animals may be able to compensate for the effects of disease so that they reach full size (Bize et al. 2003), but this may result in delayed maturation that has costs in terms of nestling or fledging mortality (Johnson et al. 1991) and a variety of other deleterious effects (Metcalfe and Monaghan 2001). In other instances, such as depressed growth in reindeer caused by biting insect harassment (Colman et al. 2003), the animals are not able to compensate and remain stunted.

The preceding discussion dealt largely with the effects of nutritional deficiency on the occurrence of other diseases, but it is equally important that various diseases place an energetic burden on wild animals experiencing a shortage of food. In many circumstances, the effects of a disease agent may only become visible in animals with restricted food supply or increased energy demands. For instance, blowfly (*Protocalliphora braueri*) larvae had no detectable effect on nestling sage thrashers except during cold, wet weather (Howe 1992). It is very difficult to separate the effects of disease from that of nutritional inadequacy, except through experimental manipulation of either the disease or the food supply. Studies by Gulland (1992), Murray et al. (1997), and Albon et al. (2002) have demonstrated the nature of interactions between intestinal parasites and food supplies in wild herbivores and provide a model for similar studies.

EFFECTS OF DISEASE ON REPRODUCTION

Reproduction is a costly activity and requires that animals make trade-offs in allocating energy. The most basic need is to maintain those body functions required for survival, and only energy in excess of that needed for survival is available for reproduction. Thus, we expect that animals in poor nutritional condition or with high survival costs, regardless of cause, will have decreased reproduction. Because disease removes energy that could be used for other purposes we should expect that disease may affect reproduction negatively. We also should expect that the detrimental effects of disease on reproduction will be highly variable. Animals in good habitat with access to abundant food may be able to compensate for the costs of disease agents, while individuals in situations with limited resources, such as in poor habitat or during poor years, may experience severe effects of disease on reproduction. Trade-offs related to reproduction may not be restricted to a single reproductive event. It is thought that future reproduction is negatively affected by current reproduction, either because of reduced survival or through reduced output in subsequent reproductive events. Both of these effects have been described in birds (Dawson et al. 2000), but the relationship of this form of trade-off to disease has not been investigated.

Activation of the immune system, even by antigens unrelated to disease, can have a measurable effect on reproduction. Female pied flycatchers injected with a nonpathogenic antigen fed their young less, produced fledglings in poorer condition, and had lower fledging success than females injected with saline (Ilmonen et al. 2000). There was no apparent effect on body condition or the amount of subcutaneous fat among the adult females, although there was reduced feather regrowth. Martin et al. (2003) estimated that the immune response to a nonpathogenic antigen by house sparrows was equivalent in energy cost to producing half an egg. These observations suggest that an animal might mount a successful immune response that results in complete

control of an infectious agent but still have reduced reproductive success and be "winning the battle but losing the war."

Disease may affect reproduction in individual animals in a variety of ways. The effects can be subdivided into those that result from a direct pathologic effect on the parents or the offspring and those in which the reproductive output is adjusted to reduce the effect of a disease on the host, for example, by altering behavior to avoid exposure or by trading reproduction for other forms of defense. The examples in table 10.3 are intended only to give a flavor of the diversity of ways in which various disease agents may affect reproduction. Gulland (1995) and Tompkins and Begon (2000) provide lists of other diseases that have been reported to cause decreased reproduction in wild animals. Most such reports are observational, and there are relatively few quantitative reports. Most studies of interactions between disease and reproduction have involved birds, particularly cavity-nesting species that can be manipulated readily.

It is easy to understand how agents that injure the reproductive organs or that cause damage to the developing embryo or fetus interfere with reproductive success. Bacteria of the genus *Brucella* act in this manner in various mammals, resulting in the disease known as brucellosis. *Brucella* spp. seldom cause the death of adult animals but establish chronic infections. The bacteria initially localize in lymphoid organs. In pregnant animals, the uterus and placenta become infected, resulting in severe inflammation and abortion of the fetus, usually late in gestation. Abortion is difficult to identify in wild animals or to quantify, because aborted fetuses are removed rapidly by scavengers. Although brucellosis is known to have been present in bison in Yellowstone National Park since 1917, the first aborted bison fetus was not recovered until 1992 (Rhyan et al. 1994). With more intense surveillance, three additional aborted calves infected with *Brucella abortus* were recovered between 1996 and 1999 (Rhyan et al. 2000). *Brucella* spp. also infect the testicles of males, resulting in severe destructive orchitis (fig. 10.2).

Infection of the uterus, placenta, or fetus with other bacteria, as well as by some fungi and viruses, may have a similar effect. Noninfectious factors can also cause in utero deaths. Female animals that are injured or stressed severely may abort, or the fetuses may die and be resorbed or mummify (fig. 10.3).

Many diseases result in reduced survival of offspring. Interactions between parental disease and survival of the offspring may be subtle, for example,

Table 10.3 Mechanisms by Which Disease Agents Affect Reproduction

Mechanism	Species	Agent
Abnormalities in offspring	Waterbirds	Selenium toxicosis[1]
	Gulls	Chlorinated hydrocarbons[2]
Death of fetus in *utero* or in *ovo*	Waterbirds	Oil contamination (egg) [3]
	Wild boar	Classical swine fever virus[4]
Decreased mating	Mice	*Trichinella spiralis*5
Delayed breeding or sexual maturity	Collared flycatcher	Disease[6]
	Sheep	Liver flukes[7]
Delayed maturation	Alpine swift	Louse-fly[8]
Direct injury to ovary, uterus, or placenta	Bison, caribou	Brucellosis[9]
	Koala	Chlamydiosis[10]
Direct injury to testes	Bison, caribou	Brucellosis[11]
Discrimination against affected animals as mates	Sage grouse	Lice[12]
Inability to establish or defend territory	Ring-necked pheasant	*Ixodes ricinus* (tick) [13]
Reduced care of young	Mallard	Dieldrin exposure[14]
	Brown pelican	Tick infestation[15]
	Bighorn sheep	Lungworm infection[16]
Reduced production of ova or fertilization	Birds	Ingested oil[17]
	Great tit	Calcium deficiency[18]
Reduced production of sperm	Mice	Tapeworm[19]
Reduced survival of offspring	Mute swans	Lead toxicosis[20]
	Purple martin	*Haemoproteus prognei*[21]

[1] Ohlendorf (1996).
[2] Fox and Weseloh (1986).
[3] Jessup and Leighton (1996).
[4] Van Campen et al. (2001).
[5] Edwards and Barnard (1987).
[6] Gustafsson et al. (1997).
[7] Hope-Cawdry (1976).
[8] Bize et al. (2003).
[9] Thorne (2001).
[10] Whittington (2001).
[11] Thorne (2001).
[12] Spurrier et al. (1991).
[13] Hoodless et al. (2002).
[14] Winn (1973).
[15] King et al. (1977).
[16] Festa-Bianchet (1988).
[17] Jessup and Leighton (1996).
[18] Tilger et al. (2002).
[19] Morales-Mentor et al. (1999).
[20] Birkhead and Perrins (1985).
[21] Davidar and Morton (1993).

ectoparasites were believed to influence reproduction in alpine marmots in two ways (Arnold and Lichtenstein 1993). Heavy infestation was thought to interfere with the ability of parents to keep infants warm during hibernation, and females that had been infested heavily during the previous winter weaned their litters later in the season with the resulting young having a lower probability of survival.

Many effects of disease on reproduction are mediated through changes in behavior. Some of these, such as the difficulty that diseased males may have in establishing or defending territory and decreased interest in mating, may be linked either to direct physiological injury or to reduced energy. Other factors that are linked to mate selection may be based on selection against mates with obvious

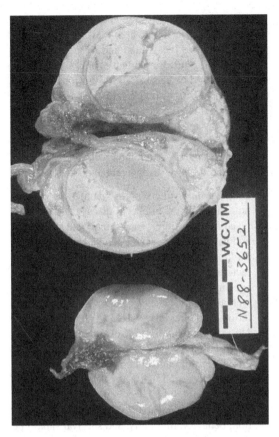

Fig. 10.2. Severe destructive inflammation of the testicles (orchitis) from a caribou infected with *Brucella suis* biovar 4.

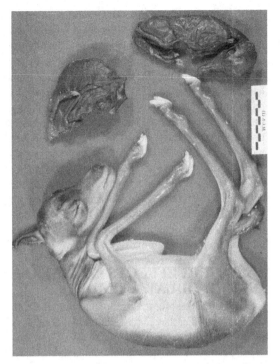

Fig. 10.3. Fetuses from the uterus of an adult female pronghorn that died of starvation. Only one fetus was alive at the time the dam died. The other two fetuses had died much earlier and the fluids had been resorbed resulting in fetal mummification. Fetal death and mummification are common in white-tailed deer and pronghorns that are in poor nutritional condition during severe winters in Saskatchewan.

physical signs of disease, such as discrimination against male sage grouse with hemorrhages caused by lice (Spurrier et al. 1991), or selection against animals with fluctuating asymmetry that has been associated with macroparasites in a variety of species (Møller 1992; Folstad et al. 1996). Diseased males also may lack resources to produce appropriate signals. Mulvey and Aho (1993) reported a negative relationship between body and antler size (both of which are related to breeding success) and liver fluke (*Fascioloides magna*) infection in male white-tailed deer. Being selected against for reproduction because of disease may be "tough luck" for the individual involved but advantageous at the population level.

Many diseases, both infectious and noninfectious, appear to interfere with care of offspring through nest abandonment, reduced feeding, and even rejection of the young. Poor fawn survival has been documented in nutritionally stressed white-tailed deer.

Under experimental conditions, postnatal fawn mortality most commonly resulted from maternal rejection by malnourished does, including failure to lick the fawn at birth, apparent fear of the neonate, failure to eat the afterbirth, and refusal to allow the fawn to nurse (Langenau and Lerg 1976).

Disease may affect lifetime reproductive output if initial reproduction is delayed or if the interval between reproductive events is extended. Cowpox virus, which is enzootic in bank voles and wood mice, had no effect on survival of these animals, but the timing of the first litter was delayed by 20–30 days by infection. This was thought to reduce fecundity by up to 25% (Feore et al. 1997).

There is a huge literature on the potential effects of endocrine-disrupting chemicals (EDC) on reproduction, particularly in birds (Crews et al. 2000; Guillette et al. 2000; Ottinger et al. 2002). Among chemicals suspected of mimicking or antagonizing the action of hormones are drugs, pesticides, herbicides, industrial chemicals, and plant phytoestrogens. These compounds are dispersed widely, and mixtures with this activity are present in municipal and landfill effluent so that many wild species are exposed. Much of the information available is from laboratory studies, and it is unclear how the results relate to the type of exposure that occurs in wild animals. Jobling et al. (2003) note, "there is little information on the relative sensitivities of different wildlife groups to these chemicals and/or mixtures of them (e.g. estrogenic effluents) and hence, there are fundamental shortfalls in our knowledge of the ecological importance of endocrine dysruption in wildlife." At this point in time, EDC are one additional factor that must be considered in evaluating reproduction in wild animals.

ASSESSING EFFECTS OF DISEASE ON INDIVIDUAL ANIMALS

Every disease has some cost to the animal (Yuill 1987). Measuring that cost for individual animals is not a trivial task except, perhaps, in a very few diseases, such as rabies, that are so damaging that infection can be regarded as a death sentence. In most diseases, including those in tables 10.1 and 10.2 that are known to cause mortality directly, the cost is modified by an ever-changing variety of stressors and challenges that interact in unpredictable ways. An experimental study of interactions among marginal malnutrition, sublethal toxicants, and infectious agents led to a conclusion that the results "suggest the possibility of added danger to humans and animals when they are malnourished and exposed to combinations of infectious agents and environmental chemicals" (Porter et al. 1984).

It is inappropriate to conclude that an agent has no significant effect on a wild species based on tests done in artificial situations in which the test animals have abundant food and are protected from other stressors. It may be equally misleading to judge the significance of a disease by comparing naturally infected and naturally uninfected animals. Munger and Karasov (1991) identified differences in nutritional state, habitat, age, immunocompetence, and infection history as factors that could confound studies that compare naturally infected and uninfected animals. For example, it would be simplistic to conclude that a parasite caused poor body condition in rabbits based on correlation between the number of parasites and body condition in a sample of wild rabbits. Equally plausible explanations for an apparent relationship might be that animals in

poor body condition (for any reason) are more vulnerable to parasites or that animals in poor habitat browse closer to the ground and so are exposed to more parasite eggs. If no effect of an agent is identified, this might be because the cost of the disease is so slight that it is insignificant, that the animal can compensate for the costs, or that the costs are significant but the methods used for measuring costs are not sufficiently sensitive.

Studies to measure the impact of disease on individuals should have several characteristics.

1. *Long-term timeline.* Fitness is a lifetime phenomenon and the effects of disease may be delayed (perhaps intergenerational) and stochastic, and have large seasonal or annual variation.
2. *Multiple factors.* Consider potential interacting factors, particularly the animals' nutrition, sex, age, and prior experience with the disease, as well as the presence of concurrent disease conditions and stressors.
3. *Disease manipulation.* Involve manipulation of the disease through experimental reduction, elimination or augmentation of the putative cause, or contributing factors such as nutrition.
4. *Variable examination.* Examine as many variables as possible. Effects on growth, reproduction, behavior, immunity, and survival should be measured.
5. *Immune system components.* Evaluate all components of the immune system (innate, humoral, cell-mediated) because different portions have different functions.

Studies of helminth parasites in red grouse (Hudson et al. 1992b), Soay sheep (Gulland 1992), snowshoe hares (Murray et al. 1997), and Svalbard reindeer (Albon et al. 2002) are models of studies of natural populations that have tried to place the effects of disease in an environmental context. I began this chapter with a quotation from Telfer et al. (2002) regarding subtle interactions of disease with other factors. Their study of cowpox virus in bank voles and wood mice is illustrative of how complex such relationships may be. Infection with the virus was associated with increased survival of rodents in summer and decreased survival in winter, and infection resulted in delayed reproduction. The researchers speculated that decreased reproductive effort as a result of infection may result in improved survival in summer but not in winter when the animals do not reproduce, and that winter survival may be compromised by limited food availability.

SUMMARY

- All disease begins with injury at the cellular level.
- Cell injury is caused by interference with energy supply to the cell or damage to cell membranes.
- Cells and tissues vary greatly in susceptibility to injury.
- A minority of diseases causes mortality directly, although these conditions are the diseases that are most obvious.

- Many diseases contribute to reduced survival by increasing susceptibility to predation, other diseases, and accidents, or by interacting with nutrition.
- Disease may reduce reproductive success directly by injuring the parent or offspring, or indirectly when reproductive output is altered to reduce the effect of disease on the host, for example, by a trade-off between reproduction and disease resistance.

11
Effects of Disease on Populations of Wild Animals

In reality, no one factor is likely to account wholly for a given population level. This is because reproduction and survival are seldom influenced by one factor alone, but by several which may act independently or in combination.
—I. Newton

Chapter 10 began with the thought that disease could be considered at any level from a single molecule to an ecosystem. In this chapter, I will discuss the impact of disease on groups of animals. Much less is known about the population biology than about the medical and physiologic aspects of most diseases. We will be concerned here "not with individuals, but with the average properties of similar (but not exactly the same) individuals belonging to the same species" (Berryman 2002).

In the same way that effects on individual cells lead to dysfunction of individuals, it is effects on the reproduction and survival of individuals that lead to population effects. The difference in approach between this chapter and chapter 10 can be illustrated by thinking about annual survival. An individual either dies during or survives for the year. At the population level, we are interested in the proportion of individuals that survives, which is similar to the probability that an "average" individual will survive. Similarly, a female Franklin's gull might raise between zero and four chicks to fledging; the fledging rate refers to the average number of chicks that fledge per female in the group. We are concerned with how abundant the animals are (population size), the population composition, the population density, and how these change over time in relation to disease. (Density is usually calculated as the number of animals in a given amount of space, but other denominators such as the number/waterhole or the number using a feeding site may be more appropriate in some situations.)

WHAT IS A POPULATION?

Defining population is not a trivial task, because the word has been used in many different manners by ecologists and disease specialists. Population was used originally to describe a group of people, but over time the use has been extended to mean a group of individuals of the same species, usually defined by some spatial limit. Thus, one finds reference to a population of mule deer in the Great Sandhills of Saskatchewan or a population of northern pintails on a wetland complex in California. In chapter 10, I noted that disease becomes important to a population when it "causes sufficient reproductive failure or mortality to reduce breeding numbers below what would otherwise occur" (Newton 1998). Use of the word "population" to describe a group of ducks wintering on a wetland presents a problem when we start to consider the effects of disease in terms of natality and mortality because none of the annual reproduction and only a fraction of the annual mortality occur on the area. The number of birds in such a group is likely determined far more by emigration and immigration than by births and deaths.

Designation of small groups as populations sometimes leads to interesting situations. For example, Beaver (1980) described the effects of DDT on an American robin "population" occupying a 71.8 ha area. In some years the recognized mortality associated with DDT "equaled or exceeded the counted population" but "prenesting population size was not depressed by DDT." This leads one to conclude that more than the entire population may have been killed by DDT, but there was no effect on the breeding population! Local population is often used for groups such as the ducks referred to earlier, but "local is a fuzzy term. In most terrestrial and marine studies its meaning is simply a matter of operational convenience" (Camus and Lima 2002). Depending on the size of the local unit, one should expect that such a group will be influenced strongly by emigration and immigration and recognize that it is only a fragment of a total population that may or may not be affected by the same disease factors.

The definition of population proposed by Berryman (2002) will be used here. A *population* is "a group of individuals of the same species that live together in an area of sufficient size to permit normal dispersal and/or migration behavior and in which numerical changes are largely determined by birth and death processes." Because there seems to be no suitable alternative word for lower levels of organization, *subpopulation* will be used for groups of organisms living in smaller areas, with the recognition that the dynamics of these will be influenced considerably by dispersion and migration. A *metapopulation* will be considered to be "a set of populations distributed over a number of patches that are connected, to a varying degree, by dispersal" (Hess 1996).

The elk that live in and around Riding Mountain National Park in Manitoba, Canada, can be used to demonstrate this categorization. (Bovine tuberculosis has been discovered recently in these animals, and defining who is who has become important.) The park is an island of natural wooded habitat in a sea of agricultural land. The elk that live there are separated from other groups of elk by many kilometers of unsuitable habitat. Habitat is used here to mean "the combination of resources, abiotic, and biotic factors that determine the presence, survival, and reproduction of a population" (Caughley and Sinclair 1994). The park is sufficiently large that the number of elk is determined by births and deaths (including predation by wolves, collisions with vehicles, and hunting immediately adjacent to the park). There appear to be three areas of elk concentration within the park with a modest amount of interchange of individuals. I consider the elk in the three groups to be subpopulations. The total of the three subpopulations in the park constitutes a population, which, together with populations of elk in the Duck Mountains to the north of Riding Mountain National Park and populations in adjacent areas of Saskatchewan, constitute a metapopulation with limited interchange. This framework is useful for thinking about disease in the elk.

The range of different diseases that affect the elk is likely to be most similar in animals within the subpopulations, and increasingly diverse as one moves to larger groups. Differences in disease status may be related to increasingly different habitat conditions in which the groups live; increased heterogeneity in disease resistance with larger group size; and because exchange of infectious diseases will be most frequent within subpopulations, less frequent among subpopulations, and infrequent among populations in the metapopulation. The concept of subpopulations, population, and metapopulation may have implications for tuberculosis, as there may be differences in prevalence among the subpopulations, and tuberculosis seems to be limited to the Riding Mountain National Park population in this area of western North America. It may also be useful when thinking about potential management of disease. For instance, if a subpopulation was reduced severely or extirpated for any reason, the area that it had occupied would likely be repopulated relatively quickly by dispersal from within the population, but extirpation of the entire population probably would be followed by limited repopulation through dispersal from the other populations. Disruption of the social "fabric" of a subpopulation by culling might have an undesirable effect if it led to increased dispersal and exchange with other groups, as occurred when local groups of badgers were culled in Great Britain (Donnelly et al. 2003).

GENERAL FEATURES OF POPULATIONS

Populations have a number of features relevant to the discussion of disease including size, spatial distribution, composition in terms of sex and age, and life history traits.

SIZE

The size of a population is determined generally by the availability of resources mediated through changes in reproduction, immigration, mortality, and emigration (the four primary population processes). (*Resource* is used here to mean something that the animal needs, including food, shelter, water, a particular range of temperature, as well as nesting sites or escape terrain, and other features peculiar to the species.) Some resources such as sunlight are nonconsumable; others such as plants eaten by ungulates are consumed and the amount available is reduced by their use. Usage of some resources is preemptive, that is, use by one animal precludes use by another. For example, if the number of tree holes available for nesting is limited, some birds will nest and others will not—there is no sharing of the resource. Space may be used preemptively by highly territorial species, and individuals unable to obtain a territory do little or no breeding. Other resources may be shared, for example, consumption of food by one individual reduces the amount available for all others, so that the misery of short supply may be shared (but not equally) by all.

If resources are unlimited, population size is likely to increase through a combination of increased reproduction and reduced mortality. The maximum (intrinsic) rate of increase is determined by the physiologic limits on reproduction of the species and by the point at which survival can no longer be increased by additional resources. The intrinsic rate of increase rarely is reached by wild species, except in the early stages of growth of a population in a new environment with abundant resources. For example, a small number of bison released in the MacKenzie Bison Sanctuary, Northwest Territories, Canada, increased at an intrinsic rate of 1.21 for some years (Gates and Larter 1990). Part of the success of newly introduced animals such as this group of bison may be that they benefit from "enemy release," that is, they are spared initially from the negative effect of predators and pathogens (Torchin et al. 2002). As the population density increases, the *per capita* availability of resources declines, the rate of increase slows, and eventually a level is reached at which population growth levels off. This level is often referred to as the "carrying capacity" (K). At this level, additions to the population through reproduction and immigration approximate losses through mortality and emigration. K is not a constant for a species nor is it static in an environment, but it represents a maximum population level consistent with the environmental conditions at the time. K is determined by limiting factors that cause the population to decline or that prevent it from increasing.

SPATIAL DISTRIBUTION

The spatial distribution of a population also is determined by the availability of resources. While we deal with averages when discussing populations, individual animals that make up the population do not live under "average" conditions. The area occupied by a species (its range) is not uniform. Some portions have abundant resources, other portions may have few resources. Usage of different parts of the range and the success of individuals that live there may be very different. This has given rise to the concept of "source" and "sink" areas. In a source area, reproduction is sufficient to more than offset mortality and extra animals disperse. In contrast, the population in a sink area may only be maintained through immigration. The spacing of animals and access to resources are influenced by social behavior. This is most obvious in highly territorial species but also occurs in less-obvious manners in which dominant individuals have greater access to resources that improve their survival and reproductive prospects. When population density is low, animals use the most favored habitat, but, as population density increases, a progressively larger proportion of the population will be forced to use less-favorable habitat.

Disease may interact with the distribution of animals in many ways. Disease may differentially affect those individuals occupying areas with marginal resources. A problem in studying the effect of disease on groups of animals, particularly on small areas, lies in knowing whether the animals being studied are in an area more typical of a source or a sink for the species. Disease may alter the social behavior of individual animals so that they are less competitive for favored areas. Occasionally, the distribution of an entire population may be limited by a single disease. For instance, Hawaiian honeycreepers are prevented from occupying lowland habitats by the presence of avian malaria (van Riper et al. 1986). Birds that try to use the lowland area die of the disease. Similarly, caribou may be prevented from repopulating areas in which *Parelaphostrongylus tenuis* is enzootic in white-tailed deer.

COMPOSITION IN TERMS OF SEX AND AGE

A population is composed of animals of both sexes and different ages. These individuals may have markedly different susceptibility to individual diseases, and the effects of disease on a population are greatly modified by its sex and age structure. In general, young animals are more susceptible than older animals to many infectious diseases, but exceptions occur, for example, juvenile European rabbits are much less susceptible than adults to rabbit hemorrhagic disease. Typically, the survival of young animals is much lower than that of adults. For example, among feral ferrets in New Zealand, the survival probability during the first year of life was 0.25, but that of animals >1 year of age was 0.55 year^{-1}, with an average life expectancy of 0.95 years (Caley et al. 2002).

In many diseases, the proportion of the population that has been exposed to the causative agent increases as a simple function of the length of exposure. For instance, moose less than 3 years of age, moose between 3 and 7 years, and moose older than 7 years had an average of 4.8, 10.6, and 34.6 hydatid cysts in their lungs, respectively (Rau and Caron 1979).

Exposure to some agents increases dramatically when animals become sexually mature because of the frequency and degree of social interaction associated with breeding. Some populations contain a large proportion of nonbreeding individuals, whereas others contain almost no nonbreeders. For instance, nonterritorial, nonbreeding individuals make up 2–4% of populations of song sparrows and >60% of mute swan populations (Newton 1998). Disease may alter the composition of a population, affecting its productivity. Dmowski et al. (2000) reported that one feature of a small mammal population exposed to heavy metal pollution was that it was "old," that is, it contained few young individuals because of heavy juvenile mortality.

The composition of a population may influence the effect and visibility of a disease. For instance, populations of seabirds are made up of many overlapping generations, and "dramatic losses due to a massive oil spill that might eliminate an entire age cohort of young birds may not be obvious if such losses are compensated by improved reproduction and survival of remaining birds, enhanced recruitment from a pool of non-breeders, or immigration from birds nesting in nearby colonies" (Burger and Gochfeld 2002).

LIFE HISTORY TRAITS

The life history of a species involves trade-offs between maximizing reproduction and maximizing survival. Wild species generally can be classified as r- or K-selected. Those that are r-selected (r = intrinsic rate of increase) emphasize high birth rates. They have a short lifespan, reproduce at an early age, and produce many offspring. They are generally but not always small, they have a high mortality rate, and individuals can be replaced rapidly through reproduction. Populations of r-selected species generally contain few nonbreeding individuals, and population size tends to be highly variable. Populations of r-selected species are generally resilient to factors that cause mortality. Moriarty et al. (2000) described a population of rabbits in Australia in which the annual mortality rate of adults was 82%. When 40% of the population disappeared during an outbreak of rabbit hemorrhagic disease, it was replaced within a few months through reproduction. The resilience of Australian rabbits to decreased reproduction will be discussed later in this chapter.

K-selected (K = carrying capacity) species emphasize survival. They have a long life span, breed for the first time at a relatively advanced age, and produce few young at each breeding. Their populations tend to have a stable age structure with many individuals that do not breed in any one season. In general, K-selected species are more vulnerable to factors that increase mortality than to factors that affect reproduction, particularly if the depression of reproduction is short term and can be "made up" later.

Even superficially similar species may have different life histories that affect their vulnerability to different diseases. For instance, among prairie-nesting ducks, mallards are r-selected and the population can increase rapidly through improved reproduction when ephemeral water conditions on the breeding grounds are suitable. Canvasbacks are K-selected and require long-term stability in wetland conditions. A disease may have very different effects on species based on their life history strategy. For example, lead poisoning acts primarily by causing mortality. Assuming equal exposure, the population effects of lead poisoning will be much greater on K-selected species such as canvasbacks (and even more so on condors) that cannot replace losses quickly than on mallards that can quickly replace birds that die.

LIMITATION, REGULATION, AND COMPENSATION

LIMITATION AND REGULATION

Populations are acted upon by many potential "limiting factors" (anything that causes the population to decline or that prevents it from increasing) including the supply of resources, climate and weather, predators, and disease agents. Usually one or a few factors are predominant. The abundance of wild animal populations in areas where breeding is not continuous is seasonally cyclic with an annual peak of numbers after the breeding season and then a decline to a minimum at the start of the next breeding season as a result of mortality (fig. 11.1). Populations could be measured at any point in the annual cycle, but the size of the breeding population (the minimum for the year) is the best measure of the combined effects of all factors that act on a population. To detect change over time, the population has to be measured at the same relative time during the annual cycle.

A population could be likened to water in a bucket. Each breeding season the bucket is filled partially or completely depending on the factors that affect reproduction that year. During the year, water trickles out through leaks (mortality factors) in the bucket. The amount of water in the bucket (the population size) depends upon when it is measured; how

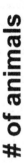

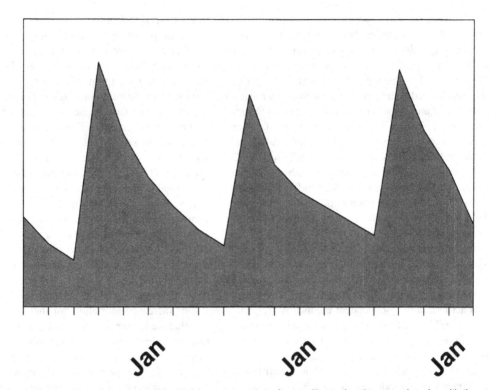

Fig. 11.1. Size of a hypothetical population of animals over a series of years illustrating the annual cycle, with the lowest population occurring just prior to breeding each year. The population might be measured at any time during the year. For example, in game animals the population size just before the hunting season might be of greatest concern, whereas the number of adults surviving to breed or the population just after breeding might be of greatest concern for conservation management and represents the outcome of all factors that act on reproduction and survival.

full the bucket was filled by reproduction to begin the year; and the number, size, and location of the leaks. The effect of one factor may be completely overshadowed by a stronger factor. If there is a very large leak located low down on the side of the bucket, that factor will be the predominant factor that limits population size and may obscure the effects of other leaks. For instance, during severe winters at northern latitudes, starvation seems to be a dominant limiting factor for deer. Winter conditions also determine the proportion of surviving does that successfully produce fawns the following spring and the subsequent survival of the fawns that are born through the following year. The relative size and location of the leaks (causes of mortality) change during the year and from year to year, and different mortality factors may be more important for males than for females, and for animals of different ages.

A limiting factor may act in an ultimate or a proximate manner, for example, if food shortage results in starvation, lack of food is both an ultimate and a proximate limiting factor. But if food shortage acts by increasing vulnerability to predation, lack of food may be the ultimate limiting factor while predation is the proximate cause of mortality. Similarly, food shortage might reduce resistance to infectious disease, which might kill animals directly, or increase their vulnerability to predation. Determining the proximate cause(s) of mortality (e.g., by examining dead animals) may not reveal the factor(s) that ultimately limit population size. Limiting factors do not act constantly or consistently, for example, food availability may be the predominant limiting factor for deer in northern latitudes during winter but not during summer, and food supply may be limiting in one winter and not in the next. Similarly, predation or parasitism may be less important in years with abundant food resources but become limiting when food is scarce.

One or a combination of limiting factors establish a population size that approximates K and the number of animals fluctuates about that level over time.

The number of some species may remain remarkably stable over decades. For example, the number of breeding pairs of golden eagles varied by only about ±15% from the mean over large areas of the United Kingdom (Newton 1979), and the number of wolves counted on a large area in Minnesota ranged between 35 and 54 (mean = 48) over 12 years (Mech and Goyal 1993). The population size of other species is remarkably variable. A population of eared grebes "collapsed" from 3.56 million in 1997 to 1.6 million in 1998 in association with an El Niño event and then rebounded to 3.27 million by 2000 (Jehl et al. 2002). The number of small-seed-eating birds may vary by a factor of 20 or more between years (Newton 1998).

Despite the variability that is evident in some species, populations do not increase indefinitely nor do they usually decrease to extinction. This has led to the concept of population "regulation" by factors that act in a density-dependent manner. A "regulating factor" is one that acts to cause population numbers to rise when they are low and to decrease when they are high. For instance, when the density of animals is low relative to food abundance, nutritional constraints on reproduction are slight and survival will likely be high. As the density of animals increases relative to the food supply, competition becomes increasingly intense and most animals suffer a degree of deprivation that affects fecundity and survival. The more dense the population becomes relative to food supply, the more intense the deprivation and the more severe the negative effects. Regulation may also occur through preemptive consumption (McPeek et al. 2001; Rodenhouse et al. 2003). At low population density, animals occupy territories in the optimal areas of habitat. As the population increases, a larger proportion of the population is forced to locate in progressively poorer habitat where it may be more vulnerable to predation or other mortality factors or have lower fecundity. Some animals are unable to establish a territory, and these individuals with "no fixed address" do not breed and have very poor survival (e.g., few nonterritorial red grouse or common shrews survive the winter) (Jenkins et al. 1963; Klok and De Roos 1998). In terms of disease, a regulating factor is one that reduces host survival or fecundity at an increasing rate as host abundance increases (Spratt 1990).

Some factors such as predation and food supply may be both limiting and regulating. Factors such as mortality of birds as a result of spraying of forest with insecticide are generally considered not to be regulatory because the *density* of birds is unlikely to affect the *proportion* of the population that is killed. However, poisoning could be limiting, at least in a local area. The effect of limiting and regulating factors on population size has been likened to temperature control in a room. The average temperature (equivalent to population size) is determined by a limiting factor (the householder who adjusts the thermostat to her taste). Regardless of whether the thermostat is set at 15°C or 25°C, the furnace is switched on when the temperature falls below the set value. The more the temperature has fallen below the set value, the longer the furnace runs. When the temperature rises above the thermostat setting, the furnace shuts off and an air conditioner might start to lower the temperature. In this analogy, the furnace and the air conditioner are regulating factors that act to return the temperature to a level set by a limiting factor.

Many diseases cause decreased reproduction and/or increased mortality, but there are relatively few that are known to have acted as a limiting factor that held a population at a level substantially lower than its usual K level for an extended period of time (table 11.1). It is interesting that the infectious diseases in table 11.1 are caused by either recently introduced agents (rinderpest in African game animals, malaria in Hawaiian birds, myxomatosis in rabbits) or multihost diseases that seem to be limiting the population of a species that is not important for maintenance of the agent (e.g., *Heterakis gallinarum* in the grey partridge). It is generally assumed that most infectious diseases act in a density-dependent manner as regulating factors, but there are few empirical data from field studies to confirm this.

If the population size and density are held below K by some factor other than resource limitation, or if the population is reduced to below K by a sudden large mortality event, such as a severe winter, the survivors may have more resources *per capita* and respond by greater reproduction and/or improved survival. The population of harbor seals in the Wadden Sea was limited by hunting at a level substantially < K until the 1960s and 1970s when hunting was prohibited (Härkönen 2003). When released from this limiting factor, the population increased exponentially until 1988, when 58% of the population died during an epizootic caused by phocine distemper virus. Subsequent to the epizootic, another period of exponential growth occurred until a second epizootic killed >50% of the population in 2002. Based on the shape of growth curve of this population, the epizootics occurred prior to the population reaching K.

Table 11.1 Diseases That Limit Size of a Wild Population Below Carrying Capacity for an Extended Period (Years)

Disease or agent	Species affected	Mechanism
Plasmodium relictum	Hawaiian honeycreepers	Increased mortality[1]
Rinderpest virus	Cape buffalo	Increased mortality[2]
Mercury from seed dressings	Gallinaceous and raptorial birds	Increased mortality[3]
Organochlorine insecticides	Peregrine falcon	Suppressed reproduction[4]
Sarcoptes scabei	Coyotes	Increased mortality[5]
Myxomatosis	European rabbit	Increased mortality[6]
Heterakis gallinarum	Grey partridge	Increased mortality, reduced fecundity[7]
Heavy metal pollution	Small mammals	Increased mortality[8]
Mycoplasma gallisepticum	House finch	Increased mortality[9]

[1]van Riper et al. (1986).
[2]Sinclair (1977).
[3]Borg et al. (1969).
[4]Cade et al. (1988).
[5]Pence and Ueckermann (2002).
[6]Kerr and Best (1998).
[7]Tompkins et al. (2000).
[8]Dmowski et al. (2000).
[9]Hochachka and Dhondt (2000).

COMPENSATION

A factor that complicates assessing the effect of disease on wild populations is the possibility of "compensation." The basic notion underlying the compensation hypothesis is that when the density of a population is reduced by one cause, the surviving members are less affected by other density-dependent factors (food limitation, predation, infection, etc.) and may enjoy better reproduction and/or survival. To illustrate the idea, assume that the "natural" annual mortality rate of a population is 50%. A specific disease enters the population and causes a mortality rate of 10%. If there were complete compensation, the total mortality rate would remain at 50%, because the mortality from other causes would be reduced to compensate for that caused by the disease. If there were no compensation, the mortality would be additive, and the total mortality rate would be 60%. (This concept is discussed more fully by Caley et al. 2002.) Compensation could take a variety of forms (table 11.2).

The concept of compensation of the type outlined above is not considered when disease in human or domestic animals is discussed. I have never heard a veterinarian say anything such as "the high mortality caused by brooder pneumonia in this chicken flock is not so bad, because it means proportionately less chickens will die of coccidiosis later." We know

Table 11.2 Compensation for the Effects of Disease at the Population Level

Effect of disease	Potential compensatory response by survivors
Increased mortality	Improved survival (reduced mortality to other causes)
	Increased reproduction
	Improved survival and increased reproduction
Decreased reproduction	Improved survival
	Increased reproduction by nonaffected adults
	Improved survival and increased reproduction

Note: The underlying hypothesis is that if the number of animals in a population is reduced by disease and resources remain constant, the surviving members of the population enjoy more resources per capita and respond by improved survival and/or reproduction.

relatively little about compensation for disease mortality, but there is evidence that mortality as a result of another factor, hunting, may be compensated for by reduced mortality from other causes in wild animals. There has been a keen search to establish how many game animals can be removed by hunting, or how many fish can be harvested, without affecting the breeding population. Density-dependent reproduction usually is not considered within the compensatory mortality theory as it relates to hunting, although Potts (1986) found that the reproductive rate increased in hunted populations of grey partridge. Although hunting is a much larger cause of mortality than disease in most hunted species, there is still controversy as to whether mortality from hunting is compensatory or additive to other causes of mortality. Ellison (1991) reviewed evidence for compensation among grouse species and concluded that compensation for hunting mortality occurs in some but not all species. For example, killing of approximately 18% of male ruffed grouse was compensated for by reduced mortality from other causes. Despite a massive amount of study, it is still unclear to what level hunting mortality in mallards should be considered compensatory (Johnson et al. 1997; Pöysä et al. 2004).

Compensation was demonstrated clearly in a study of experimentally induced reproductive dysfunction in European rabbits in Australia. Over a 5-year period, Twigg et al. (2000) surgically sterilized 0%, 40%, 60%, and 80% of free-ranging female rabbits on replicated large plots and compared the demographic effects. This might be comparable in effect to different prevalences of severe and prolonged reproductive disease. There was a marked decrease in the number of young produced on areas with a high proportion of sterilized females, but this "was overcome by increased survival of kittens and adults on the high-sterility areas, such that the base-level numbers of rabbits were maintained." The seasonal peaks in abundance were lower on the areas with high sterility, but the number of rabbits at the end of the experiment was similar across sites. Although the results were complicated somewhat by greater immigration to the sites with a high level of sterilization, there was clear evidence of a compensatory decline in "natural" mortality on areas with poor reproduction.

Some authors have considered that many conditions caused by infectious agents are subject to compensation by other mortality factors (Holmes 1982; Gregory and Keymer 1989), but empirical evidence for compensation for mortality caused by disease in wild animals is sparse. Forchhammer and Asferg (2000) compared 14 fox populations in Denmark, 7 of which were infected with sarcoptic mange. Direct density dependence was evident in all of the noninfected groups, but none of the mange-exposed populations displayed density dependence. The authors attributed this to reduced competition for territories following mortality caused by mange.

If compensation occurs, it is most likely to occur in species that have a high natural rate of mortality such as the European rabbit. Species with a low mortality rate may have less ability to compensate. The timing of mortality within the annual population cycle also may have an effect on the potential for compensation. If mortality occurs shortly after the seasonal peak of abundance, there is an extended period during which compensation might act, compared to mortality that occurred just prior to breeding.

Other factors may obscure population effects of disease. For instance, Klok and De Roos (1998) suggested that high "normal" mortality associated with competition for territory in common shrews might obscure any effect of heavy metal pollution, so long as the lifetime reproductive success of individuals was adequate to replace them. In badgers, only one female in a hierarchical group breeds. If that female died as a result of a disease, another adult female in the group replaces her, so that reproductive output of the group would remain more or less constant (Klok et al. 2000).

Some species, and particularly those at northern latitudes, including some birds, rodents, and larger mammals appear to have multiyear cyclic changes in population. The causes of many of these cyclic changes are poorly understood and may be multifactorial. However, treatment of red grouse populations with anthelmintics to reduce infection by *Trichostrongylus tenuis* prevented population crashes (Hudson et al. 1998) indicating that this agent has a role in at least some cyclic population changes. Modeling, based partially on a study of anthelmintic treatment of snowshoe hares that showed that parasitism increased vulnerability to predation, led to the conclusion that sublethal parasitism acted to destabilize population dynamics and make cycles more likely (Ives and Murray 1997). Cavanagh et al. (2004) found that the prevalence of two infections (cowpox virus and vole tuberculosis caused by *Mycobacterium microti*) increased in cyclic vole populations as the number of voles rose and peaked as the number of voles declined. They suggested that the diseases were involved in the population cycles although the mechanism was unclear.

MEASURING A POPULATION EFFECT

Except under very unusual circumstances, it is impossible to count entire populations of wild animals or to monitor them continuously. We usually are only able to estimate the number of animals on a defined area at a specific time of year. This has important implications when we come to interpret the role of various factors, including disease, in determining population size and structure. The smaller the study area, in relation to the entire area occupied by the population, the more important immigration and emigration are in determining the number of animals present. Failure to measure dispersal is more critical on small than on large areas and can lead to over or underestimation of the importance of reproduction and mortality in influencing local population trends. Many factors that influence population are not equally active at all times of year, for example, food shortage at high latitudes is usually a winter problem while in arid areas, summer drought may be important. If these seasonal effects are not considered, the effects of disease may also be over- or underestimated. Ecologists and wildlife managers may be concerned about the number of individuals in the population at different times of year (e.g., in hunted species the number of animals in autumn when animals are traditionally hunted may be important). From a population perspective, the number that survive to breed the following year is usually the critical value because it is the lowest point of the year and it determines the future additions to the population.

To understand the effect of disease on a population, the population will have to be studied over the long-term. Two studies that have demonstrated a regulatory effect of disease on a wild population were done over 6 and 8 years (Albon et al. 2002; Hudson et al. 1992b, respectively). An inherent problem of long-term studies is that the degree of variability tends to increase with the length of time a population is studied (Newton 1998). This may occur for two reasons: (1) the more years a population is followed, the greater the chance of including an unusual year, and (2) year-to-year variation may be superimposed on long-term trends in population, either up or down, perhaps related to improvement or decline in habitat quality or climate change.

DO DISEASES REALLY AFFECT POPULATIONS?

I believe that we can safely assume that disease in its plurality and various forms affects populations.

However, what we usually want to know is: Does disease X affect this population? In asking this question, we must be careful to define what we want to know. First of all, what is the population in question? Is it the group of mallards on a large staging area, the subpopulation of mallards breeding in the prairie pothole region, or the entire North American mallard population? Second, when is the effect to be measured? Is autumn prior to the hunting season, midwinter, or just prior to breeding the appropriate time to measure the population? These questions are important because a disease might affect a portion of a population but not have a detectable effect on the entire population, or might affect the dynamics of what happens in the population without affecting the end result (the size of the breeding population).

We might rephrase the question to: Would there be more animals in the population if disease X did not exist? In other words, is disease X limiting the population? This is not an academic question, because management actions are taken to reduce the effects of disease in the belief that the actions will increase wild populations. For example, about $1 million was spent each year by wildlife agencies in western Canada during the 1990s to pick up duck carcasses during botulism outbreaks in the belief that this would increase duck populations. While it is clear that many ducks die of botulism on individual wetlands, and there is some evidence to suggest that survival until the hunting season is lower among ducks from wetlands where botulism occurred than on wetlands without botulism, there currently are no data to show that botulism has an affect on spring breeding populations or on the continental duck population. In other situations, management is done to reduce or eliminate a disease for reasons other than to increase the population (such as to reduce risk to humans) without a clear understanding of the potential population effects. We might pose many questions such as:

If rabies were eliminated from fox and raccoon populations through vaccination, would the population size and density of these species increase?

If endocrine-disrupting chemicals were to be eliminated, would there be even more gulls and double-crested cormorants on the Great Lakes of North America?

If brucellosis and tuberculosis could be eliminated from bison in Wood Buffalo National Park, would there be more bison in the park?

NONINFECTIOUS DISEASES

Some noninfectious agents can have a dramatic effect on populations of wild animals (table 11.1). This may be a result of a negative effect on reproduction, such as the effect of DDT and its metabolites on certain raptorial and piscivorous birds, or of increased mortality as occurred with mercury poisoning of game birds and some raptors in Sweden (Borg et al. 1969) and small mammals near heavy metal smelters (Dmowski et al. 2000). Both depressed reproduction and increased mortality may be involved in some noninfectious conditions, for example, "massive declines in the numbers of some bird-eating and fish-eating raptors, which occurred in Europe and North America in the 1960s, were thus attributed to the combined action of DDE reducing breeding rate and HEOD (from aldrin and dieldrin) increasing mortality rate" (Newton 1998). Many other noninfectious factors either influence reproduction (e.g., calcium deficiency in small birds in acidified and naturally deficient areas; Tilgar et al. 2002) or cause mortality (e.g., lead, cholinesterase-inhibiting pesticides, neoplasia, degenerative joint disease), but their actual effect on total population size is largely unknown. This is true even for agents such as lead shot and the insecticide carbofuran that may have killed millions of birds per year. Very little is known about the effect of compensation through reduction of losses to other density-dependent factors among animals exposed to harmful compounds, although there is some evidence that it may occur. In Britain, production of young by sparrowhawks and peregrine falcons "could be reduced to less than half its normal level without causing a decline in breeding numbers" (Newton 1998) because of improved survival and earlier breeding by the remaining young.

Until recently there has been relatively little interest in trying to determine how various agents such as toxicants fit within the complex array of factors that limit and regulate populations. This will be critical for understanding factors such as endocrine-disrupting chemicals that are assumed to have sublethal effects on individuals. In the past, toxicologists have concentrated on determining the effects on individual animals, measured in terms such as the 96-hour lethal concentration for 50% of a group (LC_{50}), and on measuring residue levels without determining the effects on populations in wild animals. The existing paradigm is that individual-based findings, such as LC_{50}, accurately predict population consequences. Newman (2001) argued for a para-

digm shift to one that used population growth rate as a yardstick and that incorporated factors such as life history traits to assess the effect of toxicants. There also is a "virtual lack of long-lived species in tests of the effects of toxic chemicals on individuals and populations" (Laskowski 2000).

The general belief seems to be that factors such as toxicants operate in a non-density-dependent manner. The assumption is that exposure and susceptibility are uniform or random in the population and that these are not influenced by population density. However, at high population density, proportionately more of the population may occupy less-favorable habitat. If one feature of unfavorable habitat is elevated contaminant levels or reduced availability of a required nutrient such as calcium, the effect on the population will be, at least partially, density dependent. It also is reasonable to believe that animals disadvantaged by density-dependent features such as food deprivation or infectious agents may be more susceptible to some noninfectious agents. Noninfectious agents may interact with other factors in complex ways that make these factors either more or less important. Laskowski (2000) argued that consideration of density dependence may be of particular importance in studying the effect of sublethal toxicants on organisms with a high reproductive potential.

INFECTIOUS DISEASES

Disease caused by microparasites such as the morbilliviruses causing phocine and canine distemper and rinderpest, *Yersinia pestis*, *Francisella tularensis*, the oribiviruses causing hemorrhagic disease of deer, and the bacteria involved in pneumonia epizootics in wild sheep can cause extensive mortality with a dramatic reduction in the size of the affected group for a period of time. Some disease agents have depressed large populations below the apparent carrying capacity for an extended period of time. For instance, the number of African buffalo was maintained at very low levels for decades because of the presence of rinderpest virus (Sinclair 1977), and the number of Australian rabbits has been depressed by myxoma virus for more than half a century (Kerr and Best 1998). With many other epizootic diseases, such as avian cholera in wild waterfowl, there may be high mortality in local groups or subpopulations, but whether this translates into a reduced breeding population the following year has not been established. The effect of microparasites that occur enzootically on populations is much less clear, even though these agents may cause decreased reproduction and/or mortality of individuals. May (1994) maintained that disease can be the primary regulatory factor even when it is only responsible for a small proportion of deaths. Anderson (1995) demonstrated how a hypothetical viral infection could regulate a fox population (in a model), but there is no clearly documented field evidence of a disease caused by a microparasite in which this has occurred (Tompkins et al. 2001a). Detecting the effects of any disease at the population level will require intervention experiments in which the population can be monitored carefully before and following the reduction or removal of a disease agent. This experiment is being done across huge areas of Europe and North America through vaccination of fox populations for rabies. Although there has been no general assessment, there are indications that fox populations have increased in areas in which rabies has been eliminated (Chautan et al. 2000; Gloor et al. 2001; Damien et al. 2002) suggesting that this disease may have been limiting the population.

Ebert et al. (2000a) reported a series of experiments in which the effects of six different microparasites on a host population were assessed. The trial system used a monoclonal strain of *Daphnia magna* as the host and a constant supply of food so that the effects of genetic variability in resistance and nutrition were eliminated. The disease agents included two species of bacteria, a fungus, and three species of microsporidian parasite. One of the microsporidians was transmitted vertically, and the remainder were transmitted horizontally. Fecundity, mortality, and population abundance were measured. Some agents had severe effects on fecundity of individual hosts and others caused extensive mortality. Five of the six agents reduced host population abundance, and some of the agents drove the population to extinction. Although this study involved a situation that was highly artificial and that lacked most of the potential interacting factors that modulate the effects of any single agent, it demonstrated that the effects of microparasites seen at the individual level can be transferred to the population level.

In the past it was assumed that macroparasites did not have a regulatory influence on host populations. The aggregated distribution of most macroparasite populations (Shaw et al. 1998) has been a factor that has made it difficult to believe that a parasite can influence a population when most of the host population has few or no parasites, and only a few animals are heavily parasitized. However, Anderson and May (1978) and May and Anderson (1978) demonstrated in a simple mathematical model that regula-

tion could occur if the agent reduced host survival or host fecundity in a density-dependent manner. There have been suggestions that parasites such as the hookworm *Ancylostomum caninum* in coyotes (Pence et al. 1988) may be a regulating factor, and there are a number of experimental studies (reviewed by Tompkins et al. 2001a), in which experimental manipulation of the "parasite load" has demonstrated that parasites can affect fecundity or survival. A study of *Trichostrongylus tenuis* infection in red grouse (Hudson et al. 1998) has clearly demonstrated a regulatory effect, primarily as a result of reduced fecundity rather than increased mortality, although both effects occurred. Albon et al. (2002) found that an abomasal nematode (*Ostertagia gruehneri*) also regulated a population of reindeer through reducing fecundity rather than by decreasing survival. Declines in the population of house finches across large parts of eastern North America associated with conjunctivitis caused by *Mycoplasma gallisepticum* infection suggest that this disease acts in a density-dependent manner (Hochachka and Dhondt 2000). Aldo Leopold recognized more than 70 years ago that if infectious diseases act in a density-dependent manner, wildlife managers have a dilemma because "a high density of population—the very thing the game manager is so far seeking—must be set down as the fundamental condition favorable for disease" (Leopold 1933).

EFFECTS ON SMALL POPULATIONS

There is special concern about the effect that disease may have on small populations (Lafferty and Gerber 2002; Altizer et al. 2003) and that disease might be a factor leading to extinction. This will become an ever-greater concern in the future as continued growth of the human population puts greater pressure on natural habitats, and more and more wild species exist as isolated groups on "islands" of habitat. In considering the potential role of disease on such groups, it may be helpful to think of the factors as having a deterministic or a stochastic effect (Newton 1998). Deterministic effects result from something happening outside the animal population from which there is no escape, such as addition or loss of something from the environment. Examples might include addition of domestic animals that harbor a multihost parasite to an island situation, addition of a toxic contaminant, or decline in the availability of a required nutrient such as calcium because of acidification. Stochastic effects are those that involve an element of chance, such as a weather event. Disease could act in both manners.

Some diseases might be a direct cause of population extinction. For example, the black-footed ferret had a very close brush with extinction because of canine distemper carried by other wild carnivores from which there was no escape. Similarly, the population of the peregrine falcon disappeared from the eastern United States as a result of inability to escape the effects of DDE (Cade et al. 1988). Logiudice (2003) has presented convincing evidence that *Baylisascaris procyonis*, the roundworm of raccoons, caused or contributed to the extirpation of the Allegheny wood rat from parts of its range. Disease might also act by decreasing the ability of population to respond to other factors either by acting as a chronic stressor or by reducing resources available for coping. In general, small populations have a greater risk of extinction from stochastic events than large populations.

Certain types of infectious disease are more likely than others to cause a problem in small populations. Single-host diseases with a short infectious period are unlikely to persist in a small population because of the lack of a supply of new susceptible animals. Agents that have a long infectious period, such as *Mycobacterium bovis*, may be able to persist in small populations (which is bad news for those trying to eliminate tuberculosis in wild species). Multihost organisms that can persist in more abundant species are particularly a problem. Examples of this phenomenon include the impact of malaria carried by introduced birds on native Hawaiian birds (van Riper et al. 1986) and canine distemper carried by dogs on Ethiopian wolves (Laurenson et al. 1998) and African wild dogs (Alexander and Appel 1994). Many such problems are related to agents carried by domestic species, but Logiudice (2003) warned of the risks from disease maintained in "human-adapted" wild animals, such as raccoons, that thrive in disturbed environments.

Genetic problems in small populations might lead to or interact with disease. Inbreeding may lead to reduced fecundity or survival of young (so-called inbreeding depression). Loss of genetic variance also might result in loss of resistance to disease. Acevedo-Whitehouse et al. (2003) proposed that inbreeding increased susceptibility of California sea lions to infectious diseases, and that inbred individuals could "act disproportionately as reservoirs of infectious agents." If disease agents disappear from small populations, there is a possibility that resistance to these agents may also be lost (because they have no selective advantage in the absence of the disease), making the population highly susceptible should the agent be reintroduced. Disease might also cause a population to decline in size to the point at which genetic diversity is lost. Trudeau et al. (2004) documented reduced genetic diversity in isolated populations of black-tailed prairie dogs that were recovering from population bottlenecks caused by plague outbreaks.

SUMMARY

- A population is a "a group of individuals of the same species that live together in an area of sufficient size to permit normal dispersal and/or migration behavior and in which numerical changes are largely determined by birth and death processes" (Berryman 2002).

- Population abundance is the result of four processes: reproduction, immigration, mortality, and emigration. Disease may influence any of these.

- Most wild populations undergo seasonal changes in abundance. The breeding population may be the most useful measure of population size, as it incorporates all the components of reproductive success and survival over an entire year.

- The effect of a disease on the population might be compensated for by either reduced mortality from other causes or by increased reproduction, but the extent of compensation that occurs is unknown.

- Timing of a disease occurrence in the seasonal cycle may have a great effect on the ability for compensation to occur.

- A limiting factor is anything that causes the population to decline or prevents it from increasing.

- A regulating factor acts to cause population numbers to rise when they are low and to decrease when they are high, that is, it acts in a density-dependent manner. In terms of disease, a regulating factor reduces host survival and/or fecundity at an increasing rate as host abundance increases.

- It is assumed that most infectious diseases act in a density-dependent manner, but empirical proof of this is scant.

- Disease may cause special difficulties for small populations. The greatest risk from infectious agents is from multihost diseases maintained in other more abundant species.

- Population levels usually are not determined by one factor acting in isolation. Disease acts together with other population-limiting factors, particularly nutrition and predation.

12
Disease Shared with Humans and Domestic Animals

As the population of the world continues to expand in a logarithmic fashion, species are thrust into new environments, with all the attendant possibilities for exposure to, and dissemination of novel infectious agents.
—B. W. J. Mahy and C. C. Brown

Many infectious diseases that occur in wild animals are considered to be important because they are a risk to humans and/or domestic animals rather than because of the effect that they may have on wild animals. Rabies is a prime example of this phenomenon. For centuries rabies was thought of as a disease of domestic dogs, and it was only when dog rabies was controlled by vaccination of pets and control of stray dogs that it became evident that rabies virus also was circulating in wild animals. Rabies always had been cycling in wild animals, but this had not been recognized because the great majority of human cases could be linked to a bite from a "mad" dog. When that risk was removed, the much smaller risk of being bitten by a rabid fox, skunk, raccoon, mongoose, or bat became evident, and billions of dollars have been spent attempting to control wildlife rabies. Without the risk to humans and domestic animals, there would have been no effort to manage this disease.

The word "zoonoses" is derived from the Greek (*zoon*, animal, *noses*, disease) and is used for diseases shared by animals and humans or, more specifically, infectious diseases that are transmitted naturally between humans and animals. The singular form of the word is *zoonosis* and the adjective is *zoonotic*, as in zoonotic disease. There is no equivalent word that describes diseases that are shared between wild and domestic animals. A huge number of diseases are shared between humans and animals, and many infections that generally are thought of as uniquely human diseases developed from diseases of animals.

It has been proposed that *Mycobacterium tuberculosis*, the cause of human tuberculosis, is evolutionarily young (Sreevatsan et al. 1997) and may have evolved from *M. bovis* at approximately the time cattle were domesticated about 15,000 years ago (Stead et al. 1995; Small and Selcer 2000). However, based on analysis of the genome of *Mycobacterium* spp., Brosch et al. (2002) concluded that *M. tuberculosis* did not evolve from *M. bovis* and that both developed from a common ancestor. The human immunodeficiency viruses (HIV) that cause AIDS are of more recent animal origin, with HIV-1 having evolved from a chimpanzee variant of simian immunodeficiency virus (SIV) and HIV-2 having evolved from a SIV of the sooty mangabey monkey. Bogerd et al. (2004) suggested that "the biological barrier preventing the entry of additional SIV into the human population as zoonotic infections is potentially quite fragile." As indicated in the quotation at the beginning of this chapter, one can anticipate that many new diseases will emerge as wild animals, domestic animals, and humans come into contact in new ways. Details on individual diseases are beyond the scope of this book, but there are excellent reference texts dealing with zoonoses (Beran and Steele 1994; Palmer et al. 1998) and with the zoonotic diseases that occur in wild animals (Williams and Barker 2001; Samuel et al. 2001).

The line between humans and animals is unambiguous, although the type and intensity of contact between the two groups are constantly shifting. In contrast, the separation between wild and domestic animals is vague, uncertain, and shifting continuously. Wild animals move in and out of captivity, and domestic animals become feral. For example, in many areas there are both farmed and free-living cervids with wild animals being captured and entering the domestic pool and escapees from behind a fence becoming wild animals. Even with our traditional domestic animals, free-living animals of the same species may cohabit an area (e.g., both the fat white domestic Pekin duck and the wild mallard are *Anas platyrhynchos* and will freely interbreed). This often confuses the discussion about where a disease may have originated and in which direction transmission is proceeding.

The first step in considering any disease that wild animals may share with humans or domestic animals is to clarify the role that the different species play in the ecology of the disease. It is useful to recall a few definitions that were discussed in previous chapters. A reservoir is "one or more epidemiologically connected populations or environments in which the pathogen can be permanently maintained" (Haydon et al. 2002). The reservoir might be one or more animal species or it might be some abiotic feature of the environment, such as the soil. Animals that become infected with the disease can usually be classified into one of three types:

1. *Maintenance hosts* are those in which the disease agent is capable of cycling independently within the population in the absence of external sources of infection ($R_0 \geq 1$).
2. *Spillover hosts* are those in which the disease can be transmitted within the population but will die out without an external source of infection ($0 < R_0 < 1$).
3. *Dead-end hosts* are those in which the disease is not transmitted within the population and infections result from introductions from an external source ($R_0 = 0$) (Caley et al. 2002).

Thus, in western Canada the striped skunk is the maintenance host for rabies, domestic dogs are a potential spillover host, and cattle are a dead-end host.

It is not possible to list or discuss all the zoonoses that involve wild animals or all the diseases shared by domestic and wild animals, so I have grouped diseases and given examples of each on the basis of the role that the different species play in the ecology of the disease. Certain diseases turn up repeatedly, reflecting their ability to infect a variety of species and to be transmitted by several different routes. My general groupings are as follows:

- Shared diseases with an abiotic reservoir
- Zoonoses for which wild animals are the principal reservoir
- Zoonotic diseases maintained in both wild and domestic animals
- Zoonoses in which humans are the maintenance host
- Disease shared by wild and domestic animals

SHARED DISEASES WITH AN ABIOTIC RESERVOIR

Shared diseases with an abiotic reservoir are not transmitted among animals, but may infect many species. By most definitions, these are not truly zoonoses but they deserve mention because there is sometimes confusion as to the role that wild animals play in their ecology. Several diseases caused by fungi (including *Aspergillus* spp., *Haplosporangium* spp., *Blastomyces* spp. and *Coccidiodes* spp.) and some bacterial diseases (including tetanus and gas gangrene caused by *Clostridium* spp.) fall into this group. It is important to know that although wild animals may be infected, they play no role in transmitting these infections to humans. The fungus *Histoplasma capsulatum* is interesting. Infection occurs in dogs and humans, as well as sporadically in many other mammals, as a respiratory disease. Infection is acquired through inhalation of spores from the soil. Wild birds are not infected with the fungus, but they play a role in the ecology of the disease because the major habitat for the fungus is in soil enriched with bird droppings, such as under blackbird and starling roosts.

ZOONOSES FOR WHICH WILD ANIMALS ARE THE PRINCIPAL RESERVOIR

There are two groups within this category: diseases in which the infection is transmitted directly from wild animals to humans, and diseases in which the infection is transmitted from wild animals to domestic animals and then secondarily to humans. Although I have separated the two processes, in many diseases both routes of infection may occur.

ZOONOSES TRANSMITTED DIRECTLY FROM WILD ANIMALS TO HUMANS

There are many diseases maintained by different routes of transmission in wild animals that spill over to humans (table 12.1). These diseases are dependent upon the wildlife hosts for maintenance so that if the disease needs to be managed the management could be directed at either preventing contact between humans and the wild species or at controlling the disease in the wild animals.

More is known about many of these diseases than about almost any other type of disease in wild animals. As the diseases are studied in detail, they inevitably have been found to be more complex than initially believed. This increasing complexity is evident in our understanding of rabies. When I was a

Table 12.1 Zoonotic Diseases Maintained in Wild Animals

Human disease (agent)	Wild species involved	Major route(s) of transmission to humans
Viruses		
Australian lyssavirus infection	Bats	Bite wounds
Hantavirus Pulmonary syndrome (Sin Nombre virus)	Deer mouse	Inhalation of virus from rodent excreta
Hemorrhagic fever with renal syndrome (Puumala virus)	Bank vole	Inhalation of virus from rodent excreta
Rabies (rabies virus)	Fox, skunk, raccoon, bat plus many others	Bite wounds
West Nile fever (West Nile virus)	Birds	Mosquito
Bacteria		
Bartenellosis (Bartenella spp.)	Rodents	Fleas (?)
Chlamydia (Chlamydophila psittaci)	Birds	Inhalation of dried excrement
Ehrlichiosis (Ehrlichia chaffeensis, E. ewingii)	White-tailed deer	Ticks
Lyme borreliosis (Borrelia burgdorferi)	Rodents	Ticks
Plague (Yersinia pestis)	Rodents	Rodent fleas, direct contact
Tularemia (Francisella tularensis)	Rodents, lagomorphs	Ticks, biting flies, water, direct contact
Helminths		
Alveolar hydatid disease (Echinococcus multilocularis)	Fox	Ingestion of parasite eggs
Hydatid disease (Echinococcus granulosus)	Wolf, fox, coyote, dingo	Ingestion of parasite eggs
Metorchis conjunctus infection	Fish-eating mammals	Ingestion of inadequately cooked fish
Trichinellosis (Trichinella spiralis, T. nativa)	Bears, marine mammals	Ingestion of inadequately cooked meat
Visceral larva migrans (Baylisascaris procyonis)	Raccoons	Ingestion of parasite eggs

veterinary student, I was taught that there was one strain of rabies in nature that was usually called "street" rabies to differentiate it from vaccine strains; this strain was believed to occur wherever the disease occurred. We now know that there are many different types or strains of rabies virus that can be distinguished using monoclonal antibody and molecular techniques. The existence of these strains is of more than academic interest because each strain is maintained within the population of a single major wild animal host. For instance, in Canada one strain of rabies is maintained in striped skunks in the prairie provinces; another strain is maintained in foxes in northern Canada, Ontario, and Quebec; a third strain maintained in raccoons has recently entered Canada from the United States; and several

strains occur in insectivorous bats across Canada. All of these strains can cause fatal disease in species other than their "usual" host (including humans), but these spillover and dead-end hosts play little or no role in maintaining the disease. Similar complexity occurs in rabies in some other areas of the world. Understanding the host-specificity of the virus involved is critical for any management of rabies.

In table 12.1, Sin Nombre, Puumala, and Lassa viruses are representative of a large group of diseases called the "rodent-borne hemorrhagic fevers," a general term applied to zoonotic diseases caused by an ever-increasing collection of hantaviruses and arenaviruses carried by rodents (Mills and Childs 2001). Most of these viruses are associated with one rodent species in a particular location. The viruses generally cause chronic asymptomatic infection in the rodent host with long-term shedding of virus in secretions and excretions. Humans usually become infected through inhalation of aerosols containing virus from these secretions and excreta. Old World hantaviruses such as Hantaan and Puumala viruses cause the human disease called "hemorrhagic fever with renal syndrome." The severity of the human infection is highly variable with mortality rates ranging from <1% with Puumala virus to 15–30% with Dobrova virus (Mills and Childs 2001). New World hantaviruses, the first of which to be recognized was Sin Nombre virus, cause "hantavirus pulmonary syndrome" characterized by acute onset of severe respiratory distress and a high case fatality rate. Mills and Childs (2001) list 27 different hantaviruses, of which 14 are known to cause human disease, and only 7 of which were known to science prior to 1994. Arenaviruses also are found in both the Old and New World. Mills and Childs (2001) describe 14 arenaviruses, of which 5 are known to cause human disease. The best known is Lassa virus that causes Lassa fever in West Africa and is carried by *Mastomys* spp. rodents. Other diseases caused by arenaviruses include Argentinean, Bolivian, and Venezuelan hemorrhagic fevers, each with its own rodent host, and lymphocytic choriomeningitis, which is associated with house mice throughout the world.

West Nile fever, western equine encephalitis, Colorado tick fever, and yellow fever are representative of a very large group of zoonoses (see table 12.1) caused by agents known collectively as "arboviruses" (abbreviated from arthropod-borne viruses). As an indication of the importance and complexity of the group, Beran and Steele (1994) devote over 270 pages of text to these viruses. The group contains viruses from eight different virus families, and most use wild birds or mammals as maintenance hosts. These vertebrate hosts develop high levels of virus in their circulating blood, and blood-feeding arthropods (primarily mosquitoes and ticks) become infected and are true vectors of the viruses. The normal course is that the virus is transmitted by the arthropod back to another natural host, but, occasionally, humans and domestic animals become infected if they are fed on by infected arthropods. In many cases there is little or no detectable disease in the usual wild animal host. West Nile virus is unusual because of its high pathogenicity for some species of birds, such as corvids (Caffrey et al. 2003).

A number of important bacterial zoonoses also are transmitted by arthropods (fleas, ticks, and biting flies) including plague, tularemia, Lyme disease, Rocky Mountain spotted fever, and ehrlichiosis. Some of these diseases have been recognized for many years, and others such as infections with *Bartonella* spp. have been discovered only recently (Kosoy et al. 2003).

Wildlife workers may be at greater risk of exposure to many arthropod-borne diseases than the average member of the public because of the amount of time spent in the field as well as because they may be working in close contact with wild animals and thus have greater exposure to sessile ectoparasites such as mites and fleas.

ZOONOSES TRANSMITTED INDIRECTLY TO HUMANS THROUGH DOMESTIC ANIMALS

A number of zoonotic agents may be transmitted from a reservoir in one or more wild species to a domestic species (in which the disease cannot be maintained) and then to humans. This process occurs in rabies. Although rabies is no longer actively circulating in dogs in most developed countries, dogs and cats remain an important intermediary between rabid wild animals and humans because these pets are likely to contact sick or dead wild animals and then come into intimate contact with their owners. Most pet owners are likely to comfort a sick cat or dog, but few would allow a sick fox or skunk to come so close. Domestic cattle also may be an intermediary for rabies. Because they are curious, cattle often investigate sick animals and are bitten. Rabies is not rare in cattle in areas where the disease is enzootic in wild animals. The most common human contact with rabid cows is by veterinarians. The early signs of rabies are nonspecific, and many veterinarians have been exposed while doing a clinical examination of a cow that subsequently was found to have rabies. Pet animals in areas where rabies occurs and humans at a high risk of exposure to rabid animals should have up-to-date rabies immunization.

Another example of this type of transmission occurs with plague. The normal route of human infection is via fleas acquired from rodents or from handling rodents directly. However, pet animals can carry infected fleas from rodents into the home or become infected and sick and then transmit the disease to their owners. Eliassan et al. (2002) found an association between cat ownership and the occurrence of tularemia in humans in Sweden.

Cowpox is a good example of how the understanding of a disease may change, and a good example of a disease in which there is sequential transmission from a wildlife reservoir to domestic animals to humans. Cowpox is caused by an orthopoxvirus that is widespread in parts of Europe. As the name suggests, the virus was originally associated with cattle, and human infection was thought to occur through milking cows that had pox lesions on their teats. However, infected cattle were never common, and cases occurred among people with no direct association with cattle. It is now known that cowpox virus is enzootic and maintained in wild rodents. Infection may spread occasionally to cattle and more commonly to domestic cats that are now considered to be the most important source of infection for humans (Bennett et al. 1990; Baxby et al. 1994).

Tapeworms of the genus *Echinococcus* may be transmitted to humans either from wild or domestic carnivores. Adult *Echinococcus granulosus* occurs in the intestine of a carnivore and the larval stage occurs in the liver or lungs of a herbivore. Different animals are involved in the cycle in different areas of the world. In northern North America, the parasite has a sylvatic cycle involving wolves and moose or caribou. Humans can become infected by accidentally ingesting *Echinococcus* eggs shed by wolves (e.g., this occurs in trappers handling contaminated wolf pelts), but a greater risk occurs if infected viscera from moose or caribou are fed to dogs. The dogs become infected with adult tapeworms and contaminate the area that they share with humans with parasite eggs. (As noted in chapter 8, flies are important in transporting the eggs from carnivore feces to humans.) *Echinococcus multilocularis* cycles between smaller carnivores (particularly foxes) and wild rodents. Dogs and cats can become infected by eating infected rodents and bring the infection into the home environment. Petravy et al. (2000) observed that cats "could be ecologically intimate on one hand with infected wild rodents and on the other hand with humans." Dogs were important on St. Lawrence Island in the Bering Sea where *E. multilocularis* infection was endemic in people (Schantz et al. 1995).

Nipah and Hendra viruses are thought to be transmitted first to a domestic animal and then to humans. These viruses are in a newly created genus, *Henipavirus*, in the family Paramyxoviidae. The natural hosts appear to be wild fruit bats (*Pteropus* spp). Hendra virus infection killed horses in three incidents in Australia in which two humans also died (Westbury 2000). There was no evidence of direct transmission from bats to humans (Mackenzie et al. 2003). Nipah virus appeared suddenly in Malaysia in

1998 and 1999 as a massive outbreak in domestic pigs that resulted in the culling of 1.1 million pigs. There were 265 human cases in which 105 people died (Mackenzie et al. 2003). The affected people were pig farmers or associated with pig farming.

Avian influenza may fall within this category. Type A influenza is an important disease for domestic poultry, pigs, horses, and people worldwide. Wild waterbirds are the natural reservoir for these viruses. In waterbirds, infections are subclinical and involve the digestive tract, with virus being shed with feces into water (Liu et al. 2003). Multiple strains of virus may be present within a group of birds, and these represent a pool of genetic material within which recombination may occur (Murphy and Webster 1996). If these viruses enter a new host, such as chickens, turkeys, or pigs, there can be rapid adaptation with emergence of highly pathogenic virus that might be transmitted among domestic animals and to people (Webster et al. 1992).

ZOONOTIC DISEASES MAINTAINED IN BOTH WILD AND DOMESTIC ANIMALS

An example of zoonotic diseases maintained in wild and domestic animals is bovine tuberculosis caused by infection with *Mycobacterium bovis*. Infection of humans with this bacterium in the past occurred primarily through ingestion of unpasteurized milk from infected cows but may also occur by inhalation of bacteria expired by infected animals or through handling infected tissues. This infection is rare now in many countries where tuberculosis has been eliminated in cattle. In areas where the disease persists and is transferred among wild and domestic animals, such as in New Zealand (cattle, possums, deer, ferrets), United Kingdom (cattle, badgers), Michigan (cattle, white-tailed deer), and Manitoba (cattle, elk, white-tailed deer), human infection could occur from any of the animals involved. *Echinococcus granulosus* infection in Australia is complex. The parasite cycles between dogs and sheep. It has dingoes, dingo/domestic dog hybrids, and foxes serving as final hosts, and macropodid marsupials, feral pigs, and wombats as intermediate hosts, with "no impediment to transmission" between wildlife and domestic animals and humans (Jenkins and Morris 2003).

ZOONOSES IN WHICH HUMANS ARE THE MAINTENANCE HOST

With our anthropocentric view of the world, we are most concerned about diseases that humans contract from animals, but diseases that are clearly of human origin have been detected in wild animals. An example is infection with *Mycobacterium tuberculosis,* the cause of human tuberculosis. Most mammals are susceptible to infection by this organism, and tuberculosis caused by *M. tuberculosis* has been reported in many animals in zoological gardens and primate collections (Oh et al. 2002), often through contagion from their keepers. There are surprisingly few reports of tuberculosis caused by this organism in free-living animals considering that one-third of the world's human population is infected and that three million people die of the disease annually (Small and Selcer 2000). Alexander et al. (2002) describe epizootics of *M. tuberculosis* infection in suricates and banded mongooses in South Africa. Humans infected with tuberculosis were present in the local area, and transmission was thought to have occurred through exposure to human sputum and excreta.

Two further examples illustrate that when humans and wild animals come in contact, disease agents may be exchanged in both directions. Ferrer and Hiraldo (1995) reported occurrence of *Staphylococcus aureus* infection in 45% of nestling Spanish imperial eagles handled without gloves compared to 4% in nestlings handled with disposable gloves. They believed that the infection originated with the handlers, and they cited earlier literature describing similar infections also attributed to human contact. *Herpesvirus hominis* is a common infection of humans and has been reported in a number of species of captive primates. It usually causes transient lesions equivalent to a cold sore (King 2001) but caused disseminated fatal disease in owl monkeys (Melendez et al. 1969). More interesting is the identification of fatal encephalitis caused by this ubiquitous virus of humans in captive skunks (Emmons and Lennette 1968) and a wild striped skunk (Charlton et al. 1977). Diseases that are transmitted naturally from humans to animals are termed "anthropozoonoses." This type of disease may be more common in wild animals than is generally appreciated, because the likelihood of detecting wild animals infected with a human disease is much less than that of detecting an animal disease in humans.

DISEASE SHARED BY WILD AND DOMESTIC ANIMALS

The separation between wild and domestic animals is often blurred and the same species may be free-living on one side of a fence and domesticated on the other. This complicates deciding where disease originated and how much interchange is occurring.

There are three possible scenarios outlined below, but in some diseases the situation is far from clear. As an example, there has been considerable acrimonious debate as to whether a herpesviral disease of waterfowl, duck plague, is enzootic in wild waterfowl and spills over into captive and semicaptive birds or is maintained in birds in aviculture collections and parks and spills over into wild birds periodically. Opinions differ between Europe, where the disease is thought to be maintained in wild waterfowl, and the United States where the disease is considered to be maintained in birds associated with humans (Wobeser 1997). The three scenarios are (1) diseases maintained in wild animals that spill over into domestic animals, (2) diseases shared by wild and domestic animals with transmission in either direction, and (3) diseases maintained in domestic animals that spill over into wild animals.

DISEASES MAINTAINED IN WILD ANIMALS THAT SPILL OVER INTO DOMESTIC ANIMALS

Examples of domestic animal diseases that have a reservoir in wild animals are shown in table 12.2. Some of the diseases, such as influenza A, also appear in the discussion of zoonoses, because they may spill over to humans as well as to domestic animals. Many of the more common diseases listed in table 12.2 have been discussed in previous chapters, so I will limit my discussion to three diseases that are less well known.

Malignant Catarrhal Fever

Malignant catarrhal fever is a severe disease of cattle, some antelope, and deer caused by infection with a herpesvirus that is normally found in another species. One such virus (ovine herpesvirus-2) is found commonly in domestic sheep in which it apparently causes no disease. Another virus associated with malignant catarrhal fever is called alcelaphine herpesvirus 1 and occurs naturally in wild wildebeest. There is no evidence that it causes disease in wildebeest, but Masai tribesmen have recognized for centuries that disease occurs among cattle that have contact with calving wildebeest, and they isolate their cattle during this time (Jones 1982).

Vesicular Exanthema of Swine

During the 1930s, a disease that resembled foot-and-mouth disease occurred in domestic pigs in California. Despite eradication efforts, the disease recurred, and it was then recognized as a separate entity and given the name *vesicular exanthema of*

Table 12.2 Diseases Maintained in Wild Animals with Domestic Animals as Spillover or Dead-end Hosts

Disease agent	Type of agent	Wild animal reservoir	Domestic species most often affected
Fascioloides magna	Trematode	White-tailed deer, elk	Sheep, cattle, goats
Baylisascaris procyonis	Nematode	Raccoon	Poultry, dog, rabbits
Elaeophora schneideri	Nematode	Mule deer	Sheep, goat
Parelaphostrongylus tenuis	Nematode	White-tailed deer	Sheep, goat, llama
Cytauxzoon felis	Protozoan	Bobcat	Cat
Cowpox	Virus	Rodents	Cat, cattle
Malignant catarrhal fever	Virus	Wildebeest	Cattle
Newcastle disease	Virus	Cormorants	Poultry
Rabies	Virus	Fox, skunk, bat, raccoon, mongoose, etc.	Dog, cat, cattle
San Miguel sea lion virus infection	Virus	Pinnipeds	Pig (vesicular exanthema)
West Nile fever	Virus	Birds	Horses, dogs
Western equine encephalitis	Virus	Birds	Horses
Brucella suis biovar 2	Bacterium	European hare	Pig
Lyme disease	Bacterium	White-footed mouse	Dog, horse, cattle
Salmonellosis	Bacterium	Passerine birds at bird feeders	Cats
Tularemia	Bacterium	Rodents, lagomorphs	Sheep

swine (Lenghaus et al. 2001). The disease was associated with feeding garbage to pigs, and laws requiring that garbage fed to pigs be cooked were introduced. During the 1950s, the disease spread in swine throughout much of the United States and also occurred in Iceland. The disease disappeared in swine coincident with a slaughter program for infected herds and rigid enforcement of garbage cooking, and has not been seen since 1959. In 1972, a calicivirus was isolated during the investigation of abortions among California sea lions on San Miguel Island in the Pacific off the coast of California. In sea lions, the virus (now called San Miguel sea lion virus) causes abortion and vesicles (blisterlike lesions) on the flippers. The virus from sea lions subsequently was found to cause disease identical to vesicular exanthema in swine. In 1990, a similar calicivirus was isolated from a marine fish, and it too caused vesicular exanthema in swine. It is believed that when vesicular exanthema occurred in pigs, the original infection resulted from feeding of either fish or tissue from stranded sea lions in garbage to pigs with subsequent pig-to-pig spread. This disease is an excellent example of how human actions can circumvent a natural ecological barrier, in this case between marine and terrestrial organisms.

Newcastle Disease

The third example of domestic animal diseases that have a reservoir in wild animals is *Newcastle disease*. Newcastle disease is caused by a paramyxovirus, and virtually all birds are considered to be susceptible to infection. It also is a zoonosis, causing mild conjunctivitis or flulike signs in humans. There is a high degree of variation in virulence among strains of Newcastle disease virus. Although the virus has been detected in many wild birds, there have been very few reports of clinical disease, except in cormorants (shags). Newcastle disease has been reported in cormorants in Scotland, Russia, Canada, and the United States during the past half century (Kuiken 1999). A strain of virus that occurs in cormorants has been diagnosed on one occasion in domestic turkeys, although the route of transmission between the wild and domestic birds is unknown (Kuiken 1999).

DISEASES SHARED BY WILD AND DOMESTIC ANIMALS WITH TRANSMISSION IN EITHER DIRECTION

There are many diseases that appear to circulate between wild and domestic animal populations and that may be able to persist in either population without introduction from the other (table 12.3).

Table 12.3 Diseases That Circulate Between Wild and Domestic Animals and Persist in Either Population

Disease	Wild animal host(s)	Domestic animal host(s)
Bovine tuberculosis	Badger (United Kingdom) Brushtailed possum (New Zealand) White-tailed deer (Michigan) Elk (Manitoba)	Cattle
Paratuberculosis	Cervids, wild sheep, rabbits, hares	Cattle, sheep, goats
Canine distemper	Canids, mustelids, viverrids	Dog
Canine parvovirus	Canids	Dog
Rinderpest	African buffalo	Cattle
Classical swine fever	Boar	Pig
Brucella abortus infection	Bison, elk	Cattle
Canine heartworm (*Dirofilaria immitis*)	Coyote	Dog

Often the degree of interchange of these diseases is unknown. With more intense investigation, it may be found that slightly different strains of agent occur in the different species and that what appears as a single disease at this time actually represents different infections. For instance, canine distemper virus was thought for many years not to infect felid species. More recently, disease has been recognized in wild and captive cats that was essentially indistinguishable from canine distemper. The source of infection is unknown. Some of the morbilliviruses that have been recovered from felids have slight genetic differences from canine distemper virus, but these are considered insufficient to justify being classified as a distinct morbillivirus (Munson 2001). A virus that caused epizootic disease in Baikal seals also is considered to be a strain of canine distemper virus (Kennedy 2001). Ikeda et al. (2002) described the evolution of feline and canine parvoviruses, and the emergence of new antigenic types of canine parvovirus that have largely replaced the virus that first appeared in dogs in the mid to late 1970s. Some of these emergent "canine" strains are infectious for wild felids.

The most thoroughly investigated diseases of this type are bovine tuberculosis and brucellosis. It generally is agreed that infection with both of these agents entered wild populations from domestic cattle. Only a small proportion of the species that can become infected with *Mycobacterium bovis* can act as maintenance hosts for the agent (de Lisle et al. 2002), and defining the role of different species is both difficult and necessary if the disease is to be managed (Caley and Hone 2004). Infection with *M. bovis* that is being maintained in wild animals has interfered with elimination of the disease from cattle in several parts of the world including infection of badgers in parts of the United Kingdom (Krebs et al. 1998), brushtailed possums in New Zealand (Morris and Pfeiffer 1995), white-tailed deer in Michigan (O'Brien et al. 2002), elk in Manitoba (Lees et al. 2003), bison in northern Canada (Tessaro et al. 1990), and feral water buffalo and pigs in Australia (McInerney et al. 1995).

Maintenance of infection with *Brucella abortus* in wild animal populations in North America is limited to bison in one focus in northern Canada (Tessaro et al. 1990) and elk and bison in the vicinity of Yellowstone National Park in the United States (Ferrari and Garrott 2002). African buffalo in Kruger National Park, South Africa, are infected with both brucellosis and tuberculosis but represent little threat to cattle because the park is fenced. In at least two of these situations described above (white-tailed deer in Michigan, elk in the Yellowstone area), artificial concentration of wild animals by supplementary feeding is thought to be involved in the maintenance of disease.

DISEASES MAINTAINED IN DOMESTIC ANIMALS THAT SPILL OVER INTO WILD ANIMALS

Some of the diseases listed in table 12.3 likely fit this category under at least certain circumstances. For example, *M. bovis* undoubtedly spills over into some wild species in which it does not persist and cannot be maintained. Other diseases, including pseudorabies that is maintained in pigs (domestic and feral) and spills over into other species including raccoons (Stallknecht and Howerth 2001), *Mycoplasma con-*

junctivae that spills over from domestic sheep to chamois (Giacometti et al. 2002), and *Mannheimia haemolytica* and *Pasteurella* spp. that may spill over from domestic sheep and goats to wild sheep (Rudolph et al. 2003; Turner et al. 2004), seem to fit this category. *Toxoplasma gondii*, a protozoan whose only known final hosts are felids and particularly the domestic cat, has been recognized in an astonishing array of wild animals including marine species such as the sea otter and Indo-Pacific humpbacked dolphin (Bowater et al. 2003). Antibodies to many other infectious diseases of domestic animals have been found in wild animals indicating exposure without disease having been recognized. How these agents reach wild animals is usually unclear, and the degree of surveillance in most wild species is probably inadequate to draw firm conclusions about directions of transmission and the effect of many of the agents, or to eliminate the possibility of maintenance of the agents in wild animals.

AVOIDING ZOONOTIC DISEASES

This section is directed particularly at individuals who will be working with wild animals. I have identified particular situations in which transfer of disease from wild animals to humans is likely. The guidelines are largely common sense, the use of which is the most important preventive technique.

KNOW WHAT DISEASES OCCUR IN THE SPECIES AND HABITAT.

There is abundant information available about the diseases that occur in different wild species, although it often is necessary to extrapolate. For example, there might be no information on the prevalence of hantavirus in *Peromyscus* spp. in a particular area where you plan to work but, based on its wide geographic distribution in North America, it is safe to assume that it will be present. Do a literature search or consult with a veterinarian or wildlife health specialist before you start a project or send students or coworkers into the field. I have seen instances in which advisors have been very conscientious in training students or field assistants about the risks associated with chemicals or equipment that they will be using but failed to advise them that the wolf or arctic fox scats they were collecting for food habit studies commonly contain eggs of *Echinococcus* spp. tapeworms, and that these eggs are infectious to people.

USE PROTECTIVE CLOTHING.

People sometimes believe that a modified spacesuit, that is impractical in the field, is required to avoid

becoming infected with zoonotic agents. Except in unusual circumstances, more simple precautions are adequate. Rubber or vinyl gloves should always be used to handle animal feces, tissues, blood, and dead animals. If there is a risk that clothing will become soiled, wear protective outer clothing such as coveralls or a laboratory coat that can be removed when you are finished working with animals. For particular situations, this can be supplemented with a waterproof apron and with a mask. For diseases such as hantavirus infections, local public health officials can provide guidelines on the appropriate type of mask and eye protection that must be worn.

NEVER LET AN ANIMAL BITE OR SCRATCH YOU.

This recommendation should be obvious. Bite wounds should always be treated as a serious event, even if they are minor, because of the possibility of injection of agents. Most people are very cautious to avoid being bitten by larger animals, but become cavalier about bites by small bats or mice "that barely break the skin." Since 1980, 58% of the fatal human cases of rabies in the United States were caused by bat strain virus (McColl et al. 2000) that would have been transmitted by minor bites. While rabies is the obvious danger, many carnivores carry bacteria such as *Pasteurella multocida* in their oral cavity, and diseases such as Lyme disease and probably hantaviruses are transmitted among rodents by biting.

AVOID ANIMALS THAT ARE ACTING ABNORMALLY.

It is important that animals that are acting abnormally reach a diagnostic pathology laboratory where the cause of their illness can be determined, but the person collecting the animal must ensure that the animal is captured or killed in a manner that presents no risk to the handler. Most of the diseases that infect the nervous system and cause behavioral changes are zoonoses. Larger animals should be shot in a manner that does not damage the brain; small animals should be captured in a manner that leaves no room for human exposure.

TREAT ALL ANIMALS FOUND DEAD WITH RESPECT AND RUBBER GLOVES.

Animals found sick or dead are a rich source of information about the occurrence and distribution of disease. Whenever possible, they should be submitted to a diagnostic laboratory for investigation. Each such animal should be treated as though it is infected with a zoonotic agent. It should only be handled with gloves. Small specimens should be placed in plastic bags and packed carefully to avoid spills and leakage. Contaminated equipment should be washed thoroughly and disinfected after use.

AVOID DIRECT CONTACT WITH ABNORMAL SKIN ON WILD ANIMALS.

Many infectious agents that cause skin lesions in wild animals including sarcoptic mange, contagious ecthyma, and other diseases caused by orthopoxviruses, and fungal infections (ringworm) are zoonoses that are transmissible by direct contact with bare skin.

AVOID DIRECT CONTACT WITH FECES, ESPECIALLY THOSE OF CARNIVORES.

A great many infectious agents are transmitted through the excretions of animals. Helminth parasites carried by carnivores including *Baylisascaris procyonis* in raccoons; *Echinococcus granulosus* in wolves, dingoes, coyotes, and foxes; and *Echinococcus multilocularis* in arctic and red foxes, and coyotes are a special risk. The eggs of these parasites are shed in the droppings, and if ingested by a human, they may develop as larval parasites, some of which are a serious medical problem. The eggs in general are extremely hardy and difficult to inactivate on cages or equipment.

TREAT ALL RODENTS WITH RESPECT.

Wild rodents have been linked to a great variety of zoonotic diseases, and agents turn up in the most unexpected places. To illustrate this point, I will refer to three recent reports. Cases of typhus fever occur sporadically in humans within the range of the southern flying squirrel which is the only known reservoir for *Rickettsia prowazekki* in North America (Reynolds et al. 2003). *Bartonella washoensis*, a bacterium found in California ground squirrels, has been linked to cardiac disease in both a human (Kosoy et al. 2003) and a dog (Chomel et al. 2003). Tularemia (*Francisella tularensis* infection) occurred among wild-caught black-tailed prairie dogs at a commercial exotic pet distributor in Texas. During the month prior to identification of the disease, more than one thousand prairie dogs were shipped to ten states in the United States and seven other countries. One probable case of tularemia in an animal handler was identified (Avashia et al. 2004).

It is probable that many zoonoses remain to be discovered in rodents when one considers that at least 14 new hantaviruses have been discovered in the past decade. Excretions and secretions, nest material, and ectoparasites are all potential routes of infection. Niklasson et al. (1998) found a significant correlation in time between occurrence of three human diseases of unknown causation (myocarditis, Guillain-Barré syndrome, and insulin-dependent diabetes) and the cyclic population peaks of bank voles in Sweden. They suggested that there might be a causal relationship between these diseases and unknown infectious agents carried by voles.

THINK ABOUT THE NEXT PERSON DOWN THE LINE.

You may be conscious of disease and take care to protect yourself, but the person who does your laundry or who uses the equipment next may not be as knowledgeable. Always clean and disinfect all materials so that they do not represent a risk to anyone else.

SEEK MEDICAL ADVICE.

If you become ill after working with wild animals, you or someone with you needs to advise the physician that you may have been exposed to a zoonotic disease. Try to be as specific as possible. Zoonoses occur rarely in the general human population, and physicians have little or no experience or training in recognizing these conditions. I speak from personal experience in dealing with a physician who had no understanding that chlamydiosis (*Chlamydophila psittaci* infection) could be acquired from wild birds but was willing to do the appropriate tests on me to confirm a tentative diagnosis that I had suggested (Wobeser and Brand 1982).

SUMMARY

- Many infectious diseases that occur in wild animals also infect humans and domestic animals.
- It is important to define the role of various species as maintenance, spillover, or dead-end hosts of the disease.
- Diseases may move in all directions: from wildlife to humans, humans to wild animals, wild to domestic animals, domestic to wild animals, and wild animals to domestic animals to humans.
- Protecting yourself against zoonoses while working with wild animals consists primarily of using common sense and taking simple precautions.

13
Disease Management

Attempts to manage disease in wild animals either to prevent its occurrence or to reduce the effect to some tolerable level have become much more frequent in recent years for a variety of reasons. When management is contemplated, it is important to assess the reasons for management, to define the objectives clearly, to consider the different potential methods that may be available, to choose the most appropriate technique, and to determine how progress and success will be monitored and measured. Each of these subjects will be reviewed briefly here. For a more detailed discussion of the subject, see Wobeser (1994, 2002).

WHY ATTEMPT MANAGEMENT?

Disease in wild animals is managed for one or more of three reasons:

1. Wild animals are involved in a disease of humans.
2. Wild animals are involved in a disease affecting domestic animals.
3. Disease is having a deleterious effect on one or more wild species.

To this point in time, most attempts to manage disease have been to reduce risks to humans and domestic animals rather than to benefit wild animals per se. In some circumstances, there may be a combination of reasons for management, and a single disease may be managed for different reasons in different areas. For example, the desire to manage rabies in wild animals is usually done to reduce the risk of human infection. Reducing the rate of infection of domestic animals is a secondary benefit. The effect of rabies on wild animals has not been a major reason for management. However, in certain circumstances management of rabies may be done primarily to reduce disease in a wild species. This is currently the situation in regard to the endangered Ethiopian wolf whose existence as a species is threatened by rabies transmitted from domestic dogs. In assessing the need for management, it is important to identify the target species, that is, the species that is expected to benefit from the management. In rabies management in Europe and North America, the main target species is *Homo sapiens* and most of the management action is directed at the foxes, raccoons, and skunks that serve as reservoirs of the infectious agent. In Ethiopia, the target species is the wolf and the attempt is to use vaccination to protect the wolves from a disease reservoir in domestic dogs.

Diseases shared by humans and animals are termed *zoonoses* or *zoonotic diseases*. Zoonoses have always been important in human health, for example, more than 80% of parasitic infections in humans are caused by agents that have other animals as hosts. Many of the important infections that we think of as uniquely human, including measles and tuberculosis, are diseases that evolved from agents that we acquired from animals coincident with the domestication of livestock (Diamond 1997). Human immunodeficiency virus is considered to have originated from similar viruses in other primates. Some zoonoses such as rabies have been known to be associated with wild animals for centuries, whereas many new zoonoses related to wild animals have been discovered only very recently. Most of the "emerging diseases" of humans described in the past few decades are zoonoses, and the majority of these involve wild animals.

Many zoonotic diseases have emerged because of environmental perturbation as a direct result of human activities and increasing human population pressure, including changes in agricultural practices and water management, deforestation, wars, and domestication and movement of animals. These perturbations have resulted in closer contact between humans and wild animals, increased contact between domestic animals and wild animals, changes in populations of some species (particularly wild rodents, and species such as raccoons that thrive in human-modified environments, and some insect vectors of disease), and introduction of hosts and disease agents into novel associations. As an example, fox populations across Europe have increased greatly and foxes have moved into cities recently increasing the risk of *Echinococcus multilocularis* infection of humans (Torgerson and Budke 2003).

There has been less emphasis on the role of wild animals in diseases of domestic animals than has been directed at zoonoses, although many livestock diseases are shared with wild animals. When diseases such as bovine brucellosis and tuberculosis were widespread in domestic animals, it generally was believed that wild animals were insignificant or marginal in the ecology of the diseases. However, as control programs for tuberculosis and brucellosis, as well as for classical swine fever, foot-and-mouth disease, and swine brucellosis, resulted in near elimination of these diseases in livestock in parts of the world, residual reservoirs of these diseases in wild species have become extremely difficult to manage and have undermined eradication schemes (table 13.1). Other diseases such as Newcastle disease and avian influenza circulate in wild birds and occasionally spill over into domestic poultry causing massive outbreaks. Avian strains of influenza virus also spill over into wild seals (Stuen et al. 1994), livestock (particularly pigs), and humans as occurred in Hong Kong in 1997 when a strain from poultry spread to

humans (Bradbury 1998) and as is occurring at present in Asia. Many other diseases such as paratuberculosis (Johne's disease) occur in both wild and domestic species (Beard et al. 2001), but the amount and direction of interchange are poorly understood. Some new diseases that have emerged in domestic animals recently have originated in wild animals in a manner analogous to the emergence of zoonoses described earlier. Examples include influenza in domestic swine that probably originated in wild waterfowl and Hendra virus infection in horses and Nipah and Menangle viruses in pigs, all of which originated in fruit bats. It has been suggested that porcine respiratory and reproductive syndrome virus, a disease that appeared suddenly in North America and Europe less than two decades ago, may have originated from a virus of wild house mice that infected European wild boar initially and then spread to domestic swine (Plagemann 2003). Bengis et al. (2002) reviewed the interface area in which wild and domestic animals share diseases and predicted intensification of interaction at this interface with a need to develop innovative management strategies for dealing with shared diseases.

There have been comparatively few attempts to manage diseases for the primary benefit of wild species. When this has occurred it has usually been the result of special circumstances, including:

- increased recognition that disease is an important potential risk in translocation of wild animals or release of captive bred animals into the wild (Leighton 2002)

Table 13.1 Diseases of Domestic Livestock with a Reservoir in Wild Animals

Disease	Country	Wildlife reservoir	Domestic species
Bovine tuberculosis	New Zealand	Brushtail possum, deer, feral ferret	Cattle, farmed deer
	England, Ireland	Badger	Cattle
	United States (Michigan)	White-tailed deer	Cattle
	Canada	Bison	Cattle, bison
	(Northwest Territories, Alberta, Manitoba)	Elk, white-tailed deer	
	South Africa	African buffalo	Cattle
Brucella abortus infection	United States	Bison, elk	Cattle, bison
	Canada	Bison	
Brucella suis infection	United States	Feral swine	Pigs
Classical swine fever	Europe	Wild boar	Pigs
Pseudorabies	United States	Feral swine	Pigs

Note: These diseases have been almost eliminated from domestic livestock on a regional or national basis.

- concern that disease might imperil small or endangered populations (Scott 1988; Leön-Viscaíno et al. 1999; McCallum and Dobson 2002)
- recognition that some contaminants have serious population effects for both common and vulnerable species
- large and conspicuous outbreaks of disease that have caused public concern
- recognition that diseases may spread from domestic animals or humans with serious consequences for wild species

As an example of the latter point, canine distemper has been documented in collared peccaries in Arizona (Appel et al. 1991), lions and wild dogs in Africa (Roelke-Parker et al. 1996; Alexander and Appel 1994), seals in the Caspian Sea and Lake Baikal (Kennedy 2001), and lynx and bobcats in Canada (Canadian Cooperative Wildlife Health Centre, unpublished data). In some of these instances, it is clear that domestic dogs were the source of infection (Cleaveland et al. 2000). Similarly, *Mycoplasma conjunctivae* infection in chamois is believed to originate in domestic sheep (Giacometti et al. 2002) and staphylococcal infections in Spanish eagles were acquired through handling by humans (Ferrer and Hiraldo 1995).

OBJECTIVES OF MANAGEMENT

All forms of disease management, for both infectious and noninfectious diseases, consist of some combination of reducing exposure of the animals to harmful factors and/or increasing the ability of the animals to resist or cope with the harmful effects caused by those factors. The objective of a disease management program may be to:

1. *prevent* a disease from occurring in individual animals, in groups of animals in a particular area, or in an entire population
2. *control* a disease that is already present by reducing the frequency with which the disease occurs in the group or population or the severity of the effects of the disease or to curtail further spread
3. *eradicate* or eliminate an existing disease locally or on a larger geographic scale

Prevention is the preferable option if it is available. If disease can be prevented at the individual animal level, the cost of disease to that animal is avoided. However, to be able to use this management approach, susceptible animals need to be identified and protected prior to exposure to disease. Prevention at the population or area level is only possible for those diseases that are not already present or established. Assuming that the disease is present elsewhere, the preventive action must continue in perpetuity or so long as there is a risk of its occurring in the population of concern.

Most forms of disease management that have been attempted in wild animals have been aimed at controlling disease, with the understanding that the disease will continue to occur but that its effects can be reduced. Because the disease continues to be present, control actions must continue for as long as there is a need to reduce the effect of disease.

Eradication or elimination of a disease is a massive undertaking that may require a huge investment over a prolonged period. For instance, more than $840 million (Australian) was committed to a decades-long program to eliminate brucellosis and tuberculosis from livestock in Australia (Neumann 1997), and New Zealand was able to declare "provisional freedom" from *Echinococcus granulosus* in dogs and sheep only after a campaign that lasted for more than half a century (Pharo 2002). Because of the great difficulties, eradication is attempted only for the most serious of diseases. If eradication is successful, the effort can then cease, although energies may have to be redirected toward preventing reintroduction of the disease. Only one infectious disease, smallpox, has been eradicated in nature globally. A number of diseases, both infectious and noninfectious, have been eliminated in local or national populations of humans and domestic animals. To my knowledge, no disease management scheme in wild animals was begun with a goal of eradication of an infectious disease. Eradication of the New World screw worm (*Cochliomyia hominivora*) from the southern United States and of tsetse flies that transmit trypanosomiasis from parts of Africa were not done to benefit wild animals, but the success of these programs had major beneficial effects for wild ungulates (Reichard 2002). Current management of rabies using oral vaccination is approaching elimination of the disease in large areas of Europe and parts of North America. A few noninfectious diseases of wild animals caused by contaminants, including some forms of mercury compounds and some pesticides, have been eliminated either totally or over large areas.

OPTIONS FOR MANAGEMENT

Management actions might be directed at the disease agent, the host animal(s), or the other environ-

Table 13.2 Matrixof Management Options

	Agent	Host	Environment
Prevent			
Control			
Eradicate			

mental factors in the agent-host-environment epidemiological triangle (fig. 2.6). Manipulation of human activities can be considered as management of either the host or management of the environment, depending upon the disease. We can combine these three potential sites for management with the three management objectives described above to form a matrix containing nine potential types of intervention as shown in table 13.2.

Each cell in the matrix of table 13.2 will be reviewed briefly, with a few examples of disease management techniques that have been used in wild animals.

DISEASE PREVENTION

Measures to prevent disease are concerned primarily with reducing or averting exposure of animals to harmful factors.

Manipulation of the Disease Agent

Most diseases have a restricted geographic range. The range of infectious diseases is determined by the presence of suitable hosts and by environmental conditions suitable for transmission. These are defined by primary factors of climate, topography, and soil or bedrock and by secondary features including water bodies, vegetation, and the animals that are present. The range of some noninfectious diseases is determined by the presence of constituents such as micronutrients and toxic elements in soil or bedrock, and the range of others is determined by human activities resulting in the accumulation and/or release of contaminants. Because most diseases have a restricted distribution, a major form of disease management consists of preventing the introduction of novel agents into new areas. Regulations to prevent translocation of diseases caused by infectious agents have been used for many years in domestic livestock. Veterinarians have had considerable success in restricting the movement of diseases such as foot-and-mouth disease, classical swine fever, rinderpest,

avian influenza, and Newcastle disease around the world. There also have been notable failures such as the global dissemination of bovine tuberculosis and brucellosis in European cattle. Many of the most blatant failures to prevent spread of domestic animal diseases occurred prior to the introduction of appropriate prevention methods or before the cause and nature of the diseases were understood. However, examples, such as outbreaks of avian influenza in poultry, continue to occur despite rigid regulations.

The major technique used to prevent movement of disease agents involves placing stringent restrictions on movement of potentially infected animals and animal products by humans. The risks of disease transfer through translocation of wild animals received relatively little attention until recently, and many infectious disease agents have been moved around the world with imported wild animals. Fortunately, many disease agents that were moved to new locations either failed to become established or remained restricted to their original host species in the new environment. The examples in table 13.3 are diseases that have become established in indigenous species at the new site. This type of unintentional movement of diseases still occurs much too frequently, because of a lack of suitable regulations on animal movement or a disregard for regulations related to disease. A recent example is the translocation of monkeypox virus in African rodents imported to North America as pets with subsequent spread to pet prairie dogs and to humans (CDC 2003). This example suddenly brought the lack of regulations regarding the movement of rodents to the attention of public health officials.

A basic principle that must be recognized when trying to prevent translocation of disease agents is that "a living animal can not be readily separated from its microflora and microfauna for the purposes of translocation and it is impossible to sterilize a living animal" (Wobeser 1994). Every movement of a living animal to a new area has the potential risk of

Table 13.3 Infectious Agents That Have Spread Through Translocation of Infected Wild Animals

Agent	Origin	New site (species affected)	Animal in which the agent was translocated
Fascioloides magna	North America	Europe (red deer, fallow deer)	Elk[1]
Plasmodium relictum	Uncertain	Hawaii (endemic Hawaiian birds)	Pet birds[2]
Monkey pox	Africa	United States (prairie dogs, people)	African rodents[3]
Raccoon strain rabies	Florida	Virginia (raccoons, people)	Raccoons[4]
Elaphostrongylus cervi	United Kingdom	New Zealand (red deer, elk)	Red deer[5]
Elaphostrongylus rangiferi	Norway	Newfoundland (caribou)	Reindeer[6]
Echinococcus multilocularis	Northern United States	Southeastern United States	Red fox, coyote[7]
Angiostrongylus cantonensis	Uncertain	Australia (fruit bats)	Norway and black rats[8]
Yersinia pestis	China	North America (wild rodents)	Rats[9]

[1]Pybus (2001).
[2]van Riper et al. (1986).
[3]CDC (2003).
[4]Jenkins and Winkler (1987).
[5]Mason and McAllum (1976).
[6]Lankester (2001).
[7]Davidson et al. (1992).
[8]Barret et al. (2002).
[9]Gaspar and Watson (2001).

introducing alien disease agents. Extensive testing and treatment of animals with antibiotics and antiparasitic drugs before movement and effective quarantine after arrival help to reduce the risk of translocation of those diseases that are known and for which tests are available. Unfortunately, very few tests have been validated for use in wild animals so that the value of "negative" tests prior to translocation often is questionable. Testing and treatment do not eliminate the risk of introducing known agents and are ineffective against unrecognized diseases. The possibility of introducing an unknown agent with translocated animals is very real. It is safe to assume that a huge array of unrecognized infectious agents occur in wild animals so that unexpected risks may occur in even the best regulated translocation.

In this regard, it is instructive to recall that although both severe acute respiratory syndrome (SARS) and Ebola disease are assumed to be caused by viruses from wild animals, the actual sources are unknown, and that the many types of New World hantaviruses, Nipah virus, Hendra virus, and Australian bat lyssavirus, all of which may be fatal for humans, have been "discovered" within the past decade. Leighton (2002) reviewed how the disease risks in translocation should be considered, and Corn and Nettles (2001) provide a detailed protocol, related to movement of elk, that is an example of the rigor needed to reduce the risk of translocation of disease.

Gaydos et al. (2002a) identified another potential problem that might result from translocation of wild animals. They found marked differences in inherent susceptibility (innate resistance) to epizootic hemorrhagic disease virus among populations of white-tailed deer and suggested that similar variation in susceptibility to many diseases could occur in wild animals. Movement of animals from nonresistant groups to areas where a disease is endemic might result in failure of the translocation, or even "genetic dilution" of a resistant remnant stock if nonresistant animals are translocated to supplement an existing small population.

Preventing the release of new contaminants or the continued release of old contaminants is a logical way of preventing disease. It would be ideal if all potentially harmful compounds could be identified in advance and their release prevented; however, it is not always possible to predict in advance which compounds will become a problem for wild animals. A new substance may become very widespread before a problem is detected. For instance, there seems to have been little anticipation that second-generation anticoagulants used to control commensal rodents would cause secondary poisoning of raptorial birds and mammalian carnivores or that an anti-inflammatory drug used widely in cattle would cause fatal kidney damage in vultures (Oaks et al. 2004). There have been some notable successes in preventing disease caused by contaminants. For instance, Blus et al. (1984) described the recovery of a Canada goose population following cessation of use of the pesticide heptachlor, and Wanntorp et al. (1967) documented the cessation of mortality of granivorous game birds in Sweden when the use of alkyl mercury seed dressings was suspended. The successes have generally involved substances that were limited in distribution and in which the source and distribution were known. In contrast to the situation with mercurial seed dressings, the much more diffuse contamination of the aquatic environment with mercury has not been prevented (Evers et al. 2003).

Manipulation of the Animal(s)

The goal of this form of management is to prevent animals from being exposed to the factor(s) that cause disease or to prevent the occurrence of disease in individuals. In some circumstances, it may be possible to disperse animals away from or prevent their having access to sites where disease is occurring. This is only practical for diseases that are localized in distribution. Whooping cranes have been dispersed away from areas where avian cholera was occurring in wild waterfowl (Zinkl et al. 1977b), and ducks have been dispersed away from a site where botulism was occurring (Parrish and Hunter 1969). However, it often is very difficult to make wild animals move where they do not want to go without extensive habitat modification. Fencing has been used successfully to prevent contact and transmission of foot-and-mouth disease between African buffalo within Kruger National Park and domestic cattle outside the park (Bengis et al. 2002). Stabling horses at night and screening pig shelters have been suggested as methods to prevent contact of domestic animals with fruit bats that carry Hendra and Nipah viruses (Mackenzie et al. 2003). Gondim et al. (2004) suggested that erecting canid-proof fences about stored cattle feed, disposing of dead livestock and offal so that it was not available to coyotes, and

discouraging coyote density near barns could be used to prevent spread of *Neosporum caninum* (a protozoan that is an important cause of abortion in cattle) from coyotes to cattle. Actions to change animal distribution require continual maintenance and are prone to failure, for example, when a fence is destroyed by flood or wind, or animals become habituated and ignore repellent devices.

Another form of manipulation of the host animal is to reduce the population density in an area to prevent disease spread. Population reduction or complete depopulation around a focal area in which a disease is occurring (radial population reduction) or across the expected path of spread of an advancing disease (barrier population reduction) have been used to halt the spread of disease and prevent its movement into new areas. This form of management is appropriate only for diseases that are localized. It has been used with apparent success to prevent the spread of rabies in vampire bats in Argentina (Fornes et al. 1974), foxes in Switzerland and Denmark (Muller 1971; Wandeler et al. 1974), and striped skunks and raccoons in Canada (Gunson et al. 1978; Rosatte et al. 2001). For this form of management to be successful, there must be very effective surveillance and rapid reporting of cases so that the zone or barrier can be moved or expanded if necessary. The area of depopulation must be sufficiently wide that potentially infected individuals do not move beyond the barrier.

Occurrence of some diseases might be prevented in individual wild animals by immunization, in the same manner that you and I are protected against tetanus and many other infections. This form of immunization is practical only for small populations of highly valuable species that can be treated individually. It has been used to protect particularly valuable antelope species against anthrax in Africa and was attempted to protect wood bison from anthrax in northern Canada. The latter effort was unsuccessful because only a relatively small proportion of the population could be captured for vaccination, protective immunity was of short duration, and there was extensive mortality as a result of capture myopathy among animals captured for vaccination. Preexposure immunization for rabies in humans at elevated levels of risk, including veterinarians and wildlife workers, is a form of preventive management of this type.

Manipulation of Environmental Factors

Manipulation of environmental factors for disease prevention usually involves changing human activities. Examples include such simple actions as relocation of woodpiles at a distance from homes and other rodent-proofing activities to reduce the risk of exposure to hantaviruses carried by rodents, excluding trees favored for feeding by fruit bats from horse pens and near pig farms to reduce the risk from viruses carried by bats (Mackenzie et al. 2003), using gloves when handling nestling eagles to prevent infection of the eagles with staphylococci of human origin (Ferrer and Hiraldo 1995), and preventing wild animals from having access to point source emissions of contaminants. An important part of the management of many zoonoses is changing human behavior to reduce the risk of exposure, for example, educating people to avoid contact with wild animals that may be acting abnormally and may be infected with rabies virus, and promoting use of insect repellants to reduce the risk of being bitten by mosquitoes that transmit West Nile virus and other arboviruses from wild birds to humans.

In some circumstances, it may be possible to predict in advance that certain environmental changes will result in increased disease risk and take appropriate preventive action. Ostfeld et al. (2001) found that the abundance of nymphal ticks infected with *Borrelia burgdorferi* and, hence, the risk of Lyme disease for humans could be predicted based on acorn production 1.75 years earlier. The amount of St. Louis encephalitis virus likely to be circulating in nature can be predicted by monitoring weather (Shaman et al. 2002a), and increased rodent populations have been suggested as a predictor of risk from different hantaviruses to humans in the southwestern United States (Engelthaler et al. 1999) and Sweden (Olsson et al. 2003). If such environmental changes can be linked to disease and monitored, preventive measures such as increased public education regarding impending risk can be put in place before the increased risk occurs. In other circumstances, the environmental changes that predict disease occurrence or spread are known, but it is difficult to institute preventive action. Japanese encephalitis, a viral disease transmitted by mosquitoes, is spreading in Asia because of a combination of environmental changes including increased irrigated rice production that provides increased mosquito vector habitat, expanded pig production that provides an increased vertebrate population for the virus, and increased urban expansion that brings more people into closer contact with pig-rearing areas (Daniels 2002). Although these environmental factors favoring disease are known, they cannot be manipulated to prevent disease occurrence. However, public education

about the disease can still be done to reduce the level of human exposure.

DISEASE CONTROL
Manipulation of the Disease Agent

One method of attacking an agent to control disease is to destroy it in the environment before the animals are exposed. In the case of infectious agents, this might be done through some form of disinfection. This form of management is limited to situations in which the agent is very localized and its location is known. Disinfection using chemicals or fire has been attempted in localized occurrences of anthrax, avian cholera, and duck plague, but the effectiveness of the technique has not been assessed and the chemicals used may have serious environmental side-effects. Decontamination of raccoon latrines in urban areas has been suggested as a way of controlling human risk from the nematode *Baylisascaris procyonis* (Page et al. 1999).

Many human and domestic-animal diseases are controlled by attacking the causative agent within the host by treating infected individuals with drugs (antibiotics, anthelmintics, antifungal, and antiviral agents) that inactivate or kill the agent. The goal is to limit the damage caused by an established infection. A disadvantage of this technique is that the agent will have caused injury, and transmission may have occurred by the time of treatment. There is no reason to suspect that drug treatment would be less effective in wild animals than it has been in humans and domestic animals. However, the difficulty lies in identifying those animals that require treatment, identifying a treatment that will be effective, and delivering appropriate treatments to them. Treatment usually is only practical in special situations, such as small populations in confined areas, or for very valuable animals in which individual attention is possible. Examples of use of this technique include treatment of sarcoptic mange in foxes in Sweden (Bornstein et al. 2001) and psoroptic mange in wild sheep (Lange 1982), and anthelmintic treatment for control of *Trichostrongylus tenuis* in red grouse (Dobson and Hudson 1992), lungworms in bighorn sheep (Schmidt et al. 1979), and *Fascioloides magna* in white-tailed deer (Qureshi et al. 1994). In some of these circumstances, the treatment was effective at a local level over a short time period. Hegglin et al. (2003) demonstrated that treating foxes with anthelmintics delivered in oral baits might be possible at a citywide scale to reduce the risk of transmission of *Echinococcus multilocularis* to people. Mass medication of wild animals to destroy disease agents over a large area is probably impractical in most situations. An important disadvantage of any form of mass medication program is the likelihood that drug resistance will develop in agents exposed repeatedly to a drug or chemical.

Manipulation of the Animal(s)

Efforts to control disease by managing the host animals can be designed to reduce the level of exposure or to increase the degree of resistance. Many attempts to control infectious disease in wild animals have been based on the assumption that disease transmission is related to population density and that the rate of exposure to disease can be reduced by reducing animal density. (It must be noted that the exact nature of the relationship between population density and the rate of exposure and transmission is not known for any disease in wild animals.) This technique usually has been employed for diseases caused by microparasites (primarily viruses and bacteria) in which the host population consists of susceptible, infected, and recovered individuals (see chapter 8). There are three basic approaches to population manipulation to reduce disease exposure and transmission:

1. Reduce the density of the entire population
2. Reduce the proportion or density of infected individuals in the population
3. Reduce the proportion or density of susceptible individuals in the population

There have been attempts to reduce the overall density of animal populations to control a number of diseases (reviewed in Wobeser 1994). Some general features of such programs are evident:

1. It is difficult to reduce the density of an extensive wild population.
2. Reduction of population density without habitat modification to reduce carrying capacity is, at best, a short-term measure because populations recover quickly.
3. Population reduction that involves killing large numbers of animals is unpopular.
4. The actual degree of population reduction that is required to be effective is unknown and is probably highly disease, site, and species specific. There are no generic rules to tell one how much a population will have to be reduced to have an effect on the prevalence of a specific disease.
5. The effect of population reduction on population structure and function is usually unknown.

6. Short-term programs that tried to reduce populations over large areas have not been successful.
7. Attempts to reduce the population density on small areas without preventing immigration from surrounding areas are unlikely to be successful.

The most extensive, long-term, overall population reduction program for any disease in a wild species has been the attempt to control bovine tuberculosis in brushtail possums in New Zealand. This has been in operation for more than 40 years, has cost many millions of dollars, and has been done primarily through widespread use of poisons. The ultimate success of the program is unknown, but sustained long-term reduction of the possum population to about 22% of its precontrol density in some areas has resulted in a major reduction in the incidence of tuberculosis in cattle (Caley et al. 1999). Population reduction sometimes has unexpected results. Removing deer mice from ranch buildings resulted in an increase in the total number of mice and may have increased the risk of human exposure to hantavirus (Douglass et al. 2003).

Another approach is to reduce the density of infected individuals in the population and, hence, the probability of transmission. This approach, often called "selective culling" or "test-and-slaughter" is feasible only in situations in which infected individuals can be identified (either because the clinical features are obvious or because a sensitive live-animal test is available), individuals can be captured readily (and repeatedly) for testing, animals known to be free of the disease can be isolated from the untested population, and removal of a portion of the population is acceptable. Test-and-slaughter has been used successfully to control some livestock diseases where animals can be identified and tested relatively easily. It is not applicable to most diseases in wild populations because of the difficulty in capturing and testing animals and the lack of reliable live-animal tests. It was considered that selective culling of an urban population of mule deer to control chronic wasting disease might be feasible because a reliable test is available, at least 50% of the population could be captured, and positive animals could be removed quickly (Wolfe et al. 2004). A variation of selective culling has been used in an attempt to control tuberculosis in badgers and cattle in England. This involved "reactive culling" of badgers only in local areas that were identified on the basis of infection in cattle. The effectiveness of this technique was to have been compared in a long-term randomized trial to that of more general "proactive culling" to reduce overall badger density over large areas, and to no culling of badgers. Reactive culling was stopped as part of the program on the basis of evidence that local population reduction of badgers failed to control and may have increased the incidence of tuberculosis in cattle, compared to areas with no culling (Donnelly et al. 2003). It was thought that culling disrupted badger social organization and may have promoted long-distance dispersal of infected animals.

The third approach is to reduce the proportion or density of susceptible animals in the population through immunization. Immunization moves animals from the susceptible to the resistant group within the population and may have two effects: (1) it may increase the ability of the individual animal to resist disease, and (2) it may reduce the rate of transmission of the disease within a population. Some vaccines, such as that for rabies prevent infection, and other vaccines, such as those currently available for tuberculosis, reduce the severity of disease in the individual and the likelihood of shedding of bacteria but do not prevent infection. The aim of this form of immunization is to reduce the reproductive rate (R_0) of the disease. In some instances, it may be possible to reduce R_0 to <1 so that the disease may eventually disappear, in which case immunization becomes a technique for disease eradication. Immunization is an attractive alternative to forms of disease management that involve killing animals and has been effective in controlling many human and domestic animal diseases. However, there are a number of factors that limit the use of immunization in wild animals. The first requirement is for a suitable vaccine. Such a vaccine should produce long-lasting protective immunity (preferably as a result of a single immunization), produce no disease in the target or other species, be inexpensive and stable, and allow differentiation between immunized and recovered individuals, so that the *incidence* of disease (the number of new cases over time) can be monitored. If a suitable vaccine is available, the next requirement is for a system to deliver it to the population. The delivery system must allow immunization of a substantial proportion of the population if it is to have an effect in reducing transmission. The actual proportion of a population that must be immunized to produce effective disease control depends on many factors including the ease with which the disease is transmitted, the population density, and the rate of turnover in the population.

In a few situations, it may be practical to capture and administer vaccine directly (e.g., by syringe) to individual animals. A "trap-vaccinate-release" (TVR) program has been used in Canada to vaccinate urban raccoons, skunks, and foxes for rabies in the city of Toronto (Rosatte et al. 1992) and in Flagstaff, Arizona, to control an outbreak of bat rabies in skunks (Engeman et al. 2003). TVR also has been used to create a barrier of immunized animals to reduce the risk of spread of raccoon rabies into Ontario, and in a radial manner to form a ring of resistant animals surrounding individual cases of raccoon rabies. Kretzschmar et al. (2004) discuss the potential use of ring vaccination for control of smallpox in humans. Immunization of individuals by this method of vaccine delivery is practical only for relatively small areas. A TVR program to immunize European rabbits in Spain against myxomatosis and rabbit hemorrhagic disease was found to result in a short-term negative effect on the survival of young and subadult rabbits, with increased mortality in the first week after handling (Calvete et al. 2004). The mortality was associated with the stress of handling "in addition to the detrimental effects of vaccination," and the authors indicate the need to consider the negative effects of capture/handling in assessing the efficacy of TVR programs. Hanssen et al. (2004) found markedly reduced survival over the following year among female common eider that responded to immunization with sheep red blood cells and diphtheria/tetanus vaccine during the nesting period. They suggested that the results of their study indicate a need for caution in preventive vaccination programs that involve animals under severe nutritional stress.

The only method that has been developed for mass immunization of wild animals is distribution of vaccine in baits. This technique requires that the vaccine induces immunity by the oral route and raises many safety concerns because the vaccine is distributed in the environment where it is available to nontarget species (in contrast to TVR in which the vaccine is injected directly into the target animal). Baits containing modified live-virus rabies vaccine were first used in Switzerland in 1977, and since then millions of baits containing several different rabies vaccines have been used over wide areas of Europe and North America with a high degree of success in controlling the disease in foxes, raccoons, and coyotes over large areas (Rupprecht et al. 2001). Historical information on the early years of the rabies vaccination program in Europe is available in Müller (1997). Delahay et al. (2003) discuss the potential use of oral vaccination of badgers for tuberculosis and provide a review of the ecological factors to be considered in an immunization program in wild animals.

Manipulation of Environmental Factors

Environmental sanitation and hygiene, such as the provision of safe drinking water, adequate food, and shelter, have been extremely important in controlling many diseases of humans and domestic animals. These same principles seldom have been applied to disease management for wild animals. Many wild species are restricted to remnants of their former range in which conditions are less than optimal. Perhaps this is most evident in wild waterbirds that often are confined to crowded refuge areas with water that has been heavily used and abused before it finally becomes wildlife habitat. (It would be an interesting exercise to determine how much of the water allocated to wildlife would meet standards for drinking water or even for use for swimming by humans.) The birds have little or no option for movement to less crowded and contaminated habitat. The most obvious of the resulting disease problems relate to intoxication by contaminants such as selenium in drain water (Fairbrother et al. 1994), but contaminated or unsanitary conditions also affect many infectious diseases. This may be a direct result of accumulation of infectious agents shed by infected animals in the water or through more indirect mechanisms. Spalding et al. (1993) reported that wetlands enriched by nutrient pollution had very high populations of oligochaetes that are the first intermediate host of the nematode *Eustrongylides ignotus*. Fish containing the second intermediate stage of this parasite were found only in polluted waters, and wading birds nesting near these sites had a high prevalence of infection and of mortality attributed to the worm.

There have been few attempts to alleviate the conditions on wetlands used by waterbirds. Freshwater impounds have been proposed as a management strategy to protect ducklings on highly saline wetlands (Moorman et al. 1991) and to mitigate the effects of selenium-contaminated areas for shorebirds (Gordus 1999). Coyner et al. (2002) suggested that one way to control *Eustrongylides* infection in wading birds would be to monitor the prevalence of larval *E. ignotus* in fish and drain ponds in which fish were infected heavily. (Obviously this method would remove the habitat as well as the disease, and it would be important to assess whether habitat loss or disease does more harm to the population.)

Degradation of terrestrial habitat also may affect disease in wild animals, for example, eggshell defects in passerine birds with resulting reproductive effects have been associated with acidification (Graveland et al. 1994). Artificial calcium supplementation may alleviate the condition (Mänd and Tilgar 2003) but is not practical on a widespread or long-term basis.

One environmental manipulation that should be used wherever possible is to prevent or remove situations that artificially concentrate animals and that promote disease exchange. An example is reducing supplemental feeding to reduce transmission of bovine tuberculosis among white-tailed deer in Michigan (Miller et al. 2003). Other forms of environmental manipulation may be directed at vector species, such as draining potential mosquito breeding sites or treating these sites with larvicides as has been widely done in eastern North America in a program to reduce the local population of vector mosquitoes that may transmit West Nile virus.

DISEASE ERADICATION

Manipulation of the Disease Agent

Eradication of any disease is extremely difficult. Yekutiel (1980) described features of infectious diseases that make them more or less susceptible to eradication, and his review is useful reading for anyone contemplating eradication of an infectious disease. Use of the "sterile fly technique" to eliminate the New World screw worm and some tsetse flies has been a success story that has been of great benefit to wild populations, although the programs were not done for that purpose. Restrictions on the use of lead shot for hunting birds over large areas of the world should have the eventual effect of eliminating lead poisoning from this source, although scavenging birds such as eagles and vultures may continue to be poisoned from lead rifle bullets contained in mammalian carcasses.

Manipulation of the Animal(s)

Elimination of terrestrial (i.e., non-bat) rabies over large areas appears to be possible using intense oral vaccination campaigns, but total elimination from whole continents by this means is probably not realistic (Rupprecht et al. 2001). At present, no suitable vaccine-bait system is available for rabies in some species, such as the striped skunk, and immunization is not practical as a method to manage bat rabies. A complication of the immunization program for rabies in foxes is that fox populations have increased as mortality from rabies has been reduced. (It is not clear at this time whether this population increase is a direct effect of reduced rabies mortality.) The increased fox population density has had several effects. Among these are that if rabies reoccurs, it will be more difficult to control in the expanded fox population (Chautan et al. 2000), the risk of another zoonoses (*Echinococcus multilocularis* infection) has increased with increased fox density (Kern et al. 2003; Srèter et al. 2003), and there is concern that some endangered prey species may be at increased risk of extinction (Müller 1997). Complete elimination of the existing bison population with subsequent restocking with disease-free bison was proposed as the only feasible method of eradicating bovine tuberculosis and brucellosis from Wood Buffalo National Park in northern Canada (Connelly et al. 1990), but this met with a great deal of opposition and has not been done. Fuller (2002) provides an historical perspective on various decisions regarding management of disease in this bison population.

Manipulation of Environmental Factors

Many diseases might be eliminated by habitat manipulation, but whether this can be done for disease in wild animals and still retain a "desirable" environment that contains a diversity of species is unknown. In a few situations, a simple action such as working with farmers to change cultivation practices, as was done to eliminate mycotoxin poisoning of sandhill cranes (Windingstad et al. 1989) may be effective.

CHOOSING THE BEST TECHNIQUE AND MEASURING PROGRESS

Programs to manage disease in wild animals are experiments since there is little hard evidence to document the effectiveness of most of the techniques that have been used in the past, and there is little background on which to predict the probable success of a particular method. The more that is known about the ecology of a disease, the greater the likelihood of finding an effective method. Where possible, emphasis should be on disease prevention rather than control or eradication.

The single most important preventive technique for dealing with infectious disease is rigid control of translocation of animals to prevent introduction of novel agents and to prevent introduction of susceptible animals or strains into areas where a disease is indigenous. Introduced species also may alter the ecology of a disease already present in an area.

Introduction of the brushtail possum to New Zealand altered the ecology of bovine tuberculosis completely and made it impossible to eradicate the disease in livestock by methods that have been successful in other countries. *Echinococcus multilocularis* was undoubtedly introduced to Svalbard repeatedly by migrating arctic foxes, but the parasite did not become established there until introduction of a vole provided a suitable intermediate host so that the life cycle could be completed (Hentonnen et al. 2001).

Attempts to eliminate the causative agent once it is established are probably better suited to noninfectious diseases, such as contaminant poisoning, than to most infectious agents. The management choices that are available in any particular situation are limited by many factors, including cost and acceptability to the public. What is acceptable in one area of the world often is not acceptable elsewhere. For instance, sodium fluoroacetate (1080) has been used for many years to poison "pest" species for tuberculosis control in New Zealand, but use of this poison is prohibited in many other countries. Similarly, fencing of national parks has been used to prevent transmission of diseases from wild animals to livestock in Africa, but fencing generally is an anathema in North American parks. Immunization is attractive to the public as a gentler alternative to culling, but it only is suited for a relatively small number of diseases caused by microparasites and is most likely to succeed in diseases with a low reproductive rate, in populations with a low turnover, and in cases where the average age of infection occurs later in life. Immunization campaigns require extensive research to develop a suitable vaccine, bait delivery system and baiting plan, and a massive expenditure for baiting over a period of years.

Environmental manipulation may be the method of choice provided that the ecology of the disease is understood sufficiently to identify appropriate sites for action. An environmental manipulation that is applicable in many diseases is to reduce or eliminate factors such as artificial feeding that artificially concentrate wild animals or that promote exchange with domestic animals or humans. The potential effect of environmental manipulations, such as construction of dams or wetlands, or housing developments within forests, on disease in wild animals, humans, and domestic animals should be considered in the planning stage of such projects.

In many circumstances, no single technique may be suitable. Different techniques may be required at different stages of a management program or several methods may need to be used in combination. Modeling may be helpful in evaluating techniques, for example, Smith and Wilkinson (2003) used models to predict that a combination of culling and vaccination would be the best method for controlling local outbreaks of rabies. Control of tuberculosis in wild deer and cattle may include modification of farming practices to reduce contact between the groups, restrictions on feeding and baiting deer to reduce transmission, and reduction of the deer population. Public education and changes in human behavior form a very large part of most attempts to manage disease in wild animals.

Management programs have seldom included a system for measuring their effectiveness. It is expensive and difficult to collect the samples necessary to monitor a disease program, so that intensive surveillance is usually done only for the most important diseases, such as rabies and tuberculosis. Another difficulty lies in detecting that management is having an effect, because wild populations can only be estimated within wide confidence limits. For instance, it will be difficult to measure the success of any program to control avian cholera or botulism, given that despite more than 50 years of intensive measuring of mallard populations in North America, it is still not clear if the major mortality factor (hunting) affecting duck populations is additive or compensatory. It is particularly difficult to measure the effect of management when a disease occurs at a very low prevalence in a population. The presence of the disease can be confirmed unequivocally by finding a single case, but absence of disease can only be inferred with a degree of probability. To be relatively confident that a disease is absent, a very large sample may have to be tested. For instance, for a disease occurring at a rate of 1 per 1000 animals (prevalence = 0.1%), approximately 3000 animals would need to be examined to be 95% confident of detecting a single affected individual. In the late stages of a successful program, it may be extremely difficult to determine if a disease has been controlled or eradicated.

Despite the inherent difficulties, the effectiveness of a program should be monitored so that techniques can be adjusted or changed as needed, and so that one knows when the objective has been reached. As an example, the objective for management of avian botulism is to reduce mortality of ducks. The most commonly used technique has been to collect and dispose of duck carcasses that serve as substrate for further toxin production. Counting the number of carcasses collected is not a measure of the effectiveness of the management since it reveals nothing about the mortality rate among the ducks that are present. Effectiveness could be assessed by comparing the survival of ducks on lakes on which carcass "cleanup" was done to survival of ducks on lakes without this treatment. When this was done in western Canada, it was found that there was no difference in survival of ducks on lakes with or without treatment (Evelsizer 2002). Carcass collection was stopped, for an annual savings of about $1 million that could be applied to other areas of waterfowl management.

Pneumonia caused by *Pasteurella* spp. and related bacteria is an important disease of wild sheep in western North America. Cassirer et al. (2001) evaluated the effectiveness of immunization of bighorn sheep ewes in increasing lamb survival and concluded that "vaccinating bighorn ewes following pneumonia epidemics has little chance of increasing neonatal survival, and may be contraindicated as a management intervention."

Hegglin et al. (2003) measured the effectiveness of using anthelmintic baits to reduce the occurrence of *Echinococcus multilocularis* in Zurich, Switzerland. The objective was to reduce contamination of the environment with tapeworm eggs. Baits containing an anthelmintic drug were distributed once a month during an 18-month trial period. The effectiveness was measured by comparing the infection rate in foxes (the definitive host) and voles (the main intermediate host) on treated and untreated control sites. The study showed a pronounced reduction in environmental contamination and, by extension, a reduction in risk of human infection.

SUMMARY

- Most attempts to manage disease in wild animals have been to benefit human or domestic animal health rather than wild animals.
- The objective of management may be to prevent, control, or eradicate disease.
- All management consists of either reducing exposure to the disease agent or reducing the effect of the agent.
- Management may be directed at the causative agent, the animal, or other features of the environment.
- Preventing disease movement is an important form of disease management. Wild animals should never be translocated without a thorough assessment of the disease risks.
- Disease management through treatment of individual wild animals is impractical except in unusual circumstances.

- The distribution of wild animals may be altered to reduce exposure to disease. However, it is difficult to move wild animals and changes are short-term without habitat modification to alter carrying capacity.
- Attempts to use population reduction over large areas to control disease generally have been ineffective. Removal of factors that concentrate wild animals, such as artificial feeding, is an effective part of management of some diseases.
- Immunization of individual animals is useful only in special circumstances. Mass immunization using oral baits has been effective for control of rabies, but cost and technical difficulties limit the feasibility of this technique.
- Improvements in hygiene and sanitation, such as provision of safe drinking water, that have been extremely important in promoting human and livestock health have received little attention in wild animals.
- Many diseases can be managed through public education and alteration of human activities.
- Management programs that depend on a single technique are prone to fail because of changes in the disease, the animals, or the environment.
- Management of disease requires a long-term commitment that may be difficult to sustain, particularly if management is successful and disease becomes less visible.
- The effectiveness of very few techniques has been assessed. Programs should include a monitoring system so that new methods can be introduced if current methods are ineffective.

14
Roundup

The rôle of disease in wild-life conservation has probably been radically underestimated.
—A. Leopold

My intent in writing this book was not to discuss any specific disease in detail but to try to provide a framework for thinking about disease in wild animals in general. In this concluding chapter, I will reemphasize a few points about disease and how these relate to wildlife management.

The work and writings of Aldo Leopold generally are credited with emergence of wildlife management as a discipline in North America in the 1930s. Leopold recognized that disease was important for wild animals. He suggested that disease was involved in controlling buffer foods such as rodents for predators, delimiting the geographical distribution of some species, setting density limits for some species, causing cyclic and irruptive behavior of populations, as well as affecting sex ratios and fertility (Leopold 1933). In 1933 he published *Game Management*, which contains a chapter on disease control that is a worthwhile starting point for those interested in wildlife disease. I use it as a touchstone in courses I teach on this subject.

Wildlife managers who came after Leopold tended to either ignore disease or to have a fatalistic attitude toward disease, believing it to be a natural phenomenon that happened irrespective of human actions (Friend 1981). Disease has not been thought of in the same terms as predation, harvest, or food supply nor has it been included in basic calculations of life history other than, perhaps, as a minor item in general discussion. Friend (1981) described the evolution of response to disease die-offs by wildlife managers as a four-step process (table 14.1) and characterized the response as having stalled in the early stages of step 3 (i.e., responding in a reactive and largely unplanned manner). I have modified

table 14.1 from the original slightly by placing assessment of effectiveness of management before development of more effective management because I believe that it is not possible to develop better methods until you can measure the effectiveness of existing methods. Most of the disease-management techniques that have been used in wild animals have not been assessed objectively. It is noteworthy that Friend (1981) was concerned primarily with those diseases that cause conspicuous die-offs, because that form of disease is most obvious although not necessarily the most important.

DISEASE: MORE THAN JUST DEAD BODIES

Leopold (1933) recognized that the undervaluation of disease as an ecological factor resulted from the difficulty in observing its effects, because "diseased wild animals disappear or succumb to natural enemies." Disease is conspicuous only when many animals die over a short period and dead bodies pile up, consequently interest has centered on diseases such as avian cholera in waterfowl and morbillivirus infection in seals that cause large die-offs and on agents that cause conspicuous pathology.

Subclinical disease has received little attention, although there is abundant evidence that disease agents can affect survival and reproduction without causing obvious die-offs. For instance, subclinical infection with intestinal nematodes increased the vulnerability of snowshoe hares to predation (Ives and Murray 1997), and although cowpox virus causes no signs of clinical disease, infection caused a 25% reduction in fecundity by increasing the time to first litter by 20–30 days (Feore et al. 1997). Gunn and Irvine (2003) contrasted the situation in wild animals, in which subclinical disease is largely overlooked, with that in domestic livestock in which millions of dollars are spent annually in reducing

Table 14.1 Evolution of Responses by Wildlife Managers to Occurrence of Disease (Primarily Large Die-Offs)

Level	Response	Stage	Perspective toward disease
1	Recognition that disease exists, acceptance of disease as a natural event	Awareness	Fatalistic
2	Desire to respond to die-offs, no action because none obvious	Concern	Frustration
3	a. Response in unplanned manner	Control	Fire-fighting (reactive)
	b. Planned response		
	c. Evaluation of effectiveness of control		
	d. Development of improved methods		
4	a. Reaction well organized, prevention given attention	Prevention	Problem solving
	b. Research on control and prevention		
	c. Disease concepts integrated into routine wildlife management		

Source: Modified from Friend (1981).

subclinical effects of agents on reproduction and growth. To evaluate the effects of a disease agent on individual animals, one needs to consider all stages of development and the animal's entire life span. For instance, Cam et al. (2003) demonstrated that conditions during growth (when many infectious diseases occur) contribute to a permanent component of individual quality and fitness. In considering the effect of a disease agent on a population, the distribution of the agent and the effects of the disease on the lifetime fitness of the individuals that make up the population have to be considered.

THE COST OF DISEASE

Yuill (1987) discussed the "mayhem and subtlety" of infectious disease in wild mammals and stressed that every infection has a cost, although it may be difficult to measure the cost with the insensitive tools at our disposal. Noninfectious diseases such as those caused by nutritional deficiency, toxicants, and degenerative processes also have a cost. Disease is a relative rather than an absolute state. Disease is not like pregnancy: an animal can be a little bit or a lot diseased. Animals infected with an agent or with residues of a toxicant in their tissues may show no obvious impairment of function, although they may have made physiological or behavioral adjustments to compensate for the agent. This represents the "subtlety" of disease referred to by Yuill (1987). In such situations, it is tempting to conclude that the agent has no effect or that it is harmless, but a more accurate interpretation would be that the costs are manageable under current conditions. Under differ-

ent circumstances, the same agent may be so costly that severe impairment ("mayhem") occurs.

Although we tend to think about diseases one at a time, wild animals are affected by many different agents, often simultaneously. It is difficult to evaluate costs or to understand interactions among agents and how these relate to predation, weather, or other environmental conditions, without having some form of "currency." Energy is the best currency for measuring disease cost, although protein and other nutrients might also be the basis for trade-offs (Zuk and Stoehr 2002). Disease agents interfere with energy acquisition and reduce assimilation or retention of energy, so that energy is consumed for disease resistance and for repair of injury. The presence of a disease agent results in demands that compete for energy with growth, reproduction, resistance to other disease agents, and avoidance of predators.

I wrote this section while working in Manitoba in late March. Snow was still deep in the forest, with a heavy crust from melting and freezing. Late winter is a tough time for wild ungulates, and there was concern for moose in the area. Thinking in terms of energy costs allowed me to visualize how winter ticks (*Dermacentor albipictus*), hydatid cysts of *Echinococcus granulosus*, liver flukes (*Fascioloides magna*), and degenerative changes associated with aging might interact with each other and with weather and wolves to affect the moose. Walking in deep, crusted snow is hard work, even for a moose, and running to escape wolves consumes huge amounts of energy, so that energy demand is high at a time of year when movement and energy intake are restricted. Winter ticks occur on moose every year, but the intensity of infection is highly variable year to year. Ticks extract blood that is costly to replace, they initiate inflammation in the skin that also is costly, and they stimulate intense scratching and rubbing behavior. Heavily infested moose feed less than lightly infested animals and loss of hair increases the energy cost for thermoregulation.

Infection with *Echinococcus* hydatid cysts is common and the prevalence and intensity of infection increase with age in moose, that is, old moose are more often infected and carry more cysts than young moose. There is a mild inflammatory reaction about cysts, with a slight cost for cell turnover and replacement, and there undoubtedly is an immune response that has a cost. The liver has abundant reserve capacity so that hydatid cysts located there have little effect on liver function, but if many golf-ball-sized cysts (fig. 5.2) are located in the lungs, they reduce the capacity for gas exchange. This is not a problem for an animal moving slowly but could be critical when plunging through snow to escape wolves. Liver fluke infection is not common in this particular area, but prevalence increases with age and infection in moose results in severe inflammation and fibrosis of the liver (fig. 5.1). In my experience, moose infected with this parasite generally are in poor body condition. Degeneration of joints and attrition of teeth occur with aging in moose. Joint disease limits mobility for feeding and escape, and tooth wear reduces food acquisition and processing. Little is known about the viruses, protozoa, and intestinal worms that occur in moose except that they do occur and that they each will have a cost. Similarly, little is known about chemical residues in moose, although they may accumulate cadmium in their kidneys with age, which might affect kidney function.

When we have identified the various factors, we can begin to add up all of the costs affecting a moose. Costs related to ticks and the amount of energy required for moving through snow are highly variable from year to year. In "bad" years, individual moose may provide sustenance for more than 50,000 ticks (Samuel and Welch 1991). The cost of *Echinococcus* cysts, liver flukes, and joint disease are relatively constant from year to year. Weather is the primary underlying factor that introduces stochasticity. Weather during the previous year influenced how many ticks the moose carry and how much stored energy (fat) the animals had in the autumn. Weather during the winter determines how rapidly fat stores are depleted and how long the animals will have to wait for relief in the form of spring green-up.

In "good" years with relatively few ticks, moderate snow depth, and an early spring, the total cost is manageable and the effects of the various disease agents are "subtle" and only evident in the most disadvantaged individuals in the population, such as old bulls that entered the winter with low fat reserves because of the rut, degenerative changes in their joints, and a high probability of having hydatid cysts and liver flukes. The worst case occurs in winters when heavy tick infestation coincides with deep snow early in the fall so that fat stores are reduced, followed by severe cold and prolonged deep snow with crusting, and delayed spring breakup. Under these conditions, a larger proportion of the population will run out of energy, some will die of starvation, some will be unable to avoid or defend themselves against wolves because of lack of resources for antipredator behavior, and some that survive may have poor reproductive success. It is tempting to attribute the mortality in the bad years to the "mayhem" of winter ticks or to predation, but it is important to remember that the costs for ticks, flukes, tapeworms, joint disease, and other factors are additive and superimposed on weather and predation. This example demonstrates that disease must always be considered as a context-dependent variable (Brown et al. 2003).

EXPOSURE AND RESISTANCE

Exposure and resistance to disease agents govern the occurrence of disease. All attempts to manage or control disease consist of trying to either reduce exposure or to increase resistance. Animals do not become diseased unless they are exposed to the causative agent, and animals do not develop disease if they have adequate resistance to the agent. The "dose" of agent required to result in disease depends upon the degree of resistance of the animal, and the effectiveness of resistance depends upon the severity of the exposure challenge. Earlier I used disease caused by *Aspergillus fumigatus*, a ubiquitous saprophytic fungus growing free in the environment, to illustrate this point. Birds and mammals, including humans, are exposed frequently to the conidia (spores) of this fungus in the air (Latgé 2001) but disease is uncommon. In birds, the disease aspergillosis occurs under two circumstances: when they are exposed to an overwhelming dose of spores (e.g., by feeding on obviously moldy food) or when they have reduced resistance to infection. An extremely large exposure can overcome normal resistance, or a normal level of exposure is sufficient to overcome resistance in immunologically compromised birds. In humans, aspergillosis is uncommon except among immunosuppressed individuals in which fatal invasive infection occurs.

Exposure to disease agents is modified by many factors. Some animals are exposed to disease factors because of their ecologic niche. This is equivalent to "occupational exposure" to certain diseases, which occurs in humans. For instance, fish-eating animals often are exposed to high levels of organic mercury because methylation of mercury occurs in aquatic environments and methylmercury accumulates in fish. Thus, mercury poisoning is an occupational hazard for loons but not for geese, although they may share a wetland. I have worked for many years on Eyebrow Lake, a wetland where botulism occurs frequently in ducks. I have never found a Canada goose with botulism on this lake although the lake is used heavily by geese. However, the geese are grazing and hence not exposed to botulinum toxin in maggots from carcasses. Similarly, vultures in Pakistan are poisoned by scavenging livestock treated with an anti-inflammatory drug (Oaks et al. 2004) because of their lifestyle. Individuals within a population are exposed to more or less of an agent because of differences in food habits, movement, or behavior. For instance, young male bison are particularly at risk of infection with brucellosis because of their interest and attention to aborting animals (Rhyan 2000). Environmental conditions and animal density have a major impact on exposure, for example, *Pasteurella multocida* persists in surface water and may accumulate in wetlands used by large numbers of birds for extended periods of time.

Exposure to many infectious agents depends upon the amount and type of contact among animals. We know very little about how contact actually occurs among wild animals, although this is critical for understanding how disease is transmitted within populations. For instance, how often does an elk with tuberculosis contact another elk sufficiently intimately to transmit the disease? In some models of infectious disease, contact is assumed to occur randomly or homogenously among animals in a population. A little reflection on my own life would suggest that this model is not appropriate for me, and it is probably not appropriate for most wild animals. Most of my close contacts are not random; they are with family members, immediate neighbors, and persons of similar lifestyle and occupation. The more intimate the contact required for transmission of a disease, the less random that contact is, and the smaller

the number of effective contacts. There is consensus that contact and disease transmission among wild animals are related positively to animal abundance, but "more work is needed on understanding the mechanisms of mixing and hence disease transmission between infected and susceptible wildlife hosts, as the results of the few studies undertaken to date are somewhat contradictory" (Caley and Ramsey 2001).

Resistance involves an array of mechanisms including behavioral avoidance, physical barriers to penetration by agents, detoxification systems, and the innate and acquired immune systems. All of these may be compromised by many other factors affecting the animal. Resistance to individual agents waxes and wanes throughout an animal's life. The level of resistance among individuals within a group or population is usually highly variable. For example, Bell and Stewart (1983) observed "order-of-magnitude" differences in susceptibility to *Francisella tularensis* (the cause of tularemia) among voles reared under uniform conditions. Resistance within a population, both innate and acquired, relates to previous experience with the agent both by the population as a whole (with selection of individuals with greater innate resistance) and by the individual in the form of acquired immunity. The severe effect of many newly introduced disease agents, which cause so-called virgin soil epizootics, is the result of a lack of experience with the agent and of effective resistance.

The relationship between exposure and resistance may be complex and change rapidly. For example, cormorants of any age likely can be infected with avian paramyxovirus 1 (the cause of Newcastle disease), but clinical disease has been recognized only in hatch-year birds during a brief window of time in midsummer. This timing seems to be a result of interaction between exposure and resistance. Antibodies are transferred in the egg yolk from adult female cormorants to their offspring, so that many nestlings are resistant to infection for about 2 weeks after hatching. Hatchlings become susceptible to infection following decline of this "passive" resistance but, because they remain on the nest and have direct contact only with parents and siblings for several weeks, exposure is limited. When nestlings leave the nest and begin to wander about the colony (the cormorant equivalent of kindergarten), there is a great deal of mixing and contact. If the virus is present in the colony at this time, perhaps from adult birds, many susceptible young are exposed and develop disease with high mortality. However, if exposure does not occur during this period, the fledglings develop relative resistance as they become older. If exposed to the virus later, they may become infected but do not develop clinical disease (Kuiken et al. 1998).

DISEASE AND TRADE-OFFS

In Utopia no animal would ever be exposed to a disease agent, and, just to be on the safe side, every individual would have absolute resistance to all disease agents. In reality animals are exposed continually to disease agents, and life consists of a never-ending series of compromises and skirmishes. Life history theory suggests that organisms maximize fitness over their lifetime through physiological trade-offs between resource-demanding activities (Stearns 1992). I have identified various trade-offs that affect disease in different places in this book and will not repeat them all here, but I believe that it is critical to the understanding of disease to realize that trade-offs are being made, and that there are no absolute rules as to which competing activity will be supported. Both infectious agents and animal hosts make trade-offs. Infectious agents have to balance extracting as many resources as possible from the animal against causing so much harm that they endanger their own survival or transmission to the next host. Similarly, if the host invests heavily in resistance to one disease, it may become more susceptible to other agents as well as to predators, and it may not be able to grow or reproduce effectively.

One would assume that animals should avoid exposure to disease agents whenever possible and mount a strong resistance against those agents that cannot be avoided. But it may not always be in an animal's best interest to avoid exposure to a disease agent. For instance, the degree to which sheep avoid grazing near feces (with the attendant risk of exposure to nematode larvae) depends upon the nutritional state of the animal (Hutchings et al. 1999). For animals in a poor nutritional state, gaining high-quality nutrients apparently is more valuable than avoiding infection. It may not always be advantageous to mount a strong immune or inflammatory response to an agent if the resources required for that response limit growth, reproduction, or survival (e.g., Hanssen et al. 2004) or if the response is very damaging. (Recall that much of the damage in disease results from the response to the agent rather than from the agent itself.) Trade-offs related to disease have been studied most intensively in the relationship between parasites and reproduction in birds. Both reproduction and disease resistance are costly. Reproductive effort reduces the ability to mount an immune response (Deerenberg et al. 1997) and, conversely, immune defense can result in reduced reproductive performance (Ilmonen et al. 2000). The cost of disease in reproducing birds can be "paid" by the offspring through reduced survival or growth, or by the parents through reduced survival or reduced future reproductive performance (Møller 1994). It is clear that many diseases increase susceptibility to predation, and this may be mediated in some cases by trade-offs related to use of resources for disease resistance versus predator avoidance. Conversely, there is evidence that exposure to predators may result in reduced investment in defense against disease agents and a higher level of parasitism, also as a result of trade-offs (Navarro et al. 2004). To understand the full impact of costs and trade-offs related to disease, it may be necessary to identify the competing demands and measure these over the lifetime of the animal.

LIFE AND FAIRNESS

The initial reaction when considering disease is to think of it as a factor that acts uniformly or randomly on all members of a group or population. However, homogenous distribution of disease is probably never the case; some members of the population always bear the brunt of disease while others are spared. This unfair allocation results from differences in exposure and resistance among individuals. The uneven distribution of disease is most apparent in diseases caused by agents such as helminths. It has been known for many years that macroparasites are distributed in a clumped manner among animals (Shaw et al. 1998). Most members of any population have few or no parasites and a small number of individuals have a large number of parasites. This has important implications for understanding disease caused by these agents because severe effects are limited to a small segment of the population, and the heavily infected individuals are responsible for most of the transmission of the agent. Some authors refer to this "overdispersion" as conforming to a "20/80 rule" in which approximately 20% of the population is responsible for 80% of parasite transmission (Skorping and Jensen 2004). Why these individuals are heavily infected has received little attention. One might ask if they are genetically inferior, came from bad homes and had a troubled childhood, or got in with the wrong crowd and had unusual exposure to agents. As an alternative, could their plight be the result of trade-offs that they or their parents made in relation to other diseases? In humans, malnutrition and parasitism among children tend to occur in the same individuals with poverty as an underlying cause (Bundy and Golden 1987). In mammals, males may be more susceptible than females to infectious diseases and in some cases may be responsible for a considerable portion of the disease transmission (Ferrari et al. 2004), although the reasons for this are not clear.

There are privileged and underprivileged members in any wild population. The clearest examples of this are in highly territorial species in which the survival of non-territorial individuals is much lower than that of animals possessing territory. I am not aware of any study that has compared the overall disease status of territorial and nonterritorial individuals, but it is safe to assume that those with resources are better equipped to resist disease than those that lack resources. For instance, red grouse of low social status had larger numbers of cecal worms *(Trichostrongylus tenuis)* than did privileged grouse (Jenkins et al. 1963). Disease also may prevent individuals from competing successfully for territory and resources, for example, Delahay et al. (1995) suggested that infection with *T. tenuis* could reduce the ability of male red grouse to defend a territory. Even in nonterritorial species, there is unequal access to resources that may affect fitness (Nilsen et al. 2004). Resource shortage early in life might have consequences throughout an animal's life. Peterson (1988) suggested that nutritional stress early in life was responsible for degenerative joint disease in moose during senescence.

TRANSPECIFICS: THE PARASITES AND PATHOGENS TO WATCH OUT FOR

Caughley and Sinclair (1994) made the observation that transpecifics are the parasites and pathogens to watch out for in reference to the potential effect of disease agents on species targeted for conservation. Such species usually have small populations. In general, if an infectious agent has only a single host species, the agent cannot afford to be too damaging, because this will endanger its own existence and transmission. If the disease has a short infectious period, a large population of hosts is required to maintain sufficient susceptible animals for the disease to persist. Thus, single-species agents that are highly virulent or that must be transmitted frequently cannot persist in small host populations. The most often quoted example of this is that the measles virus (with humans as its sole host) can only persist in populations ≥300,000 to 500,000 persons.

A commonly observed phenomenon is that small host populations have a much reduced parasite community, because many of the host-specific agents have died out. This is important in the conservation of species with small numbers of individuals, because host-specific disease agents are unlikely to cause extinction (the disease will die out before the host population). However, generalist or multihost agents are not under the same constraints because they may be maintained in one or more abundant species and spill over with a severe impact on a threatened or endangered species. An example is the near extinction of the black-footed ferret by canine distemper virus, which circulated and was maintained in other abundant species including coyotes, badgers, skunks, and dogs. The distemper virus in this situation is acting in a manner directly analogous to wolves that were maintained by feeding on moose but appeared to be driving a small population of caribou to extinction (Seip 1992). The population of black-footed ferrets was inadequate to support the distemper virus and the small number of caribou could not support the wolf population, but both suffered spillover effects from more abundant animals.

Another risk associated with multihost agents is that they are often much more virulent in "alternate" or "unusual" hosts than they are in the species in which they are maintained. There are many examples of this phenomenon in wild animals including *Parelaphostrongylus tenuis* that is maintained in white-tailed deer and severely injurious in moose and caribou (Lankester 2001), *Heterakis gallinarum* that is maintained in ring-necked pheasants and injurious to grey partridge (Tompkins et al. 2000), ovine herpesvirus-2 that causes clinically silent infection in sheep and severe malignant catarrhal fever in deer, avian malaria (*Plasmodium* spp. infection) that is clinically silent in indigenous passerines but fatal in zoo penguins, Sin Nombre virus maintained in deer mice that causes fatal hantavirus pulmonary syndrome in humans, and *Brucella abortus* that usually causes mild, chronic disease in cattle and bison but causes severe, generalized disease in moose (Forbes et al. 1996).

INFLUENCE OF HUMANS ON DISEASE

As a first year university student, I had a class in English that met Saturday mornings. The earnest young instructor tried his utmost to instill a modicum of culture into unreceptive farm boys. On one occasion he gave the class a series of phrases and sentences for which we were to produce a more grammatically correct rendition. One item was the phrase "the virgin forest where the hand of man has never set foot," for which the most appreciated correction was "a virgin in the hand is worth two in the forest." I use this simply as a device to introduce the fact that there are no forests where humans have not set their foot or hand. The diseases that occur today in wild animals are different than those that occurred in pristine environments because of human activities. No wild animal is unaffected by humans and humans influence disease in many different ways (table 14.2).

The connection between humans and wildlife disease is most obvious in conditions caused by human-made toxicants and by natural poisons that have been moved about and concentrated by humans. The list of such compounds is lengthy, with the most notorious being DDT and other organo-chlorine insecticides, lead, and mercury. When Leopold wrote about disease in 1933, synthetic insecticides were still in the future and mercury poisoning had not been recognized but lead poisoning was known to occur in birds. Although in retrospect it seems that it took a long time to relate the effects of DDT to the decline of bird populations, it is important to remember that this was the first instance of widespread environmental consequences from the use of a "beneficial" chemical. The early evidence regarding DDT was correlational so that it was difficult to prove a cause:effect relationship. The DDT story exemplifies the value of long-term data in identifying problems, such as the data on eggshell thickness in British sparrowhawks. A sudden decrease in eggshell thickness followed widespread use of DDT in agriculture in 1947, with recovery occurring during the 1970s and 1980s as use of the

Table 14.2 Interrelatedness Between Disease in Wild Animals and Human Activities

Human activity	Diseases that have been influenced
Production and release of toxic materials	Insecticide, rodenticide poisoning
Movement and concentration of natural poisons	Lead, mercury, selenium poisoning
Translocation of disease agents (intentional)	Myxomatosis, rabbit hemorrhagic disease
Translocation of disease agents with domestic animals that spread to wildlife	Rinderpest, bovine tuberculosis, brucellosis
Translocation of disease agents with wild animals (unintentional)	*Elaphostrongylus rangiferi* to Newfoundland (in reindeer), *Fascioloides magna* to Europe (in elk)
Introduction of wild animals that altered the ecology of an existing disease	Brushtailed possums into New Zealand (tuberculosis), vole into Svalbard (*Echinococcus multilocularis*)
Direct spread of livestock diseases to wild animals	Chlamydial conjunctivitis from sheep to chamois
Loss of normal habitat, concentration of animals	Avian cholera in waterfowl, tuberculosis in white-tailed deer
Disease as a direct consequence of use of artificial food	Rumenitis in deer and pronghorns, mycotoxicosis in waterfowl and cranes, vitamin A deficiency in ducks
Introduction of susceptible animals into environment containing indigenous disease	Caribou into areas where *Parelaphostrongylus tenuis* had become established
Eutrophication of water with enhanced growth of toxigenic microorganisms	Cyanobacterial and domoic acid poisoning
Spread of human disease to wild animals	*Mycobacterium bovis* to suricates and mongooses
Spread of wildlife disease to humans	HIV1, HIV2 from primates
Alteration of population density	*Echinococcus multilocularis* in foxes in Europe
Spread of wildlife disease to domestic livestock	Newcastle disease from cormorants to turkeys
Climate change	Distribution of many diseases, especially those with life cycles involving invertebrates
Acidification altering availability of micronutrients and toxicants	Calcium deficiency in birds, cadmium toxicity in mammals
Removal of predators	May affect many infectious diseases

chemical was progressively restricted and then banned (Newton 1998). Without this type of data, it would have been much more difficult to link effect to cause. The story of DDT can be credited as a disease-management success as can restrictions on the use of lead shot and cessation of use of organomercurial seed dressings. But even these agents have not disappeared completely. Organochlorine insecticides, including DDT, are still used in some parts of the world (Chen and Rogan 2003), residues persist in soil and other parts of the environment, and animals still carry residues in their tissues. Accumulation of mercury continues in aquatic species and birds still die of lead poisoning. Restrictions were placed on the use of lead, mercury, and DDT because their effects were dramatic and recognizable. Wild animals are exposed to many other chemicals, such as endocrine-disrupting compounds whose effect is more subtle and difficult to prove but probably not beneficial.

Humans are inveterate translocators of animals and disease agents. In colonial times, domestic animals were moved to the colonies to establish basic agriculture. The cattle that were moved brought with them bovine tuberculosis and brucellosis, which sometimes spilled into indigenous animals. The most dramatic such introduction of disease was of rinderpest virus to Africa in cattle from India, resulting in a huge epizootic among wild ruminants (Henderson 1982). Wild animals have been moved for sport, nostalgia, industry, and trivial purposes, and these animals often have brought disease agents with them. For instance, the same phage types of *Salmonella typhimurium* occur in house sparrows in Canada and Europe (Wobeser and Finlayson 1969), and *Elaphostrongylus cervi* occurs in red deer in both Scotland and New Zealand (Mason et al. 1976). The brushtailed possum, introduced to New Zealand to establish a fur industry, became the major reservoir of bovine tuberculosis in that country. Other translocations were inadvertent: the mosquito *Aedes albopictus,* a vector for many arboviruses, was introduced to North America from Asia in used tires (Hawley et al. 1987); voles introduced to Svalbard by unknown means allowed *Echinococcus multilocularis* to become established there (Hentonnen et al. 2001). Some disease translocations can be excused because they occurred at a time when the risks were not understood, but others occurred despite abundant evidence of a disease risk. Two such instances are well documented. Tuberculosis and probably also brucellosis were moved in Canada with plains bison from Buffalo National Park to Wood Buffalo

National Park in 1926 despite knowledge that the source herd was infected with *Mycobacterium bovis* and despite strong scientific opposition to the translocation (Fuller 2002). In 1987, caribou from Newfoundland were relocated to Maine. This took place despite knowledge that Newfoundland caribou were infected with *Elaphostrongylus rangiferi,* an Old World parasite not found elsewhere in North America that causes neurological disease in caribou and moose (Lankester 1977), and that white-tailed deer in Maine were infected with *Parelaphostrongylus tenuis,* which causes fatal neurological disease in caribou. The introduction attempt failed, probably because of *P. tenuis* infection in the animals that were moved (McCollough and Connery 1990). Among other things, the latter example demonstrates a failure to recognize that disease situations now are not the same as in pristine environments. When caribou occurred naturally in Maine, white-tailed deer and *P. tenuis* were not present, and caribou on Newfoundland were not infected with *E. rangiferi,* which was introduced with reindeer from Norway in 1908 (Lankester and Fong 1989).

A third major human activity that affects disease in wild animals is habitat disruption. As natural habitat shrinks, there often is a desire to maintain populations at high density on residual areas. As Leopold observed in 1933, "a high density of population—the very thing the game manager is so far usually seeking to obtain—must be set down as the most fundamental condition favorable to disease." Waterfowl are gregarious and have always occurred in large flocks so that dense aggregation is nothing new for these species. But dense aggregations that use the same limited area of water for the entire winter, as now occurs on many refuges, is a new phenomenon. In the past, exhaustion of local food supply dictated that birds had to move frequently. The combination of abundant food in the form of agricultural crops and no where else to go now results in birds remaining in one location, together with their accumulated excreta, for months allowing wide interchange of agents such as *Pasteurella multocida.* Artificial feeding used to supplement natural habitat and to maintain a wild population at high density has the same effect and is important in the occurrence of tuberculosis in artificially fed white-tailed deer in Michigan and brucellosis in feedground elk.

Human pressure and habitat loss have brought wild and domestic animals and humans more closely together than ever before. Emergence of "new" human and livestock diseases that originate in wild animals has received attention, but the emergence of diseases such as canine distemper in wild dogs and lions and of human tuberculosis in suricates and mongooses is the mirror image of the problem. Other types of habitat modification, such as changes in the distribution and quality of water and changes in vegetation, also have dramatic effects on disease transmission.

The point of this rather depressing discussion is that we must be conscious of both the immediate and historic effects of humans on disease in the uphill battle to retain wild things in the face of an ever-increasing human population. "We manage the remaining natural habitats and fauna intensively in an effort to accommodate as much of the area's original biodiversity as possible. Our management focus is usually on making the best of the situation, while we refrain from addressing the core issue, the population explosion" (Coleman 1993).

A JOB FOR THE FUTURE

Disease in wild animals is not about to go away. It will become increasingly important and increasingly an integrated part of wildlife management (see stage 4c in table 14.1). As pointed out earlier, diseases are like weeds: they thrive in disturbed environments. Those interested in wild animals increasingly will have to deal with the effects of disease on small populations in habitat fragments, with problems related to the spillover of disease from domestic species into wild animals and from wild animals to humans and livestock, and with new chemicals and substances appearing in the "natural" environment. Who would have imagined that residues in water of birth control pills used by people might be a risk to wild animals or that a drug used to relieve pain in livestock could essentially extirpate the vulture population of a subcontinent? There will be continuing pressure to manage diseases that spill over from wild animals to humans and domestic animals. Experience in the past few years with the emergence of West Nile fever, SARS, and avian influenza should be regarded as a prelude to more of the same in the future. Often the "simple" solution proposed

to such problems is to get rid of the wild animals either partially or completely but, as demonstrated by experience with reducing badger populations in England to manage tuberculosis (Donnelly et al. 2003), this may not be the best method, even if it were ethically or morally acceptable.

There is a need to integrate those who understand what the animals are doing with those who understand the medical and physiological aspects of disease, and there is a need to use new methods to study disease. Leopold recognized that observational and correlational studies are limited in their ability to lead to an understanding of disease. Tompkins et al. (2001a) identified the same problem in trying to determine if parasites regulate populations and stated, "hosts or parasites have to be experimentally perturbed to determine if regulation occurs—experiments that few workers have undertaken." Manipulation could be done by adding agents to an uninfected host population or by removing agents from a population and observing the effect. Studies of the effects of cecal worms on red grouse (Hudson et al. 1992b), abomasal nematodes on Soay sheep (Gulland 1992), selenium deficiency in mule deer (Flueck 1994), and intestinal nematodes on snowshoe hares (Ives and Murray 1997) have demonstrated clearly that these agents have population-level effects, a fact that could not have been ascertained without experimental manipulation.

I began this book with reference to Aldo Leopold and I can think of no more apt way to conclude than by repeating the ending to his chapter on disease written more than 70 years ago.

> It should be remarked in closing this chapter that if the reader has not emerged with a clear picture of game diseases, he is no different from even the most skilled specialists, and need berate neither himself nor the book. If, however, he has built up an enlarged appreciation of the scope and complexity of the disease factor, and has caught a few convincing glimpses of its hidden mechanisms, the writer's object will have been achieved.

Appendix
Scientific Names of Species

Badger   European: *Meles meles*
North American: *Taxidea taxus*

Bat   fruit: *Pteropus* spp.
vampire: *Desmodus rotundus*

Bear   polar: *Ursus maritimus*

Beaver   *Castor canadensis*

Bison   *Bison bison*

Boar   wild: *Sus scrofa*

Bobcat   *Lynx rufus*

Buffalo   African: *Syncerus caffer*

Caribou   *Rangifer tarandus*

Canvasback   *Aythya valisneria*

Chamois   *Rupricapra rupricapra*

Chickadee   mountain: *Poecile gambeli*

Chimpanzee   *Pan troglodytes*

Cormorant   double crested: *Phalacrocorax auritius*

Condor   California: *Gymnogyps californianus*

Coot   American: *Fulica Americana*

Cougar   *Felis concolor*

Coyote   *Canis latrans*

Crab   horseshoe: *Limulus polyphemus*

Crane   sandhill: *Grus canadensis*
whooping: *Grus americana*

Crow   American *Corvus brachyrhynchos*

Deer   black-tailed: *Odocoileus hemionus columbianus*
fallow: *Dama dama*
mule: *Odocoileus h. hemionus*
red: *Cervus elaphus*
roe: *Capreolus capreolus*
white-tailed: *Odocoileus virginianus*

Dingo   *Canis familiaris dingo*

Dog   African wild: *Lycaon pictus*

Dolphin   Indo-Pacific humpbacked: *Sousa chinensis*

Duck   whistling: *Dendrocygna* spp.

Duiker   *Sylvicapra grimmia*

Eagle   bald: *Haliaeetus leucocephalus*
golden: *Aquila chrysaetos*
Imperial: *Aquila adalberti*

Eider   common: *Somateria mollisima*

Eland   *Taurotragus oryx*

Elk   (wapiti) *Cervus elaphus*

Falcon   peregrine: *Falco peregrinus*

Ferret   *Mustela furo*
black-footed: *Mustela nigripes*

Finch   house: *Carpodacus mexicanus*

Fisher   *Martes pennanti*

Flycatcher   Collared: *Ficedula albicollis*
Pied: *Ficedula hypoleuca*

Fox   red: *Vulpes vulpes*
arctic: *Alopex lagopus*

Godwit   bar-tailed: *Limosa lapponica*

Goose   lesser snow: *Anser c. caerulescens*
Canada: *Branta canadensis*

Grebe   eared: *Podiceps nigricollis*

Ground squirrel   California: *Spermophilus beechei*
Richardson's: *Spermophilus richardsoni*

Groundhog   *Marmota monax*

Grouse   red: *Lagopus lagopus*
ruffed: *Bonasa umbellus*
sage: *Centrocercus urophasianus*
sharp-tailed: *Pedioecetes phasianellus*

Guillemot   *Cepphus* spp.

Gull   Franklin's: *Larus pipixican*
glaucous: *Larus hyperboreus*

Hamster   Siberian: *Phodoptius sungorus*

Hawk   red-tailed: *Buteo jamaicensis*

Hare   European: *Lepus europus*
mountain: *Lepus timidus*
snowshoe: *Lepus americanus*

Heron	great blue: *Ardea herodias*
Ibex	*Capra pyrenaica*
Kestrel	Eurasian: *falco tinnunculus*
Knot	red: *Calidris canutus rufa*
Koala	*Phascolarctos cinereus*
Kudu	*Tragelaphus strepsiceros*
Lemming	collared: *Dicrostonyx richardsoni*
Lion	*Panthera leo*
Loon	common: *Gavia immer*
Lynx	Eurasian: *Lynx lynx*
	North American: *Lynx canadensis*
Macaque	Asian: *Macaca* spp.
Magpie	Australian: *Gymnorhina tibicen*
Mallard	*Anas platyrhynchos*
Mangabey	sooty: *Cerocerbus atys*
Marmot	alpine: *Marmota marmota*
Marten	*Martes americana*
Martin	purple: *Progne subis*
Mink	*Mustela vison*
Mongoose	banded: *Mungos mungo*
Monkey	owl: *Aotus trivergatus*
Moose	*Alces alces*
Mouse	deer: *Peromyscus maniculatus*
	house: *Mus musculis*
	northern grasshopper: *Onychomys leucogaster*
	pine: *Pitymys pinetorum*
	white-footed: *Peromyscus leucopus*
	wood: *Apodemus sylvaticus*
Muskrat	*Ondatra zibethicus*
Northern pintail	*Anas acuta*
Northern shoveler	*Anas clypeata*
Opossum	Virginia: *Didelphis virginiana*
Otter	river: *Lutra canadensis*
	sea: *Enhydra lutris*
Owl	great horned: *Bubo virginianus*
	snowy: *Nyctea scandiaca*
Partridge	grey: *Perdix perdix*
	red-legged: *Alectoris rufa*
Peccary	collared: *Tayassu tajaca*
Pelican	brown: *Pelecanus occidentalis*
Pheasant	ring-necked: *Phasianus colchicus*
Pig	feral: *Sus scrofa*
Pigeon	(rock dove) *Columba livia*
Possum	brushtail: *Trichosurus vulpecula*
Prairie dog	black-tailed: *Cynomys ludovicianus*
Pronghorn	*Antilocapra americana*

Ptarmigan	willow: *Lagopus lagopus*
Rabbit	brush: *Sylvilagus bachmani*
	cottontail: *Sylvilagus floridanus*
	European: *Oryctolagus cuniculus*
	jungle: *Sylvilagus brasiliensis*
Raccoon	*Procyon lotor*
Rat	black: *Rattus rattus*
	Norway: *Rattus norvegicus*
Redpoll	common: *Carduelis purpureus*
Redshank	*Totanus tetanus*
Reindeer	*Rangifer t. tarandus*
Robin	American: *Turdus migratorius*
Seal	Baikal: *Phoca sibirica*
	Caspian: *Phoca caspica*
	grey: *Halichoerus grypus*
	harbor: *Phoca vitulina*
	northern fur: *Callorhinus ursinus*
Sea lion	California: *Zalophus californianus*
	northern: *Eumetopias jubatus*
Sheep	bighorn: *Ovis canadensis*
	Soay: *Ovis aries*
Shrew	common: *Sorex araneus*
Sika	*Cervus nippon*
Skunk	striped: *Mephitis mephitis*
Sparrow	house: *Passer domesticus*
	song: *Melospiza melodia*
Sparrowhawk	*Accipiter nisus*
Squirrel	grey: *Sciurius carolinensis*
	southern flying: *Glaucomys volans*
Starling	*Sturnus vulgaris*
Suricate	*Suricata suricatta*
Swan	mute: *Cygnus olor*
	tundra: *Cygnus columbianus*
Swift	alpine: *Apus melba*
Teal	blue-winged: *Anas discors*
Thrasher	sage: *Oreoscoptes montanus*
Tiger	*Panthera tigris*
Tit	blue: *Parus caerulescens*
	great: *Parus major*
Vole	bank: *Clethrionomys glareolus*
	common: *Microtus arvalis*
Vulture	oriental white-backed: *Gyps bengalensis*
	turkey: *Cathartes aura*
Wildebeest	*Connochaetes taurinus*
Wolf	*Canis lupus*
	Ethiopian: *Canis simensis*
Wombat	*Vombatus* spp.
Woodrat	Allegeheny: *Neotoma magister*

Glossary

abiotic The nonliving components of the environment.

abortion Premature expulsion from the uterus of an embryo or nonviable fetus.

abscess Localized collection of pus in a cavity formed by the disintegration of tissue.

acanthocephala A phylum of parasitic animals known commonly as thorny-headed worms.

acidification To make more acid, specifically the effect of elements such as sulfur dioxide and nitrogen oxides of anthropogenic origin on rain, soils, and waters.

acidosis A serious metabolic state in which the pH of the blood drops into the acid range.

active immunity Specific acquired immunity resulting from exposure to an agent or immunization with a vaccine.

acute Having a short and relatively severe course, as in an acute infection.

adhesin A surface protein on bacteria that mediates their adhesion to host cells.

aerobic Requiring air or free oxygen for life.

aggregated distribution Used to describe the way many parasites are distributed within host populations, with most hosts having very few parasites and a few hosts having many parasites.

alopecia Loss of hair.

anaerobic Not requiring oxygen, as in organisms that live in the absence of gaseous oxygen and respiration that uses a final electron acceptor other than oxygen.

anemia A condition in which the blood is deficient in either quantity (as might occur from blood loss) or quality (as a result of deficiency of red blood cells or hemoglobin).

anorexia Lack of desire to eat.

anoxia Absence or almost total absence of oxygen in tissues (*see* **hypoxia**).

anthelmintic Drug used to treat parasitic worm (helminth) infection.

anthropogenic Produced or caused by humans.

antibody A large molecular-weight protein produced by plasma cells in response to an antigen. Antibody binds specifically to the antigen that elicited its synthesis.

anticoagulant Suppressing, delaying, or preventing blood clotting. Used in reference to rodenticides that cause death by preventing blood coagulation.

antigen Any substance, usually foreign, that can induce an immune response.

arbovirus (arthropod-borne virus) Viruses that replicate in an arthropod and are transmitted to a vertebrate in which they also replicate.

arrest (developmental) A state in which third-stage larvae of some nematodes persist in tissue of resistant hosts without development.

arthritis Inflammation of the structures of a joint.

asymptomatic Showing or causing no clinical signs of illness.

bacteriophage A virus that infects bacteria.

basement membrane A sheet of material containing glycoproteins and collagen that lies beneath epithelial and endothelial cells and supports them.

benign Used in reference to tumors that do not become invasive and do not spread to other sites in the body.

bioaccumulation Accumulation of a compound within an animal over time because the rate of intake exceeds the rate of elimination.

biomagnification (bioamplification) Increase in the concentration of a compound at successive trophic levels within a food chain.

B lymphocyte (B cell) A specific type of lymphocyte involved in humoral immunity. B cells differentiate into plasma cells that produce antibody.

body condition   Nutritional status, often measured by "condition indices" that incorporate measurement of mass and structural size.

bursa of Fabricius   Lymphoid organ located in the cloaca of birds.

cachexia   General ill health with emaciation and wasting.

capsid   The protein coat enclosing the nucleic acid of a virus.

capture myopathy   Degenerative change that may occur in skeletal muscle of wild animals following handling.

carcinogen   Substance or agent that causes neoplasia (cancer); the process is called carcinogenesis.

carrier   Individual that harbors an infectious agent within its body and although showing no clinical signs can transmit the agent to others.

carrying capacity (*K*)   Maximum sustainable density of a population under specific environmental conditions; the natural limit of a population set by the resources available in a particular environment.

case-fatality rate   Proportion of animals affected by a particular disease that die as a result of the disease.

cell-mediated immunity   Immunity affected predominantly by T lymphocytes and accessory cells (notably macrophages) rather than by antibody.

cestode   Parasitic flatworm of the class Cestoda (tapeworm).

chronic   Denoting prolonged duration (weeks, months, years).

clinical sign   Any objective evidence of disease as perceptible to an observer.

clinically silent   A disease state that does not cause perceptible clinical signs.

clone   Population of cells or organisms derived from a single precursor and having the same genetic constitution as the unit or individual from which they were derived.

cocci   Spherical bacterial cells (sing.: coccus).

coevolution   Reciprocal natural selection between two or more groups of organisms with close ecological relationships in which changes in one tend to produce changes in the other.

commensal   The species that benefits in commensalism.

commensalism   An association between organisms of two species that live together and share resources, one species benefiting from the association and the other not being harmed.

compensation   Adjust so as to offset variations. Used in relation to disease when a population reduced below carrying capacity by one factor has increased reproductive success (compensatory natality) or reduced mortality to other causes (compensatory survival).

competition   Interaction among organisms of the same or different species in which each suffers from the presence of the other, although the interaction need not be balanced.

complement   A system of serum proteins that are sequentially activated in infection, play a part in phagocytosis, and aid in clearing bacteria and other pathogens from the body.

congenital   Present at birth.

conjunctivitis   Inflammation of the ocular membranes.

connective tissue   Matrix of mucopolysaccharide ground substance, fibroblasts, collagen, and elastic fibers that surrounds and supports elements such as blood vessels, nerves, and muscles.

conspecific   Belonging to the same species.

contagious   Capable of being transmitted from one individual to another.

critical community size   Minimum population size or density required to allow an infectious agent to persist without introductions from outside.

cross-reaction   Reaction of an antibody directed against one antigen with another antigen, because the two antigens possess a common epitope. For example, *Yersinia enterocolitica* cross-reacts in some tests for *Brucella abortus,* leading to false-negative results.

cyanobacteria   A group of photosynthetic bacteria with members that produce toxins in water. Previously called blue-green algae.

cytokines   A group of proteins that mediate cellular signaling and interactions and regulate cell growth and secretion and the immune response.

cytoskeleton   Internal system of protein fibers and tubules that extend throughout the cytoplasm of eukaryotic cells, giving shape to the cell and supporting cell extensions.

dead-end host   A species that can be infected by a disease agent acquired from outside sources but that does not maintain the agent. For example, humans can be infected with West Nile virus from mosquitoes but do not transmit the disease.

definitive host   Host in an agent's life cycle in which the agent undergoes sexual replication. In general, only applicable to protozoa and metazoan parasites.

density Number of individuals in some unit of space, as in number of animals/km². Density is sometimes related to some feature such as the number of animals using a waterhole.

density-dependent Factors that limit the growth of a population, which are dependent on the existing population density. For example, the rate of predation might be higher in dense than in less-dense populations of prey.

density-independent Factors that limit the growth of a population, which are independent of the existing population density.

depopulation Deliberate reduction of the number of animals that may be partial or complete.

dermatitis Inflammation of the skin.

desquamation Shedding of the outer epithelial elements of the skin or other surfaces.

diagnosis Process of determining the nature of a case of disease; also the decision reached from this process (as in a diagnosis of lead poisoning).

direct transmission Transfer of infection from one individual to another of the same species without the requirement for involvement of another species.

disinfectant Chemical used to destroy or inhibit the growth of infectious agents, usually on inanimate surfaces.

DNA (deoxyribonucleic acid) A macromolecule that is the main component of chromosomes, and the material that transfers genetic characteristics in all life-forms.

ectoparasite A parasitic organism that lives on the outer surface of its animal host.

edema Accumulation of excessive water in the intercellular spaces of the body.

encephalitis Inflammation of the brain.

encephalopathy A degenerative disease of the brain.

endemic 1. Restricted to a particular region, as in a bird species found only on a particular island. 2. A disease that occurs with predictable regularity and rate in a human population (*see* **enzootic**).

endocrine-disrupting chemicals Exogenous compounds that mimic or antagonize the action of hormones.

endogenous Originating within the organism.

endoparasite Parasitic organism that lives within the body of its host.

endothelium Layer of specialized cells that line the interior of blood vessels and other surfaces in contact with blood such as the internal surface of the heart.

endotoxin A toxin that is part of the bacterial cell wall and is released only when the cell is degraded. Generally used for lipopolysaccharides of cell membranes of gram-negative bacteria that may induce fever, shock, and tissue destruction.

enteritis Inflammation of the intestine.

enzootic A disease of animals that occurs with predictable regularity and rate in a population or in an area.

enzyme A protein that acts as a catalyst, speeding the rate at which a biochemical reaction proceeds but not altering the direction or nature of the reaction.

eosinophil A blood leukocyte that contains granules that stain intensely with the dye eosin. Involved in inflammatory reactions, particularly those associated with parasites.

epidemiology Study of disease in populations and of the factors that determine its occurrence.

epidermis Outermost layer of the skin, composed of epithelial cells.

epithelium Sheet of cells bound tightly together that covers all external surfaces and lines internal surfaces continuous with the external environment.

epitope Region of an antigen that binds to antibody or that is recognized by the T cell receptor in association with MHC proteins.

epizootic A disease in animals that is occurring in a time or place where it is not expected, or at a rate greater than expected on past experience. (Epidemic is used for the same purpose to describe disease in humans.)

epizootic (epidemic) curve Graphic representation of the number of cases of a disease plotted over time.

eukaryote Organisms that have a membrane-bound nucleus and mitotic spindle, and in which many cellular functions are sequestered in membrane-bound organelles in the cytoplasm. Includes algae, fungi, protozoa, and all higher organisms.

eutrophication Enrichment of bodies of water by nutrients that support growth of plants and algae.

exogenous Originating outside the body.

exudate Any fluid that is exuded from a tissue or its capillaries, also fluid exuded because of injury or inflammation that has high protein and white blood cell content.

facultative agent A disease agent that may infect an animal but for which infection is not required for perpetuation of the organism. Also, opportunistic agent.

false negative   A test result that erroneously excludes an individual from a specific group. An animal that gave a negative result in a test for a feature that is actually present. For example, an animal that is infected with an agent but is not identified by a test for that disease.

false positive   A test result that erroneously includes an individual within a specific group. An animal that gave a positive result for a feature that is not actually present. For example, an animal that tests positive for a disease agent with which it is not infected.

fasciitis   Inflammation of fascia (the loose connective tissue layer beneath the skin and between muscles).

fecundity   Measure of reproduction, often expressed as a rate equal to the number of female live births per female during a unit of time (usually a year).

feral   Once domestic but readapted to the wild state.

fever   Alteration or adaptation of normal thermoregulation in which the body temperature is elevated but still under control. Fever is part of the defense system.

fibrin   Relatively insoluble protein polymer formed by conversion of a soluble plasma protein called fibrinogen. Fibrin forms the basis for blood clots. Large amounts may be formed in certain types of inflammation ("fibrinous inflammation") and be visible on the surface of organs.

fibrosis   Repair in which the injured tissue is replaced by collagen-rich scar tissue.

fibrous   Composed of or containing fibroblasts and fibrocytes.

fitness   Relative contribution by an individual of its genotype to the next generation relative to the contribution of other genotypes.

fluctuating asymmetry   Small, random deviations from bilateral symmetry in a given morphologic feature.

focal   Used to describe the distribution of lesions in tissue, and meaning a single, restricted area of involvement.

fomites   Inanimate objects that may be contaminated with infectious agent and become a vehicle for transmission (Sing.:-fomes, fomite).

fragmentation of habitat   Subdivision of extensive areas of habitat such as forests into smaller subunits separated by other types of land use.

gas gangrene   Necrosis of soft tissue with the presence of gas within the tissues liberated by bacterial fermentation caused by anaerobic, spore-forming bacteria.

genome   Complete set of genes of an organism.

gold standard (for a test)   The best evidence available to which the results of a test can be compared, e.g., identification of nematodes at necropsy might be used as a gold standard against which other tests, such as examining feces for parasite eggs, can be compared.

Golgi apparatus   Organelle in eukaryotic cells involved in directing membrane lipids and proteins and secretory proteins to the correct destination.

Gram stain   System of staining bacteria that distinguishes between groups of bacteria based on differences in cell wall composition. Gram-positive bacteria stain blue; gram-negative bacteria stain red.

habitat   Resources (food, shelter) and environmental conditions (abiotic and biotic) that determine the presence, survival, and reproduction of a population.

half-life   Time required for the activity or quantity of a substance taken into the body to decrease by half.

helper T cell   T lymphocytes that when stimulated by antigen presented in association with MHC molecules are able to enhance the function of other lymphocytes and macrophages.

hemorrhage   Escape of blood from blood vessels.

hemorrhagic   Characterized by hemorrhage.

horizontal transmission   Transfer of an infectious agent from one animal to others in the population independent of their parental relationship.

host range   Range of species susceptible to infection by an agent.

humoral immunity   Specific immunity mediated by antibodies.

hyperemia   Presence of increased blood flow to an area or tissue.

hyperthermia   Uncontrolled elevation of body temperature.

hypothermia   Subnormal body temperature.

hypotrichosis   Less than normal amount of hair on the body surface.

hypoxia   Decrease below normal level of oxygen in blood or tissues.

ichemia   Focal lack of blood flow to a tissue, usually as a result of obstruction or narrowing of arterial vessels.

icterus (jaundice) Yellow staining of tissues and excretions resulting from increased levels of bile pigments in blood.

idiopathic disease Disease whose cause is currently unknown.

immunosuppression Reduction in normal level of responsiveness of the immune system.

incidence Number of new cases of a disease occurring over a fixed period of time divided by the number of animals at risk of developing the disease during that time. Incidence is *not* synonymous with prevalence.

indigenous Belonging to the locality.

indirect transmission A form of transmission in which two or more host species are required for completion of the life cycle.

infarction Sudden death or necrosis of tissue because of interruption of blood supply.

infection Invasion and replication of an agent within a host animal.

infectious period Time period during which an infected animal is able to transmit the agent to another host.

inflammation The reaction of living vascularized tissue to injury, including changes in blood flow to the area, vascular permeability, and influx of white blood cells.

ingesta Nutrient material taken in by ingestion.

inherent Occurring as a natural part or consequence.

inherited Characteristics or qualities that are transmitted from parents to offspring by encoded cytologic data.

intensity (of infection) Number of disease agents per infected host.

intermediate host The host in indirect transmission cycles in which sexual replication of the agent does not occur (only appropriate for protozoa and helminths).

intrinsic Used in population ecology for the maximal rate of natural increase in a population having a balanced age distribution.

isolation In microbiology, to separate an organism from others, as when a particular bacterium is grown on artificial medium from a sample of diseased tissue. The viable organisms separated on a single occasion from a sample are referred to as an isolate.

K-selected Species in which selection favors maintenance of the individual and production of relatively few offspring; species with low fecundity, low mortality, and longer life span, generally associated with stable environments.

larva migrans Larval stage of a helminth that wanders for a time in host tissue but does not develop to the adult stage.

latency Persistent infection in which the agent may not be detectable and causes no detectable disease but remains capable of activation and disease production.

lesion Pathologic change in tissue.

life cycle The various stages that an organism goes through from origin to maturity and reproduction.

limitation Those factors that determine the size of the equilibrium population. Any factor that affects reproduction or causes mortality is a limiting factor.

lymph Clear, transparent fluid collected from tissues throughout the body that flows in lymphatic vessels and eventually enters the venous blood circulation.

lymphocytes White blood cells involved in the immune response, B lymphocytes mature to become plasma cells that produce antibodies, T lymphocytes are responsible for cell-mediated immunity.

lysozyme Enzyme present in some white blood cells (neutrophils, macrophages) as well as in some secretions (mucus, saliva, tears) that lyses certain bacteria and potentiates the action of complement.

macromolecule Very large polymeric organic molecules (e.g., proteins).

macroparasite An ecological classification for parasites in which direct reproduction rarely occurs in the definitive host, but asexual reproduction may occur in intermediate hosts, generation time is long, infections tend to be persistent with reinfection being common, and disease produced is usually chronic and sublethal. The organisms are generally large, they have a diversity of antigens, and host immunity is dependent on continued presence of the organisms.

macrophage Large white blood cells derived from cells in the bone marrow that are important in phagocytosis and destruction of foreign particles and cell-mediated immunity.

maintenance host Host species within which the agent can persist indefinitely without external sources of infection.

major histocompatibility complex (MHC) Chromosomal region containing the genes for histocompatibility antigens and some other genes involved in the immune response.

malaise A feeling of general discomfort and uneasiness.

mange Inflammatory disease of the skin (dermatitis) caused by any of several genera of mites.

maternal immunity Transfer of antibody from mother to the offspring through the placenta, the egg yolk (birds), or milk. (The process is called passive transfer.)

memory cell Cells generated during an immune response that survive to give an accelerated immune response on reexposure to the same antigen.

meningitis Inflammation of the membranes (meninges) that cover the brain and spinal cord.

meta-analysis Analyses that make use of published data, often from several studies, for hypothesis testing.

metapopulation A set of populations distributed over a number of patches that are connected, to some degree, by dispersal.

metazoan Animals having more than one cell and having at least two tissue layers; includes arthropods and helminths.

microaerophilic Used in reference to bacteria that require oxygen, but at concentrations less than present in air.

micronutrients Essential food items required only in small amounts (e.g., selenium, zinc).

microparasite An ecological classification of parasites that undergo rapid multiplication within their vertebrate host, have a short generation time, and have antigens that are relatively simple. Infections are generally short-lived, and host immunity following infection is long-lived.

mitochondrion Cellular organelle that is the site of aerobic respiration and ATP generation in eukaryotic cells.

morbidity rate Proportion of animals in a group that develops clinical disease attributable to a specific agent over a defined period of time.

mortality rate Proportion of animals in a group that die over a defined period of time. The cause-specific mortality rate is the proportion of the group that dies as a result of a specific cause.

multihost agent Infectious agent that is capable of infecting more than one host species.

mummification (fetal) Desiccation of a dead fetus retained in the uterus. The cause of death may be infectious or noninfectious but organisms that promote lysis must be absent and the cervix must remain closed to prevent entry of putrefactive microorganisms.

mycotic infection Infection caused by a fungus.

myelinopathy A degenerative change in the lipid-rich membranes that surround nerve fibers in the brain, spinal, and peripheral nervous system.

myiasis Disease caused by invasion of living tissue by fly (Diptera) larvae.

necropsy Postmortem examination of an animal.

necrosis Pathologic death of one or more cells, or a portion of tissue, resulting from irreversible damage. (Distinct from apoptosis, which is programmed death of cells, the mechanism by which tissues are remodeled and individual cells are deleted as a physiologic process.).

necrotic Affected by necrosis.

nematode Roundworm of the phylum Nematoda.

neoplasia Pathologic process involving uncontrolled cellular proliferation that results in formation of a tumor or neoplasm.

neoplasm Abnormal tissue that grows by cellular proliferation more rapidly than normal and continues to grow after the stimulus that initiated growth ceases.

neutrophil A type of mammalian white blood cell that is important as a phagocyte in the innate immune system responsible for killing extracellular microorganisms.

obligate parasite Organism that can only live as a parasite, that is, it requires a host animal for perpetuation and survival.

oocyst Encysted form of zygote of many protozoa that is shed from the host animal's body.

opportunistic agent A disease agent that may infect an animal but for which infection is not required for perpetuation of the organism.

orchitis Inflammation of the testicle.

organelle Subcellular units that include mitochondria, Golgi apparatus, endoplasmic reticulum.

osteomyelitis Inflammation of the bone marrow and adjacent bone.

osteoporosis Reduction in the quantity of bone.

pandemic Epidemic disease that is widespread over a large area (country, continent, globally).

parasite-mediated competition Interaction between two host species that share the same parasites in which an increase in density of one of the host species results in an increase in the density of parasites in both species. The effect may be more severe for one host species.

paratenic host Host animal in which development of a parasite does not occur but which may serve to enhance transmission or to bridge an ecological or trophic gap in a parasite's life cycle.

passive immunity Immunity resulting from transfer of preformed antibodies to a nonimmune individual, usually from a mother to offspring through the placenta or milk (mammals), or egg yolk (birds). These antibodies persist for a short time and do not provide long-lasting protection.

pathogen A disease-causing agent.

pathogenesis The chain of events and mechanisms that results in development of a disease process.

pathogenic Producing disease or pathological changes.

pathologic Diseased, resulting from disease.

pathology Branch of medical science concerned with all aspects of the nature, causes, and development of abnormal conditions, as well as the structural and functional changes that result from disease.

peristalsis Movement of the intestine and other tubular organs by which contents are propelled onward.

permeability The property of allowing passage of substances through a membrane.

phagocytosis Active process of engulfing and internalization of particulate material such as bacteria or cell fragments by cells.

plasmid Small circular portion of DNA, physically separate and replicating independently from the chromosome of bacteria. Often confers some advantage to the bacterium such as resistance to antibiotics.

pneumonia Inflammation of the lung.

poikilothermic Used to describe animals whose body temperature varies with that of the surrounding medium.

population Group of individuals of the same species that live together in an area of sufficient size to permit normal dispersal and/or emigration behavior and in which numerical changes are largely determined by birth and death processes (Berryman 2002).

predation Trophic relationship in which one species, the predator, kills and consumes many prey animals during its lifetime.

pregnancy toxemia A metabolic disease of sheep precipitated by dietary deficiency of net energy during the extreme energy demands of late pregnancy.

prepatent period Time interval from infection until infectious stages are shed by a host. (Usually reserved for infections caused by metazoan parasites.)

prevalence A measure of how many animals have a condition at a specific point in time. The number of animals with the condition as a proportion of the total number in the group at that time.

primary immune response The immune response that follows the first contact of an animal with an antigen.

prion Derived from "proteinaceous infectious particle" to describe contagious agents composed of abnormally folded protein with no nucleic acid, believed to be the cause of spongiform encephalopathies.

prokaryote Cells lacking a nuclear membrane, large complex chromosomes, mitotic/meiotic spindle, and intracellular organelles. Bacteria are prokaryotes.

pseudovertical transmission Transmission that occurs from any member of a group to neonatal animals early in their life, for example, before they emerge from the den.

purulent Containing or forming pus.

pus Semiliquid product of inflammation containing leukocytes, dead cell debris, and tissue liquefied by enzymes produced by neutrophils.

pustule Small pimplelike swelling containing purulent material.

receptor Structure on the surface of a cell that is recognized by a specific extracellular molecule or agent that binds to it.

regeneration Regrowth of functional cells or parts of an organ so that function is restored.

regulation Process by which a density-dependent factor tends to return a population to its equilibrium following a perturbation.

reproductive rate (R_0) For microparasites, R_0 is the average number of secondary infections that arise from introduction of one infected individual into a totally susceptible population. For macroparasites, R_0 is the average number of female offspring that live to reproduce and are produced by a single female introduced into a totally susceptible population.

reservoir One or more epidemiologically connected population or environment in which an infectious agent can be permanently maintained (Haydon et al. 2002).

rickets Nutritional bone disease of growing animals caused by nutritional deficiency of phosphorus or vitamin D, characterized by overproduction and deficient calcification of bone.

r-selected Species in which production of many young is favored at the expense of maintaining the individual. Tendency toward high fecundity, high mortality, and shorter life span and usually associated with unstable environments.

salinization Accumulation and deposition of excessive amounts of soluble mineral salts in soil or water.

saprophyte An organism that gains its nourishment directly from dead or decaying organic matter.

scarring Repair of injury in which functional tissue is replaced by less-specialized connective tissue resulting in diminished function.

scavenger A species that gains nutrients by feeding on animals that died for other reasons.

secondary poisoning Poisoning resulting from toxic residues being passed from one vertebrate to another. This includes residues that have been assimilated into the tissues of the first animal (such as insecticides in fat) and residues in the digestive tract that have not been assimilated by the first animal.

secondary response Rapid rise in antibody or cell-mediated immunity following second or subsequent exposure to an antigen (also called amnestic response).

sensitivity (of a test) Ability of a test to correctly identify those animals that are actually positive; the proportion of affected animals that are identified as positive by the test.

septicemia Presence of pathogenic bacteria in the blood stream.

serology Science concerned with measuring antibodies or antigens in blood serum.

sexual transmission A form of direct transfer of infection between individuals through sexual contact.

sink habitat A habitat in which reproduction is inadequate to replace mortality and the population is only maintained through immigration from more favorable areas.

source habitat A habitat in which reproduction is more than sufficient to offset mortality and extra animals disperse.

specificity (in relation to the immune system) Ability to recognize and react to a particular antigen epitope.

specificity (of a test) Ability of a test to correctly identify those animals that are negative; the proportion of the animals that are not affected that test negative.

spillover host A host species within which a multiple-host disease agent can persist for some

time (there is some intraspecific transmission) but will eventually die out without an external source of infection.

spongiform Descriptive term for spongelike texture or appearance.

sterile fly technique (sterile male technique) Disease management technique used for certain parasitic flies in which females breed only once a season. Artificially reared, sterile males that are sexually active are released to compete with wild males and reduce reproduction.

stochastic A process in which there is an element of randomness or chance.

stress A system or process for receiving, evaluating, and responding to stimuli that threaten to disturb the homeostatic equilibrium of an animal. The response is a cascade of reactions under neuroendocrine control that involves catecholamines, glucocorticosteroids, and other mediators.

stressor Stimulus that elicits the stress response.

surveillance Organized collection, collation, and analysis of data on disease occurrence.

survival In populations, survival is usually calculated as a rate: the number of animals alive at the end of a period of time (often 1 year) divided by the number alive at the beginning of the time unit.

T cell A subgroup of lymphocytes involved in the cell-mediated immune response and as helper cells in the humoral immune response.

test-and-slaughter Selective removal (culling) of affected individuals from a population following testing. The term comes from use in control of livestock diseases in which animals that tested positive were sent to slaughter.

tetanus A disease characterized by tonic muscular contractions caused by a toxin produced by the bacterium *Clostridium tetani* acting on the central nervous system.

thrombosis Formation of a blood clot or thrombus within a blood vessel as a result of coagulation that may lead to partial or complete obstruction of blood flow.

titre A measure of the amount of antibody present in serum, usually expressed as the reciprocal of the highest dilution of the serum that produces an antibody-mediated response.

translocation Movement or transfer from one place to a different place.

transmissible Capable of being transmitted.

transmission Process by which an agent is shed from one host and infects another.

transovarial transmission Transmission of an agent from one generation of host to the next through the egg.

transport host An animal that may be contaminated by an infectious agent and carry it to another host but in which the agent does not complete a required part of its life cycle or multiply.

transstadial transmission Transmission of an agent from one developmental stage of an invertebrate to the next stage (e.g., from larval to nymphal stage).

trematode Flatworm of the class Trematoda (fluke).

trophic level Level in a food chain defined by the method of obtaining food and in which all organisms are the same number of energy transfers from the original source of energy (e.g., herbivore).

trophic relationship Connected by nutrition or feeding, as in predator and prey.

validity (of a test) Ability to distinguish between those that have the feature (such as a disease) and those that do not.

vascular Relating to or containing blood vessels.

vector An invertebrate that transmits an infectious agent among vertebrates and in which the agent multiplies or completes some required portion of its life cycle.

verminous Adjective used to describe conditions caused by worm parasites (e.g., verminous pneumonia).

vertical transmission Transmission of an infectious agent from parent to offspring.

vesicle Fluid-filled space within the epithelium of the skin or a mucous membrane (a blister).

viremia Presence of virus in the blood.

virion A complete virus particle.

virulence The ability of a disease agent to cause harm or injury.

virulent With a marked ability to cause disease or damage.

xenobiotic Foreign to a living organism; also a synthetic chemical not occurring naturally.

zoonosis Infectious disease that is transmitted naturally between animals and humans (plural: zoonoses)

Bibliography

Abbot, K., T. Ksiazek, and J. Mills. 1999. Long-term hantavirus persistence in rodent populations in central Arizona. *Emerging Infectious Diseases* 5:102–112.

Acevedo-Whitehouse, K., F. Gulland, D. Greig, and W. Amos. 2003. Disease susceptibility in California sea lions. *Nature* 422:35.

Actor, J. K., M. Shirai, M. C. Kullberg, M. L. Buller, A. Sher, and J. A. Berzofsky. 1993. Helminth infection results in decreased virus-specific CD8+ cytotoxic T-cell and TH1 cytokine responses as well as delayed virus clearance. *Proceedings of the National Academy of Science of the United States of America* 90:948–952.

Adrian, W. J., T. R. Spraker, and R. B. Davies. 1978. Epornitics of aspergillosis in mallards (*Anas platyrhynchos*) in north central Colorado. *Journal of Wildlife Diseases* 14:212–217.

Albon, S. D., A. Stien, R. J. Irvine, R. Langvatn, E. Ropstad, and O. Halvorsen. 2002. The role of parasites in the dynamics of a reindeer population. *Proceedings of the Royal Society, London B* 269:1625–1632.

Alexander, K. A., and M. J. G. Appel. 1994. African wild dogs (*Lycaon pictus*) endangered by a canine distemper epizootic among domestic dogs near the Masai Mara National Reserve, Kenya. *Journal of Wildlife Diseases* 30:481–485.

Alexander, K. A., E. Playdell, M. C. Williams, E. P. Lane, J. F. C. Nyange, and A. L. Michel. 2002. *Mycobacterium* tuberculosis: an emerging disease of free-ranging wildlife. *Emerging Infectious Diseases* 8:598–601.

Altizer, S., C. L. Nunn, P. H. Thrall, J. L. Gittleman, J. Antonovics, A. A. Cunningham, A. P. Dobson, V. Ezenwa, K. E. Jones, A. B. Petersen, M. Poss, and J. R. C. Pilliam. 2003. Social organization and parasite risk in mammals: integrating theory and empirical studies. *Annual Review of Ecology and Evolutionary Systematics* 34:517–47.

Anderson, R. C. 1992. *Nematode Parasites of Vertebrates: Their Development and Transmission*, Wallingford: CAB International.

Anderson, R. M. 1991. Populations and infectious diseases: ecology or epidemiology. *Journal of Animal Ecology* 60:1–50.

————. 1995. Evolutionary processes in the spread and persistence of infectious agents in vertebrate populations. *Parasitology* 111:S15–S31.

Anderson, R. M., and R. M. May. 1978. Regulation and stability of host-parasite population interactions. I. Regulatory processes. *Journal of Animal Ecology* 47:219–247.

————. 1979. Population biology of infectious disease: Part 1. *Nature* 280:361–367.

————. 1982. Coevolution of hosts and parasites. *Parasitology* 85:411–426.

————. 1986. The invasion, persistence and spread of infectious diseases within animal and plant communities. *Philosophical Transactions of the Royal Society, London B* 314:533–570.

Anderson, R. M., and W. Trewhalla. 1985. Population dynamics of the badger (*Meles meles*) and the epidemiology of bovine tuberculosis (*Mycobacterium bovis*). *Philosophical Transactions of the Royal Society, London B* 310:327–381.

Anderson, R. M., H. C. Jackson, R. M. May, and A. M. Smith. 1981. Population dynamics of fox rabies in Europe. *Nature* 289:765–781.

Anderson, S. H., and E. S. Williams. 1997. Plague in a complex of white-tailed prairie dogs and associated small mammals in Wyoming. *Journal of Wildlife Diseases* 33:720–732.

Apanius, V. 1998. Stress and immune defense. *Behavior* 27:133–153.

Apanius, V., and G. A. Schad. 1994. Host behaviour and the flow of parasites through host populations. In *Parasitic and Infectious Diseases: Epidemiology and Ecology,* edited by M. E. Scott and G. Smith, pp. 115–128. San Diego: Academic Press.

Appel, M. J. C., C. J. Reggiardo, B. A. Summers, S. Pearce-Kelling, C. J. Maré, T. H. Noon, R. E. Reed, J. N. Shively, and C. Orwell. 1991. Canine distemper virus infection and encephalitis in javelinas (collared peccaries). *Archives of Virology* 119:147–152.

Arneberg, P., I. Folstad, and A. J. Karter. 1996. Gastrointestinal nematodes depress food intake in naturally infected reindeer. *Parasitology* 112:213–219.

Arnold, W., and A. V. Lichtenstein. 1991. Ectoparasite loads decrease the fitness of alpine marmots (*Marmota marmota*) but are not a cost of sociality. *Behavioral Ecology* 4:36–39.

Atkinson, C. T., K. L. Woods, R. J. Dusek, L. S. Sileo, and W. M. Iko. 1995. Wildlife disease and conservation in Hawaii: pathogenicity of avian malaria (*Plasmodium relictum*) in experimentally infected Iiwi (*Vestiaria coccinea*). *Parasitology* 111:S59–S69.

Avashia, S. B., J. M. Petersen, C. M. Lindley, M. E. Schriefer, K. L. Gage, M. Cetron, T. A. DeMarcus, D. K. Kim, J. Buck, J. A. Montenieri, J. L. Lowell, M. F. Antolin, M. Y. Kosoy, L. G. Carter, M. C. Chu, K. A. Hendricks, D. T. Dennis, and J. L. Kool. 2004. First reported prairie dog-to-human tularemia transmission, Texas, 2002. *Emerging Infectious Diseases* 10: 483–486.

Baker, A. J., P. M. González, T. Piersma, L. J. Niles, I. de lima Serrano do Nascimento, P. W. Atkinson, N. A. Clark, C. D. T. Minton, M. K. Peck, and G. Aarts. 2004. Rapid population decline in red knots: fitness consequences of decreased refuelling rates and late arrival in Delaware Bay. *Proceedings of the Royal Society, London B* 271:875–882.

Baker, R. J., A. M. Bickham, M. Bondarkov, S. P. Gaschak, C. W. Matson, B. E. Rodgers, J. K. Wickliffe, and R. K. Chesser. 2001. Consequences of polluted environments on population structure: the bank vole (*Clethrionomys glareolus*) at Chornobyl. *Ecotoxicology* 10:211–216.

Bakker, T. C, M. D. Mazzi, and S. Zali. 1997. Parasite induced changes in behavior and color make *Gammarus pulex* more prone to fish predation. *Ecology* 78: 1098–1104.

Ball, G. H. 1943. Parasitism and evolution. *American Naturalist* 77:345–364.

Banks, P. B. and F. Powell. 2004. Does maternal condition or predation risk influence small animal population dynamics? *Oikos* 106:176–184.

Barker, I. K., and C. R. Parrish. 2001. Parvovirus infections. In *Infectious Diseases of Wild Mammals*, edited by E. S. Williams and I. K. Barker, pp. 131–146. Ames: Iowa State University Press.

Barnard, C. J. 1984. *Producers and Scroungers: Strategies of Exploitation and Parasitism*. London: Chapman and Hall.

Barnes, A. M. 1982. Surveillance and control of bubonic plague in the United States. In *Animal Disease in Relation to Animal Conservation*, edited by A. Edwards and U. McDonnell, pp. 237–270. London: Academic Press.

Barret, J. L., M. S. Carlisle, and P. Prociv. 2002. Neuroangiostrongylosis in wild black and grey-headed flying foxes (*Pteropus* spp.). *Australian Veterinary Journal* 80:554–558.

Bartlett, M. S. 1960. The critical community size for measles in the US. *Journal of the Royal Statistical Society A* 123:37–44.

Baxby, D., M. Bennett, B. Getty. 1994. Human cowpox 1969–1993: a review based on 54 cases. *British Journal of Dermatology* 131:598–607.

Beard, P. M., M. J. Daniels, D. Henderson, A. Pirie, K. Rudge, D. Buxton, S. Rhind, A. Greig, M. R. Hutchings, I. McKendrick, K. Stevenson, and J. M. Sharp. 2001. Paratuberculosis infection of nonruminant wildlife in Scotland. *Journal of Clinical Microbiolology* 39:1517–1521.

Beaver, D. L. 1980. Recovery of an American robin population after earlier DDT use. *Journal of Field Ornithology* 51:220–228.

Bedhomme, S., P. Agnew, C. Sidobre, and Y. Michalakis. 2004. Virulence reaction norms across a food gradient. *Proceedings of the Royal Society, London B* 271: 739–744.

Begon, M., and R. G. Bowers. 1995. Beyond host-pathogen dynamics. In *Ecology of Infectious Diseases in Natural Populations*, edited by B. T. Grenfell and A. P. Dobson, pp. 478–509. Cambridge: Cambridge University Press.

Begon, M., S. M. Hazel, S. Telfer, K. Brown, R. Carslake, J. Chantry, T. Jones, and M. Bennett. 2003. Rodents, cowpox virus and islands: densities, numbers and thresholds. *Journal of Animal Ecology* 72:343–355.

Belay, E. D., R. A. Maddox, E. S. Williams, M. W. Miller, P. Gambetti, and L. B. Schonberger. 2004. Chronic wasting disease and potential transmission to humans. *Emerging Infectious Diseases* 10:977–984.

Bell, J. F., and S. S. Stewart. 1975. Chronic shedding tularemia nephritis in rodents: possible relation to occurrence of *Francisella tularensis* in lotic waters. *Journal of Wildlife Diseases* 11:421–430.

———. 1983. Quantum differences in oral susceptibility of voles, *Microtus pennsylvanicus*, to virulent *Francisella tularensis* type B, in drinking water: implications to epidemiology. *Ecology of Disease* 2:151–155.

Bellrose, F. C., Jr. 1959. Lead poisoning as a mortality factor in waterfowl populations. *Illinois Natural History Survey Bulletin* 27:235–288.

Bengis, R. G., R. A. Kock, and J. Fischer. 2002. Infectious animal diseases: the wildlife/livestock interface. *Revue Scientifique et Technique OIE* 21:53–65.

Bennett, M., C. J. Gaskell, D. Baxby, R. M. Gaskell, D. F. Kelly, and J. Naidoo. 1990. Feline cowpox virus infection. A review. *Journal of Small Animal Practice* 14: 167–173.

Beran, G. W., and J. L. H. Steele. 1994. *Handbook of Zoonoses*, 2d ed. Boca Raton: CRC Press.

Berdoy, M., J. P. Webster, and D. W. MacDonald. 1995. Parasite-altered behaviour: is the effect of *Toxoplasma gondii* on *Rattus norvegicus* specific? *Parasitology* 111:403–409.

Bergelson, J. L., and C. B. Purrington. 1996. Surveying patterns in the cost of resistance in plants. *American Naturalist* 148:536–558.

Bergerud, A. T., 1971. The population dynamics of Newfoundland caribou. *Wildlife Monographs* 25:1–55.

Beringer, J., L. P. Hansen, and D. E. Stallknecht. 2000. An epizootic of hemorrhagic disease in white-tailed deer. *Journal of Wildlife Diseases* 36:588–591.

Berryman, A. A. 2002. Population: a central concept for ecology? *Oikos* 97:439–442.

Bethel, W. M., and J. C. Holmes. 1973. Altered evasive behavior and responses to light in amphipods harboring acanthocephalan cystacanths. *Journal of Parasitology* 59:945–956.

———. 1974. Correlation of development of altered evasive behavior in *Gammarus lacustris* (Amphipoda) harboring cystacanths of *Polymorhus paradoxus* (Acanthocephala) with the infectivity to the definitive host. *Journal of Parasitology* 60:272–274.

Beyer, W. N., D. J. Audet, G. H. Heinz, D. J. Hoffman, and D. Day. 2000. Relation of waterfowl poisoning to sediment lead concentrations in the Coeur d'Alene River basin. *Ecotoxicology* 9:207–218.

Beyer, W. N., G. H. Heinz, and A. W. Redmon-Norwood. 1996. *Environmental Contaminants in Wildlife: Interpreting Tissue Concentrations.* Boca Raton: Lewis Publishers.

Birkhead, M., and C. Perrins. 1985. The breeding biology of the mute swan *Cygnus olor* on the River Thames with special reference to lead poisoning. *Biological Conservation* 32:1–11.

Biser, J. A., L. A. Vogel, J. Berger, B. Hjelle, and S. S. Loew. 2004. Effects of heavy metals on immunocompetence of white-footed mice (*Peromyscus leucopus*). *Journal of Wildlife Diseases* 40:173–184.

Bize, P., A. Roulin, L.-F. Bersier, D. Pfluger, and H. Richner. 2003. Parasitism in Alpine swift nestlings. *Journal of Animal Ecology* 72:633–639.

Black, F. L. 1966. Measles endemicity in insular populations: critical community size and its evolutionary implication. *Journal of Theoretical Biology* 11:207–211.

Blus, L. J. 1982. Further interpretation of the relation of organochlorine residues in brown pelican eggs to reproductive success. *Environmental Pollution* 28A:15–33.

Blus, L. J., C. J. Henny, D. J. Lenhardt, and T. E. Kaiser. 1984. Effects of heptachlor- and lindane-treated seed on Canada geese. *Journal of Wildlife Management* 48:1097–1111.

Blus, L. J., S. N. Wiemeyer, and C. J. Henny. 1996. Organochlorine pesticides. In *Noninfectious Diseases of Wildlife.* 2d ed., edited by A. Fairbrother, L. N. Locke, and G. L. Hoff, pp. 61–70. Ames: Iowa State University Press.

Boag, B. 1988. Observations on the seasonal incidence of myxomatosis and its interactions with helminth parasites in the European rabbit (*Oryctolagus cuniculus*). *Journal of Wildlife Diseases* 24:450–455.

Bogerd, H. P., B. P. Doehle, H. L. Wiegand, and B. R. Cullen. 2004. A single amino acid difference in the host APOBEC3G protein controls the primate species specificity of HIV type 1 virion infectivity factor. *Proceedings of the National Academy of Science of the United States of America* 101:3770–3774.

Bolin, C. 2000. Leptospirosis. In *Emerging Diseases of Animals,* edited by C. Brown and C. Bolin, pp. 185–200. Washington, D.C.: ASM Press.

Bolker, B. M., and B. T. Grenfell. 1995. Space, persistence and the dynamics of measles epidemics. *Philosophical Transactions of the Royal Society, London B* 348:309–320.

Boonstra, R. 1977. Effect of the parasite *Wohlfahrtia vigil* on *Microtus townsendii* populations. *Canadian Journal of Zoology* 55:1057–1060.

Boots, M., and R. G. Bowers. 2004. The evolution of resistance through costly acquired immunity. *Proceedings of the Royal Society, London B* 271:715–723.

Borg, K., H. Wanntorp, K. Erne, and E. Hanko. 1969. Alkyl mercury poisoning in terrestrial Swedish wildlife. *Viltrevy* 6:301–379.

Borg, K., K. Erne, E. Hanko, and H. Wanntorp. 1970. Experimental methyl mercury poisoning in the goshawk (*Accipiter g. gentilis* L.). *Environmental Pollution* 1:91–104.

Bornstein, S., T. Mörner, and W. M. Samuel. 2001. *Sarcoptes scabei* and sarcoptic mange. In *Parasitic Diseases of Wild Mammals,* 2d ed., edited by W. M. Samuel, M. J. Pybus, and A. A. Kocan, pp. 107–119. Ames: Iowa State University Press.

Botkin, D. B., P. A. Jordan, A. S. Dominski, and G. E. Zhutchison. 1973. Sodium dynamics in a northern ecosystem. *Proceedings of the National Academy of Science of the United States of* America 70:2745–2748

Bowater, R. O., J. Norton, S. Johnson, B. Hill, P. O'Donoghue, and H. Prior. 2003. Toxoplasmosis in Indo-Pacific humpbacked dolphins (*Sousa chinensis*) from Queensland. *Australian Veterinary Journal* 81:627–632.

Bowyer, R. T., G. M. Blundell, M. Ben-David, S. C. Jewett, T. A. Dean, and L. K. Duffy. 2003. Effects of the *Exxon Valdez* oil spill on river otters: injury and recovery of a sentinel species. *Wildlife Monographs* 153:1–53.

Boyce, W., A. Fisher, H. Provencio, E. Rominger, J. Thilsted, and M. Ahim. 1999. Elaeophorosis in bighorn sheep in New Mexico. *Journal of Wildlife Diseases* 35:786–789.

Braack, L. E. O., and V. de Vos. 1990. Feeding habits and flight range of blow-flies (*Chrysomyia* spp.) in relation to anthrax transmission in the Kruger National Park, South Africa. *Onderstepoort Journal of Veterinary Research* 57:141–142.

Bradbury, J. 1998. Hong Kong avian influenza characterized. *Lancet* 351:189.

Brosch, R., S. V. Gordon, M. Marmiesse, P. Brodin, C. Buchrieser, K. Eiglmeier, T. Garner, C. Gutierrez, G. Hewinson, K. Kremer, L. M. Parsons, A. S. Pym, S. Samper, D. Van Soolingen, and S. T. Cole. 2002. A new evolutionary scenario for the *Mycobacterium tuberculosis* complex. *Proceedings of the National Academy of Science of the United States of America* 99:3684–3689.

Brown, M. J. F., R. Schmid-Hempel, and P. Schmid-Hempel. 2003. Strong context-dependent virulence in a host-parasite system: reconciling genetic evidence with theory. *Journal of Animal Ecology* 72:994–1002.

Bryant, J., H. Wang, C. Cabezas, G. Ramirez, D. Watts, K. Russell, and A. Barrett. 2003. Enzootic transmission of yellow fever virus in Peru. *Emerging Infectious Diseases* 9:926–933.

Bundy, D. A. P., and M. H. N. Golden. 1987. The impact of host nutrition on gastrointestinal helminth populations. *Journal of Parasitology* 95:623–635.

Burger, J. 1997. Effects of oiling on feeding behavior of sanderlings and semipalmated plovers in New Jersey. *Condor* 99:290–298.

Burger, J., and M. Gochfeld. 2002. Effects of chemicals and pollution on seabirds. In *Biology of Marine Birds*, edited by E. A. Schreiber and J. Burger, pp. 485–525. Boca Raton: CRC Press.

Burgess, E. C., and T. M. Yuill. 1981. Vertical transmission of duck plague virus (DPV) by apparently healthy DPV carrier waterfowl. *Avian Diseases* 25:795–800.

Bustnes, J. O., K. E. Erikstad, V. Bakken, F. Mehlum, and J. U. Skaare. 2000. Feeding ecology and the concentration of organochlorines in glaucous gulls. *Ecotoxicology* 9:179–186.

Buttgereit, F., G.-R. Burmeister, and M. D. Brand. 2000. Bioenergetics of immune functions: fundamental and therapeutic aspects. *Immunology Today* 21:192–199.

Cade, T. J., J. H. Enderson, C. G. Thelander, and C. M. White. 1988. *Peregrine Falcon Populations: Their Management and Recovery*. Boise: The Peregrine Fund.

Caffrey, C., T. J. Weston, and S. C. R. Smith. 2003. High mortality among marked crows subsequent to the arrival of West Nile virus. *Wildlife Society Bulletin* 31:870–872.

Caley, P., and D. Ramsey. 2001. Estimating disease transmission in wildlife, with emphasis on leptospirosis and bovine tuberculosis in possums, and effects of fertility control. *Journal of Applied Ecology* 38:1362–1370.

Caley, P., and J. Hone. 2004. Disease transmission between and within species, and the implications for disease control. *Journal of Applied Ecology* 41:94–104.

Caley, P., G. J. Hickling, P. E. Cowan, and D. U. Pfeiffer. 1999. Effects of sustained control of brushtail possums on *Mycobacterium bovis* infection in cattle and brushtail possum populations in Hohotaka. *New Zealand Veterinary Journal* 47:133–142.

Caley, P., J. D. Coleman, and G. J. Hickling. 2001. Habitat-related prevalence of macroscopic *Mycobacterium bovis* infection in brushtail possums *(Trichosurus vulpecula)* Hohonu Range, Westland, New Zealand. *New Zealand Veterinary Journal* 49:82–87.

Caley, P., L. M. McElrea, and J. Hone. 2002. Mortality rates of feral ferrets *(Mustela furo)* in New Zealand. *Wildlife Research* 29:323–328.

Caley, P., N. J. Spencer, R. A. Cole, and M. G. Efford. 1998. The effect of manipulating population density on the probability of den-sharing among common brushtail possums, and the implications for transmission of bovine tuberculosis. *Wildlife Research* 25:383–392.

Calisher, C. H., J. N. Mills, W. P. Sweeney, J. R. Choate, D. E. Sharp, K. M. Canestorp, and B. J. Beaty. 2001. Do unusual site-specific population dynamics of rodent reservoirs provide clues to the natural history of hantaviruses? *Journal of Wildlife Diseases* 37:280–288.

Calvete, C., R. Estrada, J. J. Osacar, J. Lucientes, and R. Villafuerte. 2004. Short-term negative effects of vaccination campaigns against myxomatosis and viral hemorrhagic disease (VHD) on the survival of European wild rabbits. *Journal of Wildlife Management* 68:198–205.

Cam, E., J-Y. Monnat, and J. E. Hines. 2003. Long-term fitness consequences of early conditions in the kittiwake. *Journal of Animal Ecology* 72:411–424.

Camus, P. A., and M. Lima. 2002. Populations, metapopulations, and the open-closed dilemma: the conflict between operational and natural population concepts. *Oikos* 97:433–438.

Carey, A. B., R. G. McLean, and G. O. Maupin. 1980. The structure of a Colorado tick fever ecosystem. *Ecological Monographs* 50:131–151.

Carmichael, J. 1938. Rinderpest in African game. *Journal of Comparative Pathology* 51:264–268.

Carmichael, W. W. 1994. The toxins of cyanobacteria. *Scientific American* 270(1):78–86.

Carney, W. P. 1969. Behavioral and morphological changes in carpenter ants harboring dicrocoelid metacercariae. *American Midland Naturalist* 82:605–611.

Caron, A., P. C. Cross, and J. T. du Toit. 2003. Ecological implications of bovine tuberculosis in African buffalo herds. *Ecological Applications* 13:1338–1345.

Cassirer, E. F., K. M. Rudolph, P. Fowler, V. L. Coggins, D. L. Hunter, and M. W. Miller. 2001. Evaluation of ewe vaccination as a tool for increasing bighorn lamb survival following pasteurellosis epizootics. *Journal of Wildlife Diseases* 37:49–57.

Caughley, G., and A. R. E. Sinclair. 1994. *Wildlife Ecology and Management*. Malden: Blackwell Science, Inc.

Cavanagh, R., M. Begon, M. Bennett, T. Ergon, I. M. Graham, P. E. W. de Haas, C. A. Hart, M. Koedam, K. Kremer, X. Lambin, P. Ruholl, and D. van Soolingen. 2002. *Mycobacterium microti* infection (vole tuberculosis) in wild rodent populations. *Journal of Clinical Microbiology* 40:3281–3285.

Cavanagh, R., X. Lambin, T. Ergon, M. Bennett, I. M. Graham, D. van Soolingen, and M. Begon. 2004. Disease dynamics in cyclic populations of field voles *(Microtus agrestis)*: cowpox virus and vole tuberculosis *(Mycobacterium microti)*. *Proceedings of the Royal Society, London B* 271:859–867.

CDC. 2003. Update: multistate outbreak of monkeypox—Illinois, Indiana, Kansas, Missouri, Ohio, and Wisconsin, 2003. *Mortality and Morbidity Weekly Reports* 52:589–590.

Charlton, K. M., G. C. Dulac, F. C. Thomas, and H. K. Mitchell. 1977. Necrotizing encephalitis in skunks caused by *Herpes simplex* virus. *Canadian Journal of Comparative Medicine* 41:460–465.

Chautan, M., D. Pontier, and M. Artois. 2000. Role of rabies in recent demographic changes in red fox (*Vulpes vulpes*) populations in Europe. *Mammalia* 64:391–410.

Chen, A., and W. J. Rogan. 2003. Nonmalarial infant deaths and DDT use for malarial control. *Emerging Infectious Diseases* 9:960–964.

Chomel, B. B., A. C. Wey, and R. W. Kasten. 2003. Isolation of *Bartonella washoensis* from a dog with mitral valve endocarditis. *Journal of Clinical Microbiology* 41:5327–5332.

Christe, P., A. Oppliger, and H. Richner. 1994. Ectoparasite affects choice and use of roost sites in the great tit, *Parus major. Animal Behavior* 47:895–898.

Cichoń, M., M. Chadzińska, A. Ksiazek, and M. Konarzewski. 2002. Delayed effect of cold stress on immune response in laboratory mice. *Proceedings of the Royal Society, London B* 269:1493–1497.

Claessen, D., and A. M. de Roos. 1995. Evolution of virulence in a host-pathogen system with local pathogen transmission. *Oikos* 74:401–413.

Clark, L., and J. R. Mason. 1988. Effect of biologically active plants used as nest material and the derived benefit to starling nestlings. *Oecologia* 77:174–180.

Clayton, D. H., and D. M. Tompkins. 1995. Comparative effects of mites and lice on the reproductive success of rock doves (*Columba livia*). *Parasitology* 110:195–206.

Cleaveland, S., M. G. J. Appel, W. S. K. Chalmers, C. Chillingworth, M. Kaare, and C. Dye. 2000. Serological and demographic evidence for domestic dogs as a source of canine distemper virus infection for Serengeti wildlife. *Veterinary Microbiology* 72:217–227.

Cleaveland, S. C., M. K. Laurenson, and L. H. Taylor. 2001. Diseases of humans and their domestic mammals; pathogen characteristics, host range and the risk of emergence. *Philosophical Transactions of the Royal Society, London B* 356:991–999.

Cliplef, D. J., and G. Wobeser. 1993. Observations on waterfowl carcasses during a botulism epizootic. *Journal of Wildlife Diseases* 29:8–14.

Clubb, S. L., and J. K. Frenkel. 1992. *Sarcocystis falculata* of opossums: transmission by cockroaches with fatal pulmonary disease in psittacine birds. *Journal of Parasitology* 78:116–124.

Colburn, T., and C. Clement. 1992. *Chemically-induced Alterations in Sexual and Functional Development: The Wildlife/Human Connection*. Princeton: Princeton Scientific Publishing.

Coleman, R. A. 1993. San Francisco Bay—an urban/wildlife shuffle. *Transactions of the North American Wildlife and Natural Resources Conference* 58:137–142.

Collins, S. J., V. A. Lawson, and C. L. Masters. 2004. Transmissible spongiform encephalopathies. *Lancet* 363:51–62.

Colman, J. E., C. Pedersen, D. O. Hjermann, O. Holand, S. R. Moe, and E. Reimers. 2003. Do wild reindeer exhibit grazing compensation during insect harassment? *Journal of Wildlife Management* 67:11–19.

Combes, C. 2000. Parasites, hosts, questions. In *Evolutionary Biology of Host-parasite Relationships: Theory meets Reality,* edited by R. Poulin, S. Morand, and A. Skorping, pp.1–62. Amsterdam: Elsevier.

Connelly, R., W. A. Fuller, B. Hubert, R. A. Mercredi, and G. Wobeser. 1990. *Northern Diseased Bison, Report of the Environmental Assessment Panel*. Ottawa: Federal Environmental Assessment Review Office, Environment Canada.

Conner, M. M., C. W. McCarty, and M. W. Miller. 2000. Detection of bias in harvest-based estimates of chronic wasting disease prevalence in mule deer. *Journal of Wildlife Diseases* 36:691–699.

Cooch, E. G. 2002. Fledgling size and survival in snow geese: timing is everything (or is it?). *Journal of Applied Statistics* 29:143–162.

Cooke, J. A., and M. S. Johnson. 1996. Cadmium in small mammals. In *Environmental Contaminants in Wildlife*, edited by W. N. Beyer, G. H. Heinz, and A. W. Redman-Norwood, pp.377–388. Boca Raton: Lewis Publishers.

Cooke, P. S., R. E. Peterson, and R. A. Hess. 2002. Endocrine disruptors. In *Handbook of Toxicologic Pathology*, 2d ed., Vol. 1, edited by W. M. Haschek, C. M. Rousseaux, and M. A. Wallig, pp. 501–528. San Diego: Academic Press.

Cook, M. I., S. R. Beissinger, G. A. Toranzos, R. A. Rodriguez, and W. J. Arendt. 2003. Trans-shell infection by pathogenic micro-organisms reduces the shelf life of non-incubated bird's eggs: a constraint on the onset of incubation? *Proceedings of the Royal Society, London B* 270:2230–2240.

Cook, W. E., E. S. Williams, and S. A. Dubay. 2004. Disappearance of bovine fetuses in northwestern Wyoming. *Wildlife Society Bulletin* 32:254–259.

Coop, R. L., and I. Kyriazakis. 1999. Nutrition-parasite interaction. *Veterinary Parasitology* 84:187–204.

Corn, J. L., and V. F. Nettles. 2001. Health protocol for translocation of free-ranging elk. *Journal of Wildlife Diseases* 37:413–426.

Couvilion, C. E., V. F. Nettles, C. A. Rawlings, and R. L. Joyner. 1986. Elaeophorosis in white-tailed deer: Pathology of the natural disease and its relation to oral food impaction. *Journal of Wildlife Diseases* 22:214–223.

Coyner, D. F., M. G. Spalding, and D. J. Forrester. 2002. Epizootiology of *Eustrongylides ignotus* in Florida: distribution, density, and natural infections in intermediate hosts. *Journal of Wildlife Diseases* 38:483–499.

Coyner, D. F., S. R. Schaack, M. G. Spalding, and D. J. Forrester. 2001. Altered predation susceptibility of mosquitofish infected with *Eustrongylides ignotus*. *Journal of Wildlife Diseases* 37:556–560.

Cransac, N., A. J. M. Hewison, J. M. Gaillard, J. M. Cugnase, and M. L. Maublanc. 1997. Patterns of mouflon (*Ovis gmelin*) survival under moderate environmental conditions: effects of sex, age, and epizootics. *Canadian Journal of Zoology* 75:1867–1875.

Crews, D., E. Willingham, and J. K. Skipper. 2000. Endocrine disruptors: present issues, future directions. *Quarterly Review of Biolology* 75:243–260.

Cromie, R. L., N. J. Ash, M. J. Brown, and J. L. Stanford. 2000. Avian immune responses to *Mycobacterium avium*: the wildfowl example. *Developmental and Comparative Immunology* 24:169–185.

Cunningham, A. A., J. K. Kirkwood, M. Dawson, Y. I. Spencer, R. B. Green, and G. A. H. Wells. 2004. Distribution of bovine spongiform encephalopathy in greater kudu (*Tragelaphus strepsiceros*). *Emerging Infectious Diseases* 10:1044–1049.

Curry, A. J., K. J. Else, F. Jones, A. Bancroft, R. K. Grencis, and D. W. Dunne. 1995. Evidence that cytokine-mediated immune interactions induced by *Schistoma mansoni* alter disease outcome in mice concurrently infected with *Trichuris muris*. *Journal of Experimental Biology* 181:769–774.

Damien, B. C., B. E. E. Martina, S. Losch, J. Mossong, A. D. M. E. Osterhaus. 2002. Prevalence of antibodies against canine distemper virus among red foxes in Luxembourg. *Journal of Wildlife Diseases* 38:856–858.

Daniels, M. J., M. R. Hutchings, P. M. Beard, D. Henderson, A. Grig, K. Stevenson, and J. M. Sharp. 2003. Do non-ruminant wildlife pose a risk of paratuberculosis to domestic livestock and vice versa in Scotland? *Journal of Wildlife Diseases* 39:10–15.

Daniels, P. W. 2002. Emerging arboviral diseases. *Australian Veterinary Journal* 80:216.

Daoust, P. Y., D. G. Busby, L. Ferns, J. Goltz, S. McBurney, C. Poppe, and H. Whitney. 2000. Salmonellosis in songbirds in the Canadian Atlantic provinces during winter-summer 1997–98. *Canadian Veterinary Journal* 41:54–59.

Daszak, P., A. A. Cunningham, and A. D. Hyatt. 2000. Emerging infectious diseases of wildlife— threats to biodiversity and human health. *Science* 287:443–450.

Davidar, P., and E. S. Morton. 1993. Living with parasites: prevalence of a blood parasite and its effect on survivorship in the purple martin. *Auk* 110:109–116.

Davidson, W. R., F. A. Hayes, V. F. Nettles, and F. E. Kellogg. 1981. *Diseases and Parasites of White-tailed Deer.* Tallahassee: Tall Timbers Research Station.

Davidson, W. R., M. J. Appel, F. L. Doster, O. E. Baker, and J. F. Brown. 1992, Diseases and parasites of red foxes, gray foxes, and coyotes from commercial sources selling to fox-chasing enclosures. *Journal of Wildlife Diseases* 28:581–58

Davies, R. W., and J. Wilkialis. 1981. A preliminary investigation on the effects of parasitism of domestic ducklings by *Theromyzon rude* (Hirudinoidea: Glossiphonidae). *Canadian Journal of Zoology* 59:1196–1199.

Dawson, A., S. A. Hinsley, P. N. Ferns, R. H. C. Bonser, and L. Eccleston. 2000. Rate of moult affects feather quality: a mechanism linking current reproductive effort to future survival. *Proceedings of the Royal Society, London B* 267:2093–2097.

Day, J. F., and J. D. Edman. 1983. Malaria renders mice susceptible to mosquito feeding when gametocytes are most infective. *Journal of Parasitology* 69:163–170.

Deerenberg, C., V. Apanius, S. Daan, and N. Bos. 1997. Reproductive effort decreases antibody responsiveness. *Proceedings of the Royal Society, London B* 264:1021–1029.

Delahay, R. J., G. J. Wilson, G. C. Smith, and C. L. Cheeseman. 2003. Vaccinating badgers (*Meles meles*) against *Mycobacterium bovis*: the ecological considerations. *Veterinary Journal* 166:43–51.

Delahay, R. J., J. R. Speakman, and R. Moss. 1995. The energetic consequences of parasitism: effects of a developing infection of *Trichostrongylus tenuis* (Nematoda) on red grouse (*Lagopus lagopus scoticus*) energy balance, body weight and condition. *Parasitology* 110:473.

De Lisle, G. W., R. G. Bengis, S. M. Schmitt, and D. J. O'Brien. 2002. Tuberculosis in free-ranging wildlife: detection, diagnosis and management. *Revue Scientifique et Technique OIE* 21:317–334.

de Roode, J. C., R. Culleton, S. J. Cheesman, R. Carter, and A. F. Read. 2004. Host heterogeneity is a determinant of competitive exclusion or coexistence in genetically diverse malaria infections. *Proceedings of the Royal Society, London B* 271:1073–1080.

De Solla, S. R., M. L. Fletcher, and C. A. Bishop. 2003. Relative contributions of organochlorine contaminants, parasitism, and predation to reproductive success of eastern spiny softshell turtles (*Apalone spiniferus spiniferus*) from southern Ontario, Canada. *Ecotoxicology* 12:261–270.

Dhondt, A. A., D. L. Tessaglia, and R. L. Slothower. 1998. Epidemic mycoplasmal conjunctivitis in house finches from eastern North America. *Journal of Wildlife Diseases* 34:265–280.

Diamond, J. M. 1997. *Guns, Germs, and Steel: The Fates of Human Societies.* New York: W. W. Norton.

Diefenbach, D. R., C. S. Rosenberry, and R. C. Boyd. 2004. From the field: efficacy of detecting chronic wasting disease via sampling hunter-killed white-tailed deer. *Wildlife Society Bulletin.* 32:267–272.

Dieterich, R. A. 1981. Brucellosis. In *Alaskan Wildlife Diseases*, edited by R. Dieterich, pp. 53–58. Fairbanks: University of Alaska.

Dieterich, R. A., J. K. Morton, and R. L. Zarnke. 1991. Experimental *Brucella suis* biovar 4 in a moose. *Journal of Wildlife Diseases* 27:470–472.

DiGiacomo, R. F., and T. D. Koepsell. 1986. Sampling for detection of infection or disease in animal populations. *Journal of the American Veterinary Medical Association* 89:22–23.

Dmowski, K., M. Kozakiewicz, and A. Kozakiewicz. 2000. Small mammal response at population and community level to heavy metal pollution (Pb, Cd, Tl). In *Demography in Ecotoxicology*, edited by J. Kammenga and R. Laskowsi, pp. 113–125. Chichester: John Wiley & Sons.

Dobson, A. P. 1985. The population dynamics of competition between parasites. *Parasitology* 91:317–347.

Dobson, A. P., and P. J. Hudson. 1992. Regulation and stability of a free-living host-parasite system: *Trichostrongylus tenuis* in red grouse. II. Population models. *Journal of Animal Ecology* 61:487–498.

———. 1995. Microparasites: Observed patterns. In *Ecology of Infectious Diseases in Natural Populations*, edited by B. T. Grenfell and A. P. Dobson, pp. 52–89. Cambridge: Cambridge University Press.

Donaldson, A. I., J. Gloster, L. D. J. Harvey, and D. H. Deans. 1982. Use of prediction models to forecast and analyse airborne spread during the foot-and-mouth disease outbreak in Brittany, Jersey and the Isle of Wight, 1981. *Veterinary Record* 110:53–57.

Donnelly, C. A., R. Woodroffe, D. R. Cox, J. Bourne, G. Gettinby, A. M. Le Fevre, J. P. McInerney, and W. I. Morrison. 2003. Impact of localized badger culling on tuberculosis incidence in British cattle. *Nature* 426:834–837.

Dorland, W. A. N. 2000. *Dorland's Illustrated Medical Dictionary*, 29th ed. Philadelphia: W. B. Saunders Co.

Douglass, R. J., A. J. Kuenzi, C. Y. Williams, S. J. Douglass, and J. N. Mills. 2003. Removing deer mice from buildings and the risk for human exposure to Sin Nombre virus. *Emerging Infectious Diseases* 9:390–392.

Dragon, D. C., and R. P. Rennie. 1995. The ecology of anthrax spores: tough but not invincible. *Canadian Veterinary J.* 36:295–301.

Duncan, J., H. W. Reid, R. Moss, J. D. P. Phillips, and A. Watson. 1978. Ticks, louping ill and red grouse on moors in Speyside, Scotland. *Journal of Wildlife Management* 42:500–505.

Dyer, N. W. 2001. *Haemophilus somnus* bronchopneumonia in American bison (*Bison bison*). *Journal of Veterinary Diagnostic Investigation* 13:419–421

Eason, C. T., E. C. Murphy, G. R. C. Wright, and E. B. Spurr. 2002. Assessment of risks of brodifacoum to non-target birds and mammals in New Zealand. *Ecotoxicology* 11:35–48.

Ebedes, H. 1976. Anthrax epidemics in Etosha National Park. *Madoqua* 10:99–118.

Ebert, D. 1999. The evolution and expression of parasite virulence. In *Evolution in Health and Disease*, edited by S. C. Stearns, pp. 161–172. Oxford: Oxford University Press.

Ebert, D., and J. J. Bull. 2003. Challenging the trade-off model for the evolution of virulence: is virulence management feasible? *Trends in Microbiology* 11:15–20.

Ebert, D., C. D. Zschokke-Rohringer, and H. J. Carius. 2000b. Dose effects and density-dependent regulation of two microparasites of *Daphnia magna*. *Oecologia* 122:200–209.

Ebert, D., M. Lipsitch, and K. L. Mangin. 2000a. The effect of parasites on host population density and extinction: experimental epidemiology with *Daphnia* and six microparasites. *American Naturalist* 156:459–477.

Edwards, J. C., and C. J. Barnard. 1987. The effects of *Trichinella* infection on intersexual interactions in mice. *Animal Behavior* 35:533–540.

Eldridge, M. D. B., J. M. King, A. K. Loupis, P. B. S. Spencer, A. C. Taylor, L. C. Pope, and G. P. Hall. 1999. Unprecedented low levels of genetic variation and inbreeding depression in an island population of the black-footed rock-wallaby. *Conservation Biology* 13:531–541.

Eliasson, H., J. Lindbäck, J. P. Nuorti, M. Arneborn, J. Giesecke, and A. Tegneli. 2002. The 2000 tularemia outbreak: a case-control study of risk factors in disease-endemic and emergent areas, Sweden. *Emerging Infectious Diseases* 8:956–960.

Ellison, L. N. 1991. Shooting and compensatory mortality in tetraonids. *Ornis Scandinavica* 22:229–240.

Elton, C. 1931. The study of epidemic disease among wild animals. *Journal of Hygiene* 31:435–456.

Emmons, R. W., and E. H. Lennette. 1968. Isolation of herpesvirus hominis from naturally infected pet skunks. *Health and Laboratory Science* 5:31–37

Engelthaler, D. M., D. G. Mosley, J. E. Cheek, C. E. Levy, K. K. Komatsu, P. Ettestad, T. Davis, D. T. Tanda, L. Miller, J. W. Frampton, R. Porter, and R. T. Bryan. 1999. Climatic and environmental patterns associated with hantavirus pulmonary syndrome, Four Corners region, United States. *Emerging Infectious Diseases* 5:87–94.

Engeman, R. M., K. L. Christensen, M. J. Pipas, and D. L. Bergman. 2003. Population monitoring in support of a rabies vaccination program for skunks in Arizona. *Journal of Wildlife Diseases* 39:746–750.

Errington, P. L. 1946. *Special Report on Muskrat Diseases*. Iowa Cooperative Wildlife Research Unit Quarterly Report July, August, September: 34–51.

———. 1963. *Muskrat Populations*. Ames: Iowa State University Press.

Escutinaire, S., P. Chalon, F. De Jaegere, L. Karelle-Bui, G. Mees, B. Brochier, F. Rozenfeld, and P.-P. Pastoret. 2002. Behavioral, physiologic, and habitat influences on the dynamics of Puumala virus infection in bank voles (*Clethrionomys glareolus*). *Emerging Infectious Diseases* 8:930–936.

Evans, A. S. 1977. Limitations to Koch's postulates. *Lancet* 2:1277–1278.

Evelsizer, D. D. 2002. *Management of Avian Botulism and Survival of Molting Mallards*. MSc Thesis, University of Saskatchewan, Saskatoon.

Evers, D. C., K. M. Taylor, A. Major, R. J. Taylor, R. H. Poppenga, and A. M. Scheuhammer. 2003. Common loon eggs as indicators of methylmercury availability in North America. *Ecotoxicology* 12:69–81.

Ewald, P. W. 1983. Host-parasite relations, vectors, and the evolution of disease severity. *Annual Review of Ecology and Systematics* 14:465–485.

———. 1994. *Evolution of Infectious Disease*. Oxford: Oxford University Press.

———. 1995. The evolution of virulence: a unifying link between parasitology and ecology. *Journal of Parasitology* 81:659–669.

Ezenwa, V. O. 2003. Interactions among host diet, nutritional status and gastrointestinal parasite infection in wild bovids. *International Journal of Parasitology* 34:535–542.

Fair, J. M., E. S. Hansen, and R. E. Ricklefs. 1999. Growth, developmental stability and immune response in juvenile Japanese quails (*Coturnix coturnix japonica*). *Proceedings of the Royal Society, London B* 266:1735–1742.

Fairbrother, A. 1994. Immunotoxicology of captive and wild birds. In *Wildlife Toxicology and Population Modeling: Integrated Studies of Agroecosystems,* edited by R. J. Kendall and T. E. Lachter, Jr., pp. 251–261. Boca Raton: Lewis Publishers.

Fairbrother, A., M. Fix, T. O'Hara, and C. A. Ribic. 1994. Impairment of growth and immune function of avocet chicks from sites with elevated selenium, arsenic, and boron. *Journal of Wildlife Diseases* 30:222–233.

Fallis, A. M., and G. F. Bennett. 1966. On the epizootiology of infections caused by *Leucocytozoon simondi* in Algonquin Park, Ontario. *Canadian Journal of Zoology* 44:101–112.

Fancy, S. G., and R. G. White. 1985. Energy expenditure of caribou while cratering in snow. *Journal of Wildlife Management* 49:987–993.

Farrgalo, J. A., T. Laaksonen, V. Povri, and E. Korpimaki. 2002. Inter-sexual differences in the immune response of Eurasian kestrels under food shortage. *Ecology Letters* 5:95–101.

Fenner, F., and J. Ross. 1994. Myxomatosis. In *The European Rabbit. The History and Biology of a Successful Colonizer*, edited by H. V. Thompson and C. M. King, pp. 205–240. Oxford: Oxford University Press.

Feore, S. M., M. Bennett, J. Chantrey, T. Jones, D. Baxby, and M. Begon. 1997. The effect of cowpox virus infection on fecundity in bank voles and wood mice. *Proceedings of the Royal Society, London B* 264:1457–1461.

Ferrari, M. J., and R. A. Garrott. 2002. Bison and elk: brucellosis seroprevalence on a shared winter range. *Journal of Wildlife Management* 66:1246–1254.

Ferrari, N., I. M. Cattadori, J. Nespereira, A. Rizzoli, and P. J. Hudson. 2004. The role of host sex in parasite dynamics: field experiments on the yellow-necked mouse *Apodemus flavicollis. Ecology Letters* 7:88–94.

Ferrer, M., and F. Hiraldo. 1995. Human-associated staphylococcal infection in Spanish imperial eagles. *Journal of Wildlife Diseases* 31:534–536.

Festa-Bianchet, M. 1988. Nursing behaviour of bighorn sheep: correlates of ewe age, parasitism, lamb age, birth date and sex. *Animal Behavior* 36:1445–1454.

Fielder, P. C. 1986. Implications of selenium levels in Washington mountain goats, mule deer, and Rocky Mountain elk. *Northwest Science* 60:15–20

Finkenstädt, B., and B. Grenfell. 1998. Empirical determinants of measles metapopulation dynamics in England and Wales. *Proceedings of the Royal Society, London B* 265:211–220.

Finkenstädt, B., M. Keeling, and B. Grenfell. 1998. Patterns of density dependence in measles dynamics. *Proceedings of the Royal Society, London B* 265:753–762.

Fischer, J. R., L. A. Lewis-Weis, and C. M. Tate. 2003. Experimental vacuolar myelinopathy in red-tailed hawks. *Journal of Wildlife Diseases* 39:400–406.

Fix, A. S., C. Waterhouse, E. C. Greiner, and M. K. Stoskopf. 1988. *Plasmodium relictum* as a cause of avian malaria in wild-caught Magellanic penguins (*Spheniscus magellanicus*). *Journal of Wildlife Diseases* 24:610–619.

Flueck, W. T. 1994 Effect of trace elements on population dynamics: selenium deficiency in free-ranging black-tailed deer. *Ecology* 75:807–812.

Flynn, A., and A. W. Franzmann. 1974. Manifestation of copper deficiency in a nonrestricted wild animal: the Alaskan moose (*Alces alces gigas*). In *Trace Substances in Environmental Health*, edited by D. D. Hemphill, pp. 95–99. Columbia: University of Missouri Press.

Folstad, I., P. Arneberg, and A. J. Karter. 1996. Antlers and parasites. *Oecologia* 105:556–558.

Forbes, L. B., S. V. Tessaro, and W. Lees. 1996. Experimental studies of *Brucella abortus* in moose (*Alces alces*). *Journal of Wildlife Diseases* 32:94–104.

Forbus, W. D. 1943. *Reactions to Injury: Pathology for Students of Medicine*. Baltimore: Williams and Wilkins.

Fornes, A., R. D. Lord, M. L. Kums, O. P. Larghi, E. Fuenzalida, and L. Lazaera. 1974. Control of bovine rabies through vampire bat control. *Journal of Wildlife Diseases* 10:310–316.

Forchhammer, M. C., and T. Asferg. 2000. Invading parasites cause a structural shift in red fox dynamics. *Proceedings of the Royal Society, London B* 267:779–786.

Forrester, D. J. 1971. Bighorn sheep lungworm-pneumonia complex. In *Parasitic Diseases of Wild Mammals*, edited by J.W. Davis and R.C. Anderson, pp. 158–173, Ames: Iowa State University Press.

Forrester, D. J., and M. Spalding. 2002. *Parasites and Diseases of Wild Birds in Florida*. Gainesville: University Press of Florida.

Fowler, M. E. 1983. Plant poisoning in free-living wild animals: a review. *Journal of Wildlife Diseases* 19:34–43

Fox, G. A., and D. V. Weseloh. 1986. Colonial waterbirds as bio-indicators of environmental contamination in the Great Lakes. *ICBP Technical Publication* 6:209–215.

Frank, S. A., and J. S. Jeffrey. 2000. The probability of severe disease in zoonotic and commensal infections. *Proceedings of the Royal Society, London B* 268:53–60.

Franklin, C. L., S. L. Motzel, C. L. Besch-Williford, R. R. Hook, Jr., and L. K. Riley. 1994. Tyzzer's infection: Host specificity of *Clostridium piliforme* isolates. *Laboratory Animal Science* 44:568–572.

Frederick, S., M. McGhee, and M. G. Spalding. 1996. Prevalence of *Eustrongyloides ignotus* in mosquitofish (*Gambusia holbrooki*) in Florida: historical and regional comparisons. *Journal of Wildlife Diseases* 32:552–555.

Friend, M. 1981. Waterfowl management and waterfowl disease: independent or cause and effect relationships? *Transactions of the North American Wildlife and Natural Resources Conference* 46:94–103.

Friend, M., and J. C. Franson. 1999. *Field Manual of Wildlife Disease: General Field Procedures and Diseases of Birds.* Washington, D.C.: U.S. Department of the Interior, U.S. Geolological Survey, Biolological Research Division, Information Technical Report 1999–001.

Fuller, W. A. 2002. Canada and the "Buffalo," *Bison bison*: a tale of two herds. *Canadian Field-Naturalist* 116:141–159.

Furniss, P. R., and B. D. Hahn. 1981. A mathematical model of an anthrax epizootic in the Kruger National Park. *Applied Mathematical Modeling* 5:130–136.

Gage, K. L., and J. A. Montenieri. 1994. The role of predators in the ecology, epidemiology, and surveillance of plague in the United States. In *16th Vertebrate Pest Conference*, edited by W. S. Halverson and A. H. Crabb, pp. 200–206. Davis: University of California.

Galloway, T., and R. Handy. 2003. Immunotoxicity of organophosphorus pesticides. *Ecotoxicology* 12:345–363.

Ganz, T. 2002. Epithelia: not just physical barriers. *Proceedings of the National Academy of Sciences of the United States of America* 99:3357–3358.

Gaspar, P. W., and R. P. Watson. 2001. Plague and yersiniosis. In *Infectious Diseases of Wild Mammals*, 3d ed., edited by E. S. Williams and I. K. Barker, pp. 313–329. Ames: Iowa State University Press.

Gates, C. C., and N. C. Larter. 1990. Growth and dispersal of an erupting large herbivore population in Northern Canada: the Mackenzie wood bison (*Bison bison athabascae*). *Arctic* 43:231–238.

Gates, C. C., B. Elkin, and D. Dragon. 2001. Anthrax. In *Infectious Diseases of Wild Mammals.* 3d ed., edited by E. S. Williams and I. K. Barker, pp. 396–412. Ames: Iowa State University Press.

Gaydos, J. K., D. E. Stallknecht, D. Kavanaugh, R. J. Olsen, and E. G. Fuchs. 2002a. Dynamics of maternal antibodies to hemorrhagic disease viruses (Reoviridae: Oribivirus) in white-tailed deer. *Journal of Wildlife Diseases* 38:253–257.

Gaydos, J. K., W. R. Davidson, F. Elvinger, D. G. Mead, E. W. Howerth, and D. E. Stallknecht. 2002b. Innate resistance to epizootic hemorrhagic disease in white-tailed deer. *Journal of Wildlife Diseases* 38:743–749.

Gemmell, M. A. 1959. Hydatid disease in Australia. IV. Observations on the incidence of *Echinococcus granulosus* on stations and farms in endemic regions of New South Wales. *Australian Veterinary Journal* 35:396–402.

Gemmell, M. A., J. R. Lawson, and M. G. Roberts. 1986. Population dynamics in echinococcosis and cysticercosis: biological parameters of *Echinococcus granulosus* in dogs and sheep. *Parasitology* 92:599–620.

Gemmill, A. W., and A. F. Read. 1998. Counting the cost of disease resistance. *Trends in Ecology and Evolution* 13:8–9.

Getz, L. L., J. E. Hofmann, B. J. Klatt, L. Verner, F. R. Cole, and R. D. Lindroth. 1987. Fourteen years of population fluctuations of *Microtus ochragaster* and *M. pennsylvanicus* in east central Illinois. *Canadian Journal of Zoology* 65:1317–1325.

Giacometti, M., M. Janovsky, H. Jenny, H. Nicolet, L. Belloy, E. Goldschmidt-Clermont, and J. Frey. 2002. *Mycoplasma conjunctivae* infection is not maintained in alpine chamois in eastern Switzerland. *Journal of Wildlife Diseases* 38:297–304.

Gibbs, E. P. J. 1991. Epidemiology of orbiviruses—bluetongue: Towards 2000 and the search for patterns. In *Bluetongue, African Horse Sickness, and Related Orbiviruses,* edited by T. E. Walton and B. I. Osburn, pp. 65–75, Boca Raton: CRC Press.

Gilbert, L., R. A. Norman, M. K. Laurenson, H. W. Reid, and P. J. Hudson. 2001. Disease persistence and apparent competition in a three-host community: an empirical and analytical study of large scale, wild populations. *Journal of Animal Ecology* 70:1053–1061.

Gill, C. E., and J. E. Elliott. 2003. Influence of food supply and chlorinated hydrocarbon contaminants on breeding success of bald eagles. *Ecotoxicology* 12:95–111.

Glines, M. V., and W. M. Samuel. 1984. The development of the winter tick, *Dermacentor albipicus*, and its effect on the hair coat of moose, *Alces alces*, of central Alberta, Canada. *Acarology* 6:1208–1214.

Gloor, S., F. Bontadina, D. Hegglin, P. Deplazes, and U. Breitenmoser. 2001. The rise of urban fox populations in Switzerland. *Mammalian Biology* 66:155–164.

Gloster, J., R. F. Sellers, and A. I. Donaldson. 1982. Long distance transport of foot-and-mouth disease virus over the sea. *Veterinary Record* 110:47–52.

Gondim, L. F. P., M. M. McAllister, W. C. Pitt, and D. E. Zemlicka. 2004. Coyotes (*Canis latrans*) are definitive hosts of *Neospora caninum*. *International Journal of Parasitology* 34:159–161.

Gordus, A. G. 1999. Selenium concentrations in eggs of American avocets and black-necked stilts at an evaporation basin and freshwater wetland in California. *Journal of Wildlife Management* 63:497–501.

Graham, G. L. 1966. The behavior of beetles, *Trilobium confusum*, parasitized by the larval stage of a chicken tapeworm, *Raillietina cesticillus*. *Transactions of the American Microscopical Society* 85:163.

Grasman, K. A., and G. A. Fox. 2001. Associations between altered immune function and organochlorine contamination in young Caspian terns (*Sterna caspia*) from Lake Huron, 1997–1999. *Ecotoxicology* 10:101–114.

Graveland, J., and R. H. Drent, 1997, Calcium availability limits breeding success of passerines on poor soils. *Journal of Animal Ecology* 66:279–288.

Graveland, J., R. van der Wall, J. H. van Balen, and A. J. van Noordwijk. 1994. Poor reproduction in forest passerines from decline of snail abundance on acidified soils. *Nature* 368:446–448.

Greenwood, R. J., W. E. Newton, G. L. Pearson, and G. J. Schamber. 1997. Population and movement characteristics of radio-collared striped skunks in North Dakota during an epizootic of rabies. *Journal of Wildlife Diseases* 33:226–241.

Gregory, R. D., and A. E. Keymer. 1989. The ecology of host-parasite interactions. *Scientific Progress* 73:67–80.

Grenfell, B. T., and A. P. Dobson. 1995. *Ecology of Infectious Diseases in Natural Populations*. Cambridge: Cambridge University Press.

Gubler, D. J., P. Reiter, K. L. Ebi, W. Yap, R. Nasci, and J. A. Patz. 2001. Climate variability and change in the United States: Potential impacts on vector-and rodent-borne diseases. *Environmental Health Perspectives* 109:223–233.

Guerra, M., E. Walker, C. Jones, S. Paskewitz, M. R. Cortinas, A. Stancil, L. Beck, M. Bobo, and U. Kitron. 2002. Predicting the risk of Lyme disease: habitat suitability for *Ixodes scapularis* in the north central United States. *Emerging Infectious Diseases* 8:289–297.

Guillette, L. J., D. A. Crain, M. P. Gunderson, S. A. E. Kools, M. R. Milnes, E. F. Orlando, A. A. Rooney, and A. R. Woodward. 2000. Alligators and endocrine disrupting contaminants: A current perspective. *American Zoologist* 40:438–452.

Gulland, F. M. D. 1992. The role of nematode parasites in Soay sheep (*Ovis aries* L.) mortality during a population crash. *Parasitology* 105:493–503.

———. 1995. Impact of infectious diseases on wild animal populations: a review. In *Ecology of Infectious Diseases in Natural Populations,* edited by B. T. Grenfell and A. P. Dobson, pp. 20–51. Cambridge: Cambridge University Press.

Gunn, A., and R. J. Irvine. 2003. Subclinical parasitism and ruminant foraging strategies—a review. *Wildlife Society Bulletin* 31:117–126.

Gunson, J. R., W. J. Dorward, and D. B. Schowalter. 1978. An evaluation of rabies control in Alberta. *Canadian Veterinary Journal* 19:214–220.

Gustafsson, L., D. Nordling, M. S. Andersson, B. C. Sheldon, and A. Qvarnström. 1997. Infectious diseases, reproductive effort and the cost of reproduction in birds. In *Infection, Polymorphism and Evolution*, edited by W. D. Hamilton and J. C. Howard, pp 53–115. London: Chapman & Hall.

Hadju, V., L. S. Stephenson, K. Abadi, H. O. Mohammed, D. D. Bowman, and R. S. Parker. 1996. Improvements in appetite and growth in helminth-infected schoolboys three and seven weeks after a single dose of pyrantel pamoate. *Parasitology* 113:497–504.

Hanley, J. A., and A. Lippman-Hand. 1983. If nothing goes wrong, is everything all right? Interpreting zero numerators. *Journal of the American Medical Association* 249:1743–1745.

Hanley, T. A., and J. D. McKendrick. 1985. Potential nutritional limitations for black-tailed deer in a spruce-hemlock forest, southeastern Alaska. *Journal of Wildlife Management* 49:103–114.

Hansen, F., F. Jeltsch, K. Tackmann, C. Staubach, and H.-H. Thulke. 2004. Processes leading to a spatial aggregation of *Echinococcus multilocularis* in its natural intermediate host *Microtus arvalis*. *International Journal of Parasitology* 34:37–44.

Hanson, R. P. 1969. Koch is dead. *Bulletin of the Wildlife Disease Association* 5:150–156.

Hanssen, S. A., D. Hasselquist, I. Folstad, and K. E. Eriksta. 2004. Costs of immunity: immune responsiveness reduces survival in a vertebrate. *Proceedings of the Royal Society, London B* 271:925–930.

Hanssen, S. A., I. Folstad, and K. E. Erikstad. 2003. Reduced immunocompetence and cost of reproduction in common eiders. *Oecologia* 136:457–464

Härkönen, T. 2003. Development of populations of harbour seals and grey seals in the Wadden Sea and the North Sea since 1988. In *Management of North Sea Harbour and Grey Seal Populations, pp. 13–18.* Proceedings of an International Symposium, EcoMare, Texel, The Netherlands, November 29–30, 2002. Wadden Sea Ecosystem No. 17. Wilhelmshaven: Common Wadden Sea Secretariat.

Hart, B. L. 1988. Biological basis of the behaviour of sick animals. *Neurosciences and Behavior Reviews* 14: 273–294.

———. 1997. Behavioural defence. In *Host-Parasite Evolution. General Principles and Avian Models*, edited by D. H. Clayton and J. Moore, pp. 59–77. Oxford: Oxford University Press.

Hartung, R. 1967. Energy metabolism in oil-covered ducks. *Journal of Wildlife Management* 31:798–804.

Hartup, B. K., A. A. Dhondt, K. V. Sydenstricker, W. M. Hochachka, and G. V. Kollias. 2001. Host range and dynamics of mycoplasmal conjunctivitis among birds in North America. *Journal of Wildlife Diseases* 37:72–81.

Harvell, C. D., C. E. Mitchell, J. R. Ward, S. Altizer, A. P. Dobson, R. S. Ostfeld, and M. D. Samuel. 2002. Climate warming and disease risks for terrestrial and marine biota. *Science* 296:2158–2162.

Harwood, C. L., I. S. Young, D. L. Lee, and J. D. Altringham. 1996. The effect of *Trichinella spiralis* infection on the mechanical properties of the mammalian diaphragm. *Parasitology* 113:535–543.

Haschek, W. M., C. G. Rousseaux, and M. A. Wallig. 2002. *Handbook of Toxicologic Pathology*, 2d ed. San Diego: Academic Press.

Hasselquist, D., J. A. Marsh, P. W. Sherman, and J. C. Wingfield. 1999. Is avian humoral immunocompetence suppressed by testosterone? *Behavioral Ecology and Sociobiology* 45:167–175.

Hawley, W. A., P. Reiter, R. S. Copeland, C. B. Pumpuni, and G. B. Craig, Jr. 1987. *Aedes albopictus* in North America: probable introduction in used tires from northern Asia. *Science* 236:1114.

Haydon, D. T., S. Cleaveland, L. H. Taylor, and M. K. Laurenson. 2002. Identifying reservoirs of infection: a conceptual and practical challenge. *Emerging Infectious Disease* 8:1468–1473.

Hayes, M. A., and G. A. Wobeser. 1983. Subacute toxic effects of dietary T-2 toxin in young mallard ducks. *Canadian Journal of Comparative Medicine* 47:180–187.

Heesterbeek, J. P., and M. G. Roberts. 1995. Mathematical models for microparasites of wildlife. In *Ecology of*

Infectious Diseases in Natural Populations, edited by B. T. Grenfell and A. P. Dobson, pp. 90–122. Cambridge: Cambridge University Press.

Hegglin, D., P. I. Ward, and P. Deplazes. 2003. Anthelmintic baiting of foxes against urban contamination with *Echinococcus multilocularis*. *Emerging Infectious Diseases* 9:1266–1272

Helmby, H., M. Kuillberg, and M. Troye-Blomberg. 1998. Altered immune responses in mice with concomitant *Schistosoma mansoni* and *Plasmodium chabaudi* infections. *Infection and Immunity* 66:5167–5174.

Henderson, W. M. 1982. The control of disease in wildlife when a threat to man and farm livestock. In *Animal Disease in Relation to Animal Conservation*, edited by M. A. Edwards and U. McDonell, pp. 287–297. London: Academic Press.

Henke, S. E., D. B. Pence, and F. C. Bryant. 2002. Effect of short-term coyote removal on populations of coyote helminths. *Journal of Wildlife Diseases* 38:54–67.

Henny, C. J., L. J. Blus, E. J. Kolbe, and R. E. Fitzner. 1985. Organophosphate insecticides (famphur) topically applied to cattle kills magpies and hawks. *Journal of Wildlife Management* 49:648–658.

Henriksen, P., H. H. Dietz, S. A. Henriksen, and P. Gjelstrup. 1993. Sarcoptic mange in red fox in Denmark. A short report. *Dansk Veterinaertidsskrift* 76: 12–13.

Hentonnen, H., E. Fuglei, C. N. Gower, V. Haukisalmi, R. A. Ims, Niemimaa, and N. G. Yoccoz. 2001. *Echinococcus multilocularis* on Svalbard: introduction of an intermediate host has enabled the local life-cycle. *Parasitology* 123:547–552.

Herman, C. M., and W. J. L., Sladen. 1958. Aspergillosis in waterfowl. *Transactions of the North American Wildlife Conference* 23:187–191.

Herman, T. B. 1981. *Capillaria hepatica* (Nematoda) in insular populations of the deer mouse *Peromyscus maniculatus*: cannibalism or competition for carcasses? *Canadian Journal of Zoology* 59:776–784.

Hess, G. 1996. Disease in metapopulation models: implications for conservation. *Ecology* 77:1617–1632.

Hester, R. E., and R. M. Harrison. 1999. *Endocrine Disrupting Chemicals, Issues in Environmental Science and Technology 12*. Cambridge: Royal Society of Chemistry.

Heuschele, W. P., and H. W. Reid. 2001. Malignant catarrhal fever. In *Infectious Diseases of Wild Mammals*, 3d ed., edited by E. S. Williams and I. K. Barker, pp. 157–164. Ames: Iowa State University Press.

Hibler, C., and J. L. Adcock. 1971. Elaeophorosis. In *Parasitic Diseases of Wild Mammals*, edited by J. W. Davis and R. C. Anderson, pp. 263–278. Ames: Iowa State University Press.

Hibler, C. P., T. R. Spraker, and E. T. Thorne. 1982. Protostrongylosis in bighorn sheep. In *Diseases of Wildlife in Wyoming,* edited by E. T. Thorne, N. Kingston, W. R. Jolly, and R. C. Bergstrom, pp. 208–213. Cheyenne: Wyoming Game and Fish Department.

Hibler, C. P., T. R. Spraker, and R. L. Schmidt. 1977. Treatment of bighorn sheep for lungworms. *Transactions of the 1977 Desert Bighorn Council*: 12–14

Hill, A. B. 1965. The environment and disease: association or causation. *Proceedings of the Royal Society, London* 58:295–300.

Hochachka, W. M., and A. A. Dhondt. 2000. Density-dependent decline of host abundance resulting from a new infectious disease. *Proceedings of the National Academy of Science of the United States of America* 97:5303–5306.

Hochberg, M. E., and M. van Baalen. 2000. *A geographical perspective of virulence*. In *Evolutionary Biology of Host-parasite Relationships: Theory meets Reality,* edited by R. Poulin, S. Morand, and A. Skorping, pp. 81–96. Amsterdam: Elsevier.

Hoffmann, J. A., F. C. Kafatos, C. A. Janeway, Jr., and R. A. B. Ezekowitz. 1999. Phylogenetic perspectives in innate immunity. *Science* 284:1313–1318.

Holmes, J. C. 1982. Impact of infectious disease agents on the population growth and geographical distribution of animals. In *Population Biology of Infectious Diseases*, edited by R. M. Anderson and R. M. May, pp. 37–51. Berlin: Springer-Verlag.

Holmes, J. C., and W. M. Bethel. 1972. Modification of intermediate host behavior by parasites. In *Behavioral Aspects of Parasite Transmission*, edited by E. U. Canning and C. A. Wright, pp. 123–149. London: Academic Press.

Holmstad, P. R., A. Anwar, T. Iezhova, and A. Skorping. 2003. Standard sampling techniques underestimate prevalence of avian hematozoa in willow ptarmigan (*Lagopus lagopus*). *Journal of Wildlife Diseases* 39: 354–358.

Holt, J. G., N. R. Krieg, P. H. A. Sneath, J. T. Staley, and S. T. Williams. 1994. *Bergey's Manual of Determinative Bacteriology*. 9th ed. Baltimore: Williams and Wilkins.

Homan, R. N., J. V. Regosin, D. M. Rodrigues, J. M. Reed, B. S. Windmiller, and L. M. Romero. 2003. Impacts of varying habitat quality on the physiological stress of spotted salamanders (*Ambystoma maculatum*). *Animal Conservation* 6:11–18.

Honour, S. M., S. Kennedy, S. Trudeau, and G. Wobeser. 1995. Vitamin A status of wild mallards (*Anas platyrhynchos*) wintering in Saskatchewan. *Journal of Wildlife Diseases* 31:289–298.

Hoodless, A. N., K. Kurtenbach, P. A. Nuttall, and S. E. Randolph. 2002. The impacts of ticks on pheasant territoriality. *Oikos* 96:245–250.

Hoogenbloom, I., and C. Dikstra. 1987. *Sarcocystis cernae*: a parasite increasing the risk of predation of its intermediate host *Microtus arvalis*. *Oecologia* 74:86–92.

Hope-Cawdry, M. J. 1976. The effects of fascioliasis on ewe fertility. *British Veterinary Journal* 132:568–575.

Howe, F. P. 1992. Effects of *Protocalliphora braueri* (Diptera: Calliphoridae) parasitism and inclement weather on nestling sage thrashers. *Journal of Wildlife Diseases* 28:141–143.

Howerth, E. W., D. E. Stallknecht, and P. E. Kirkland. 2001. Bluetongue, epizootic hemorrhagic disease, and other orbivirus-related diseases. In *Infectious Diseases of Wild Mammals*, edited by E. S. Williams and I. K. Barker, pp. 77–97. Ames: Iowa State University Press.

Hoy, J. B., and J. R. Anderson. 1978. Behavior and reproductive physiology of blood-sucking snipe flies (Diptera: Rhagionidae: Symphoromyia) attacking deer in northern California. *Hilgardia* 46:113–168.

Hudson, P. J., and A. P. Dobson. 1995. Macroparasites: Observed patterns in naturally fluctuating animal populations. In *Ecology of Infectious Diseases in Natural Populations,* edited by B. T. Grenfell and A. P. Dobson, pp. 144–176. Cambridge: Cambridge University Press.

Hudson, P. J., A. P. Dobson, and D. Newborn. 1992a. Do parasites make prey more vulnerable to predation? Red Grouse and parasites. *Journal of Animal Ecology* 61:681–692.

————. 1998. Prevention of population cycles by parasite removal. *Science* 282:2256–2258.

Hudson, P. J., A. Rizzoli, B. T. Grenfell, H. Heesterbeek, and A. P. Dobson. 2001. *The Ecology of Wildlife Diseases*. Oxford: Oxford University Press.

Hudson, P. J., D. Newborn, and A. P. Dobson. 1992b. Regulation and stability of a free-living host-parasite system: *Trichostrongylus tenuis* in red grouse. I. Monitoring and parasite reduction experiments. *Journal of Animal Ecology* 61:477–486.

Hugh-Jones, M. E., and V. de Vos. 2002. Anthrax and wildlife. *Revue Scientifique et Technique OIE* 21: 359–383.

Humberg, D. D., D. Graber, S. Sheriff, and T. Miller. 1986. Estimating autumn-spring nonhunting mortality in southern Missouri. In *Lead Poisoning in Wild Waterfowl*, edited by J. S. Feierabend and A. B. Russell, pp. 77–87. Washington, D.C.: National Wildlife Federation.

Hunt, E. G., and A. I. Bischoff. 1960. Inimical effects on wildlife of periodic DDD applications to Clear Lake. *California Fish and Game* 46:91–106.

Hunter, P. R. 2003. Climate change and waterborne and vector-borne disease. *Journal of Applied Microbiology* 94:37S–46S.

Hurd, H., and S. Fugo. 1991. Changes induced by *Hymenolepsis diminuta* (Cestoda) in the behaviour of the intermediate host *Tenebrio molitor* (Coleoptera). *Canadian Journal of Zoology* 69:2291–2294.

Hutchings, M. R., I. Kyriazakis, I. J. Gordon, and F. Jackson. 1999. Trade-offs between nutrient intake and faecal avoidance in herbivore foraging decisions: the effect of animal parasite status, level of feeding motivation and sward nitrogen content. *Journal of Animal Ecology* 68:310–323.

Ikeda, Y., K. Nakamura, T. Miyazawa, Y. Tohya, E. Takahashi, and M. Mochizuki. 2002. Feline host range of canine parvovirus: recent emergence of new antigenic types in cats. *Emerging Infectious Diseases* 8:341–352.

Ilmonen, P., T. Taarna, and D. Hasselquist. 2000. Experimentally activated immune defence in female pied flycatchers results in reduced breeding success. *Proceedings of the Royal Society, London B* 267:665–670.

Ives, A. R., and D. L. Murray. 1997. Can sublethal parasitism destabilize predator-prey population dynamics? A model of snowshoe hares, predators and parasites. *Journal of Animal Ecology* 66:265–278.

Jackson, W. B., and Ashton, A. D., 1986, Case histories of anticoagulant resistance. In *Pesticide Resistance: Strategies and Tactics for Management*, pp. 355–369. Washington, D.C.: National Academy Press.

Jansen, J., Jr. 1964. Some problems related to the parasite inter-relationship of deer and domestic animals. *Transactions of the International Union for Game Biology* 6:127–132.

Jehl, J. R. Jr., W. S. Boyd, D. S. Paul, and D. W. Anderson. 2002. Massive collapse and rapid rebound: population dynamics of eared grebes (*Podiceps nigricollis*) during an ENSO event. *Auk* 119:1162–1166.

Jenkins, D., A. Watson, and G. R. Miller. 1963. Population studies on Red Grouse *Lagopus lagopus scoticus* (Lath.) in north-east Scotland. *Journal of Animal Ecology* 32:317–376.

Jenkins, D. J., and B. Morris. 2003. *Echinococcus granulosus* in wildlife in and around the Kosciuszko National Park, south-eastern Australia. *Australian Veterinary Journal* 81:81–85

Jenkins, S. R., and W. G. Winkler. 1987. Descriptive epidemiology from an epizootic of raccoon rabies in the Middle Atlantic States, 1982–1983. *American Journal of Epidemiology* 126:429–437.

Jensen, T., M. van de Bildt, H. H. Dietz, T. H. Andersen, A. S. Hammer, T. Kuiken, and A. Osterhaus. 2002. Another phocine distemper outbreak in Europe. *Science* 297:209.

Jessup, D. A., and F. A. Leighton. 1996. Oil pollution and petroleum toxicity to wildlife. In *Noninfectious Diseases of Wildlife*, 2d ed., edited by A. Fairbrother, L. N. Locke, and G. L. Hoff, pp. 141–156. Ames: Iowa State University Press.

Jobling, S., D. Casey, T. Rodgers-Gray, J. Oehlmann, U. Schulte-Oehlmann, S. Pawlowski, T. Baunbeck, A. P. Turner, and C. R. Tyler. 2003. Comparative responses of molluscs and fish to environmental estrogens and an estrogenic effluent. *Aquatic Toxicology* 65:205–220.

Johnson, D. H., C. T. Moore, W. L. Kendall, J. A. Dubrovsky, D. F. Caithamer, J. R. Kelley, Jr., and B. K. Williams. 1997. Uncertainty and the management of mallard harvests. *Journal of Wildlife Management* 61:202–216.

Johnson, L. S., M. D. Eastman, and L. H. Kermott. 1991. Effect of ectoparasitism by larvae of the blowfly *Protocalliphora parorum* (Diptera: Calliphoridae) on nestling house wrens, *Troglodytes aedon*. *Canadian Journal of Zoology* 69:1441–1446.

Jones, C. G., R. S. Ostfeld, M. P. Richard, E. M. Schauber, and J. O. Wolff. 1998. Chain reactions linking acorns to gypsy moth outbreaks and Lyme disease risk. *Science* 279:1023–1025.

Jones, D. M. 1982. Conservation in relation to animal disease in Africa and Asia. In *Animal Disease in Relation to Animal Conservation,* edited by M. A. Edwards and U. McDonnell, pp. 271–285. London: Academic Press.

Jones, L., M. Gaunt, R. Hails, K. Laurenson, P. J. Hudson, H. W. Reid, and E. Gould. 1987. Amplification of louping-ill virus infection during co-feeding of ticks on mountain hares (*Lepus timidus*). *Medical and Veterinary Entomology* 11:172–176.

Jonzén, N., P. Lundberg, E. Ranta, and V. Kaitala. 2002. The irreducible uncertainty of the demography-environment interaction in ecology. *Proceedings of the Royal Society, London B* 269:221–223.

Joubert, L., P. Duclos, and P. Toaillen. 1982. La myxomatose des garennes dans le Sud-Est. La myxamatose amyxamateuse. *Revue de Medicine Vétérinaire* 133: 739–753.

Kalmbach, E. R. 1939. American vultures and the toxin of Clostridium botulinum. *Journal of the American Veterinary Medical Association* 94:187–191.

Kalmbach, E. R., and M. F. Gunderson. 1934. *Western Duck Sickness—a Form of Botulism.* Washington, D.C.: U.S. Department of Agriculture Technical Bulletin, No. 411.

Karstad, L., P. Lusis, and D. Wright. 1971. Tyzzer's disease in muskrats. *Journal of Wildlife Diseases* 7:96–99.

Kavaliers, M., and D. D. Colwell. 1995a. Decreased predator avoidance in parasitized mice: neuromodulatory correlates. *Parasitology* 111:257–263.

———. 1995b. Reduced spatial learning in mice infected with the nematode, *Heligmosomoides polygyrus.* *Parasitology* 110:591–597.

Kazacos, K. R. 2001. *Baylisascaris procyonis* and related species. In *Parasitic Diseases of Wild Mammals,* 2d ed., edited by W. M. Samuel, M. J. Pybus, and A. A. Kocan, pp. 301–341. Ames: Iowa State University Press.

Kelsey, J. L., A. S. Whittemore, A. S. Evans, and W. D. Thompson. 1996. *Methods in Observational Epidemiology.* Oxford: Oxford University Press.

Kemper, H. E. 1938. Filarial dermatosis of sheep. *North American Veterinarian* 19:36–41.

Kennedy, S. 1990. A review of the 1988 European seal morbillivirus epizootic. *Veterinary Record* 127:563–567.

———. 2001. Morbillivirus infections in aquatic mammals. In *Infectious Diseases of Wild Mammals.* 3d ed., edited by E. S. Williams and I. K. Barker, pp. 64–76. Ames: Iowa State University Press.

Kermack, W. O., and A. G. McKendrick. 1927. A contribution to the mathematical theory of epidemics. *Proceedings of the Royal Society A* 115:700–721.

Kern, P., K. Bardonnet, E. Renner, H. Auer, Z. Pawlowski, R. W. Ammann, D. A. Vuitton, P. Kern, and the European Echinococcosis Registry. 2003. European echinococcosis registry: human alveolar echinococcosis, Europe, 1982–2000. *Emerging Infectious Diseases* 9:343–349.

Kerr, P. J., and S. M. Best. 1998. Myxoma virus in rabbits. *Revue Scientifique et Technique OIE* 17:256–268.

Keusch, G. T. 1993. Nutrition and infection. In *Mechanisms of Microbial Disease,* 2d ed., edited by M. Schaechter, G. Medoff, and B. L. Eisenstein, pp. 891–898. Baltimore: Williams & Wilkins.

Khoury, M. J. 1985. *A Genealogic Study of Inbreeding and Prereproductive Mortality in the Old Order Amish.* Baltimore: s.n.

Kida, H. 2003. Distribution and circulation of influenza viruses in nature. *Nippon Rinsho* 61:1865–1871.

King, C. M. 1976. The fleas of a population of weasels in Wytham Woods, Oxford. *Journal of Zoology, London* 180:525–535.

King, K. A., D. R. Blankinship, R. T. Paul, and R. C. A. Rice. 1977. Ticks as a factor in the 1975 nesting failure of Texas brown pelicans. *Wilson Bulletin* 89:157–158.

King, N. W., 2001, Herpesviruses of nonhuman primates. In *Infectious Diseases of Wild Mammals,* 3d ed., edited by E. S. Wiliams and I. K. Barker, pp. 147–157. Ames: Iowa State University Press.

Kinsey, S. G., B. J. Prendergast, and R. J. Nelson. 2003. Photoperiod and stress affect wound healing in Siberian hamsters. *Physiology and Behavior* 78:205–211.

Klok, C., and A. M. De Roos. 1998. Effects of habitat size and quality on equilibrium density and extinction time for *Sorex araneus* populations. *Journal of Animal Ecology* 67:195–209.

Klok, C., A. De Roos, S. Broekhuizen, and R. Van Apeldoorn. 2000. Effects of heavy metals on the badger *Meles meles*: interaction between habitat quality and fragmentation. In *Demography in Ecotoxicology*, edited by J. Kammenga and R. Laskowski, pp. 73–89. Chichester: John Wiley & Sons.

Kluger, M. J. 1979. *Fever, Its Biology, Evolution and Function.* Princeton: Princeton University Press.

Klurfeld, D. M. 1993. *Nutrition and Immunology.* New York: Plenum Press.

Kocan, A. A. 2001. Blood-inhabiting protozoans. In *Parasitic Diseases of Wild Mammals,* 2d ed., edited by W. M. Samuel, M. J. Pybus, and A. A. Kocan, pp. 520–536. Ames: Iowa State University Press.

Koella, J. C., and M. J. Packer. 1996. Malaria parasites enhance blood-feeding of their naturally infected vector *Anopheles punctulatus. Parasitology* 113:105–109.

Kosoy, M., M. Murray, R. D. Gilmore, Jr., Y. Bai, and K. L. Gage. 2003. *Bartonella* strains from ground squirrels are identical to *Bartonella washoensis* isolated from a human patient. *Journal of Clinical Microbiology* 41:645–650.

Kosoy, M. Y., R. L. Regnery, O. I. Kosaya, D. C. Jones, E. L. Marston, and J. E. Childs. 1998. Isolation of *Bartonella* spp. from embryos and neonates of naturally infected rodents. *Journal of Wildlife Diseases* 34:305–308.

Kraaljeveld, A. R., and H. C. J. Godfray. 1997. Trade-offs between parasitoid resistance and larval competitive ability in *Drosophila melanogaster. Science* 389:278–280.

Krebs, J. R., R. M. Anderson, T. Clutton-Brock, C. A. Donnelly, S. Frost, W. I. Morrison, R. Woodroffe, and D. Young. 1998. Badgers and bovine TB: conflicts between conservation and health. *Science* 279:817–818.

Kretzschmar, M., S. van den Hof, J. Wallinga, and J. van Wijgaarden. 2004. Ring vaccination and smallpox control. *Emerging Infectious Diseases* 10:832–841.

Kuiken, T. 1999. Review of Newcastle disease in cormorants. *Waterbirds* 22:333–347.

Kuiken, T., F. A. Leighton, G. Wobeser, K. L. Danesik, J. Riva, and R. A. Heckert. 1998. An epidemic of Newcastle disease in double-crested cormorants from Saskatchewan. *Journal of Wildlife Diseases* 34:457–471.

Kültz, D. 2003. Evolution of cellular stress proteome: from monophyletic origin to ubiquitous function. *Journal of Experimental Biology* 206:3119–3124.

Lafferty, K. D. 1999. The evolution of trophic transmission. *Parasitology Today* 15:111–115.

Lafferty, K. D., and A. K. Morris. 1996. Altered behavior of parasitized killifish increases susceptibility to predation by bird final hosts. *Ecology* 77:1390–1397.

Lafferty, K. D., and L. R. Gerber. 2002. Good medicine for conservation biology: the intersection of epidemiology and conservation theory. *Conservation Biology* 16:593–604.

Lafferty, K. D., and R. D. Holt. 2003. How should environmental stress affect the population dynamics of disease? *Ecology Letters* 6:654–664.

Landys-Ciannelli, M. M., T. Piersma, and J. Jukema. 2003. Strategic changes of internal organs and muscle tissue in the bar-tailed godwit during fat storage on a spring stopover site. *Functional Ecology* 17:151–159.

Lange, R. 1982. *Management of Psoroptic Mange in Desert Bighorn Sheep of New Mexico.* Stillwater: Wildlife Disease Association, Educational Aid.

Langelier, K. M. 1993. Barbiturate poisoning in twenty-nine bald eagles. In *Raptor Biomedicine,* edited by P. T. Redig, J. Cooper, J. D. Remple, and D. B. Hunter, pp. 231–232. Minneapolis: University of Minnesota.

Langenau, E. E., Jr., and J. M. Lerg. 1976. The effects of winter nutritional stress on maternal and neonatal behavior in penned white-tailed deer. *Applied Animal Ethology* 2:207–233.

Lankester, M. W. 1977. Neurologic disease in moose caused by *Elaphostrongylus cervi* Cameron, 1931 from caribou. *Proceedings of the North American Moose Conference* 13:177–190.

———. 2001. Extrapulmonary lungworms of cervids. In *Parasitic Diseases of Wild Mammals,* 2d ed., edited by W. M. Samuel, M. J. Pybus, and A. A. Kocan, pp. 228–278. Ames: Iowa State University Press.

———. 2002. Low-dose meningeal worm (*Parelaphostrongylus tenuis*) infections in moose (*Alces alces*). *Journal of Wildlife Diseases* 38:789–795.

Lankester, M. W., and D. Fong. 1989. Distribution of elaphostrongyline nematodes (Metastrongyloidea: Protostrongylidae) in cervidae and possible effects of

moving *Rangifer* spp. into and within North America. *Alces* 25:133–145.

Lashley, F. R., and J. D. Durham. 2002. Preface. In *Emerging Infectious Diseases. Trends and Issues,* edited by F. R. Lashley and J. D. Durham, pp. xv–xviii. New York: Springer Publishing Inc.

Laskowski, R. 2000. Shochastic and density-dependent models in ecotoxicology. In *Demography in Ecotoxicology,* edited by J. Kammenga and R. Laskowski, pp. 57–71. Chichester: John Wiley & Sons.

Latgé, J.-P. 2001. The pathobiology of *Aspergillus fumigatus. Trends in Microbiology* 9:382–389.

Laurenson, K., C. Sillero-Zubiri, H. Thompson, F. Shiferaw, S. Thergood, and J. Malcolm. 1998. Disease as a threat to endangered species: Ethiopian wolves, domestic dogs and canine pathogens. *Animal Conservation* 1:273–280.

Laurenson, M. K., R. A. Norman, L. Gilbert, H. W. Reid, and P. J. Hudson. 2003. Identifying disease reservoirs in complex systems: mountain hares as reservoirs of ticks and louping-ill virus, pathogens of red grouse. *Journal of Animal Ecology* 72:177–185.

Lawson, R. J., and M. A. Gemmell. 1983. Hydatosis and cysticercosis: the dynamics of transmission. *Advances in Parasitology* 22:261–308.

———. 1985. The potential role of blowflies in the transmission of taeniid tapeworm eggs. *Parasitology* 91:129–143.

Lederberg, J. 1997. Foreword. In *Emerging Infections 1,* edited by W. M. Scheld, D. Armstrong, and J. M. Hughes, pp xiii. Washington, D.C.: ASM Press.

Lees, V. W., S. Copeland, and P. Rousseau. 2003. Bovine tuberculosis in elk (*Cervus elaphus manitobensis*) near Riding Mountain National Park, Manitoba from 1992 to 2002. *Canadian Veterinary Journal* 44:830–831.

Legname, G., I. V. Baskakov, H. O. Nguyen, D. Reisner, F. E. Cohen, S. J. DeArmond, and S. B. Prusiner. 2004. Synthetic mammalian prions. *Science* 305:673–676.

Leiby, P. D., and W. G Dyer. 1971. Cyclophyllidean tapeworms of wild carnivores. In *Parasitic Diseases of Wild Mammals,* edited by J. W. Davis and R. C. Anderson, pp. 175–234. Ames: Iowa State University Press.

Leighton, F. A. 1993. The toxicity of petroleum oils to birds. *Environmental Research* 1:92–103.

———. 2002. Health risk assessment of the translocation of wild animals. *Revue Scientifique et Technique OIE* 21:187–195.

Leighton, F. A., H. A. Artsob, M. C. Chu, and J. G. Olson. 2001. A serological survey of rural dogs and cats on the southwestern Canadian prairie for zoonotic pathogens. *Canadian Journal of Public Health* 92:67–71.

Leighton, F. A., M. Ferguson, A. Gunn, E. Henderson, and G. Stenhouse. 1988. Canine distemper in sled dogs. *Canadian Veterinary Journal* 29:299.

Le Maho, Y. 1983 Metabolic adaptations to long-term fasting in Antarctic penguins and domestic geese. *Journal of Thermal Biology* 8:91–96.

Lenghaus, C., M. J. Studdert, and D. Gavier-Widen. 2001. Calicivirus infections. In *Infectious Diseases of Wild Mammals*, 3d ed., edited by E. S. Williams and I. K. Barker, pp. 280–291. Ames: Iowa State Press.

Lenski, R. E., and R. M. May. 1994. The evolution of virulence in parasites and pathogens: reconciliation between two competing hypotheses. *Journal of Theoretical Biology* 169:253–265.

León-Viscaíno, L., M. R. Ruíz de Ybáñez, M. J. Cubero, J. M. Ortiz, J. Espinosa, L. Pérez, M. A. Simón, and F. Alonso. 1999. Sarcoptic mange in Spanish ibex. *Journal of Wildlife Diseases* 35:647–659.

Leopold, A. 1933. *Game Management*. New York: Charles Scribner's Sons.

Levav, M., A. F. Mirsky, P. M. Schantz, S. Castro, and M. E. Cruz. 1995. Parasitic infection in malnourished school children: effects on behaviour and EEG. *Parasitology* 110:103–111.

Levin, B. R. 1996. The evolution and maintenance of virulence in microparasites. *Emerging Infectious Diseases* 2:93–192.

Levin, B. R., and C. Svanborg-Eden. 1990. Selection and evolution of virulence in bacteria: an ecumenical excursion and modest suggestion. *Parasitology* 100:S103–115.

Levin, B. R., and R. Antia. 2001. Why we don't get sick: the within-host population dynamics of bacterial infections. *Science* 292:1112–1115.

Levine, S., and H. Ursin. 1991. What is stress? In *Stress Neurobiology and Neuroendocrinology*, edited by M. R. Brown, G. F. Koob, and C. Rivier, pp. 3–21. New York: Marcel Dekker Inc.

L'Heureux, N., M. Festa-Blanchet, and J. T. Jorgenson. 1996. Effects of visible signs of contagious ecthyma on mass and survival of bighorn lambs. *Journal of Wildlife Diseases* 32:286–292.

Lindström, A., and T. G. T. Jaenson. 2003. Distribution of the common tick, *Ixodes ricinus* (Acari: Ixodidae), in different vegetation types in southern Sweden. *Journal of Medical Entomolology* 40:375–378.

Liu, M., Y. Guan, M. Peiris, S. He, R. J. Webby, D. Perez, and R. G. Webster. 2003. The quest of influenza A viruses for new hosts. *Avian Diseases* 47:849–856.

Lochmiller, R. I., and C. Deerenberg. 2000. Trade-offs in evolutionary immunology: just what is the cost of immunity? *Oikos* 88:87–98

Logiudice, K. 2003. Trophically transmitted parasites and the conservation of small populations: raccoon roundworm and the imperiled Allegheny woodrat. *Conservation Biology* 17:258–266.

Loisin, A., J-M. Gaillard, and J-M. Julien. 1996. Demographic patterns after an epizootic of keratoconjunctivitis in a chamois population. *Journal of Wildlife Management* 60:517–527.

Lord, R. D. 1992. Seasonal reproduction of vampire bats and its relationship to the seasonality of bovine rabies. *Journal of Wildlife Diseases* 28:292–294.

Lugton, I., G. Wobeser, R. S. Morris, and P. Caley. 1997. Epidemiology of *Mycobacterium bovis* infection in feral ferrets (*Mustela furo*) in New Zealand. II. Routes of infection and excretion. *New Zealand Veterinary Journal* 45:161–167.

Lumeij, J. T. 1996. Syphilis in European brown hares (*Lepus europus*). *Veterinary Quarterly* 18:151–152.

Lyons, E. T., and M. C. Keyes. 1978. Observations on the infectivity of parasitic third-stage larvae of *Uncinaria lucasi* Stiles 1901 (Nematoda: Ancylostomatidae) of northern fur seals *Callorhinus ursinus* Linn., on St. Paul Island, Alaska. *Journal of Parasitology* 64:454–48.

Mackenzie, J. S., H. E. Field, and K. J. Guyatt. 2003. Managing emerging diseases borne by fruit bats (flying foxes), with particular reference to henipaviruses and Australian bat lyssavirus. *Journal of Applied Microbiology* 94:59S–69S.

Mahy, B. W. J., and C. C. Brown. 2000. Emerging zoonoses: crossing the species barrier. *Revue Scientifique et Technique OIE* 19:33–40.

Malkinson, M., C. Banet, Y. Weisman, S. Pokamunski, R. King, M.-T. Drouet, and V. Deubel. 2002. Introduction of West Nile virus in the Middle East by migrating white storks. *Emerging Infectious Diseases* 8:392–397.

Mamaev, L. V., N. N. Denikina, S. I. Belikov, V. E. Volichikov, I. K. G. Visser, M. Fleming, C. Kai, T. C. Harder, B. Liess, A. D. M. E. Osterhaus, and T. Barrett. 1995. Characteristics of morbilliviruses isolated from Lake Baikal seals (*Phoca sibirica*). *Veterinary Microbiology* 40:251–259.

Mänd, R., and V. Tilgar. 2003. Does supplementary calcium reduce the cost of reproduction in the Pied Flycatcher *Ficedula hypoleuca*. *Ibis* 145:67–77.

Marchandeau, S., J. Chantal, Y. Portejoie, S. Barraud, and Y. Chaval. 1998. Impact of viral hemorrhagic disease on a wild population of European rabbits in France. *Journal of Wildlife Diseases* 34:429–435.

Marchlewska-Koj, A., J. Kapusta, and M. Kruczek. 2003. Prenatal stress modifies behaviour in offspring of bank voles (*Clethrionomys glareolus*). *Physiology and Behavior* 79:671–678.

Martin, L. B, II, A. Scheuerlein, and M. Wikelski. 2003. Immune activity elevates energy expenditure of house sparrows: a link between direct and indirect costs? *Proceedings of the Royal Society, London B* 270: 153–158.

Mason, P. C., and H. J. F. McAllum. 1976. *Dictyocaulus viviparus* and *Elaphostrongylus cervi* in wapiti. *New Zealand Veterinary Journal* 24:23.

Mason, P. C., N. R. Kiddey, R. J. Sutherland, D. M. Rutherford, and A. P. Green. 1976. *Elaphostrongylus cervi* in red deer. *New Zealand Veterinary Journal* 24:22–23.

Massey, R. C., A. Buckling, R. French-Constant. 2004. Interference competition and parasite virulence. *Proceedings of the Royal Society, London B* 271: 785–788.

Matumoto, M. 1969. Mechanisms of perpetuation of animal viruses in nature. *Bacteriological Reviews* 33: 404–418.

May, R. M. 1994. Disease and the abundance and distribution of bird populations: a summary. *Ibis* 137: S85–S86.

May, R. M., and R. M. Anderson. 1978. Regulation and stability of host-parasite population interactions. II Destabilizing processes. *Journal of Animal Ecology* 47:249–267.

———. 1983. Parasite-host coevolution. In *Coevolution,* edited by D. J. Futuyama and M. Slatkin, pp. 186–206. Sunderland: Sinuaer Associates.

Mazet, J. K., W. M. Boyce, J. Mellies, I. A. Gardner, R. K. Clark, and D. A. Jessup. 1992. Exposure to *Psoroptes* sp. mites is common among bighorn sheep (*Ovis canadensis*) populations in California. *Journal of Wildlife Diseases* 28:542–547.

McCallum, H., and A. Dobson. 2002. Disease, habitat fragmentation and conservation. *Proceedings of the Royal Society, London B* 269:2041–2049.

McCarty, C. W., and M. W. Miller. 1998. A versatile model of disease transmission applied to forecasting bovine tuberculosis dynamics in white-tailed deer populations. *Journal of Wildlife Diseases* 34:722–730.

McColl, K. A., N. Tordo, and A. A. Setién. 2000. Bat lyssavirus infections. *Revue Scientifique et Technique OIE* 19:177–196.

McCollough, M., and B. Connery. 1990. *An Evaluation of the Maine Caribou Reintroduction Project, Maine Caribou Project Report.* Orono: University of Maine.

McCoy, G. W. 1911. The susceptibility to plague of the weasel, the chipmunk, and the pocket gopher. *Journal of Infectious Diseases* 8:42–46.

McCoy, G. W., and C. W. Chapin. 1912. Bacterium tularense the cause of a plague-like disease of rodents. *United States Public Health Marine Hospital Bulletin* 53:17–23.

McInerney, J., K. J. Small, and P. Caley. 1995. Prevalence of *Mycobacterium bovis* infection in feral pigs in the northern territory. *Australian Veterinary Journal* 72:448–451.

McLandress, M. R. 1983. Sex, age, and species differences in disease mortality of Ross' and lesser snow geese in California: implications for avian cholera research. *California Fish and Game* 69:196–206.

McPeek, M. A., N. L. Rodenhouse, R. T. Holmes, and T. W. Sherry. 2001. A general model of site-dependent population regulation: population-level regulation without individual-level interactions. *Oikos* 94:417–424.

Meagher, M., W. J. Quinn, and L. Stackhouse. 1992. Chlamydial-caused infectious keratoconjunctivitis in bighorn sheep of Yellowstone National Park. *Journal of Wildlife Diseases* 28:171–176.

Mech, L. D., and S. M. Goyal. 1993. Canine parvovirus effect on wolf population change and pup survival. *Journal of Wildlife Diseases* 29:330–333.

Melendez, L. V., C. Espana, R. D. Hunt, and M. D. Daniel. 1969. Natural *Herpes simplex* infection in the owl monkey (*Aotus trivirgatus*). *Laboratory Animal Care* 19:38–45.

Metcalfe, N. B., and P. Monaghan. 2001. Compensation for a bad start: grow now, pay later? *Trends in Ecology and Evolution* 16:254–260.

Meteyer, C. U., R. R. Dubielzig, F. J. Dein, L. A. Baeten, M. K. Moore, J. R. Jehl, Jr., and K. Wesenberg. 1997. Sodium toxicity and pathology associated with exposure of waterfowl to hypersaline playa lakes of southeast New Mexico. *Journal of Veterinary Diagnostic Investigation* 9:269–280.

Mellor, P. S., and C. J. Leake. 2000. Climate and geographic influences on arboviral infections and vectors. *Revue Scientifique et Technique OIE* 19:41–54.

Miller, M. A., M. E. Grigg, C. Kreuder, E. R. James, A. C. Melli, P. R. Crosbie, D. A. Jessup, J. C. Boothroyd, D. Brownstein, and P. A. Conrad. 2004a. An unusual genotype of *Toxoplasma gondii* is common in California sea otters (*Enhydra lutra nereis*) and is a cause of mortality. *International Journal of Parasitology* 34:275–284.

Miller, M. W., and E. S. Williams. 2003. Horizontal prion transmission in mule deer. *Nature* 425:35–36.

Miller, M. W., E. S. Williams, C. W. McCarty, T. R. Spraker, T. J. Kreeger, C. T. Larsen, and E. T. Thorne. 2000. Epizootiology of chronic wasting disease in free-ranging cervids in Colorado and Wyoming *Journal of Wildlife Diseases* 36:676–690.

Miller, M. W., E. S. Williams, N. T. Hobbs, and L. L. Wolfe. 2004b. Environmental sources of prion transmission in mule deer, *Emerging Infectious Diseases* 10:1003–1007.

Miller, R., J. B. Kaneene, S. D. Fitzgerald, and S. M. Schmitt. 2003. Evaluation of the influence of supplemental feeding of white-tailed deer (*Odocoileus virginianus*) on the prevalence of bovine tuberculosis in the Michigan wild deer population. *Journal of Wildlife Diseases* 39:84–95.

Mills, J. N., and J. E. Childs. 2001. Rodent-borne hemorrhagic fever viruses. In *Infectious Diseases of Wild Mammals.* 3d ed., edited by E. S. Williams and I. K. Barker, pp. 254–270. Ames: Iowa State University Press.

Mills, J. N., T. G. Ksiazek, C. J. Peters, and J. E. Childs. 1999. Long-term studies of hantavirus reservoir populations in the southwestern United States: a synthesis. *Emerging Infectious Diseases* 5:95–101.

Mims, C. A., A. Nash, and J. Stephen. 2001. *Mims' Pathogenesis of Infectious Disease,* 5th ed. San Diego: Academic Press.

Mineau, P. 1993. *The Hazard of Carbofuran to Birds and Other Vertebrate Wildlife.* Technical Report No. 177. Ottawa: Canadian Wildlife Service, Wildlife Toxicology Section, Environment Canada.

Mocarski, E. S., Jr. 2002. Virus self-improvement through inflammation: no pain, no gain. *Proceedings of the National Academy of Science of the United States of America* 99:3362–3364.

Møller, A. P. 1992. Parasites differentially increase the degree of fluctuating asymmetry in secondary sexual characters. *Journal of Evolutionary Biology* 5:691–699.

————. 1994. Parasites as an environmental component of reproduction in bird as exemplified by the swallow *Hirundo rustico*. *Ardea* 82:161–172.

Møller, A. P., and N. Saino. 2004. Immune response and survival. *Oikos* 104:299–304.

Moore, J. 2002. *Parasites and the Behavior of Animals.* Oxford: Oxford University Press.

Mooring, M. S., and B. L. Hart. 1992. Animal grouping for protection from parasites: selfish herd and encounter-dilution effects. *Behaviour* 123:173–193.

Moorman, A. M., T. E. Moorman, G. E. Baldassarre, and D. M. Richard. 1991. Effects of saline water on growth and survival of mottled duck ducklings in Louisiana. *Journal of Wildlife Management* 55:471–476.

Morales-Mentor, J., A. Gamboa-Dominguez, M. Rodriguez-Dorantes, and M. A. Cerbon. 1999. Tissue damage in the male murine reproductive system during experimental *Taenia crassiceps* cysticercosis. *Journal of Parasitology* 85:887–890.

Moriarty, A., G. Saunders, and B. J. Richardson. 2000. Mortality factors acting on adult rabbits in central-western New South Wales. *Wildlife Research* 27: 613–619.

Morris, R. S., and D. U. Pfeiffer. 1995. Directions and issues in bovine tuberculosis epidemiology and control in New Zealand. *New Zealand Veterinary Journal* 43:256–265.

Mörschel, F. H., and D. R. Klein. 1997. Effects of weather and parasitic insects on behavior and group dynamics of caribou of the Delta Herd, Alberta. *Canadian Journal of Zoology* 75:1659–1670.

Morse, S. S. 1995. Factors in the emergence of infectious diseases. *Emerging Infectious Diseases* 1:7–15.

Moss, R., A. Watson, I. B. Trenholm, and R. Parr. 1993. Cecal threadworms *Trichostrongylus tenuis* in red grouse *Lagopus lagopus scoticus*: effects of weather and host density upon estimated worm burden. *Parasitology* 107:199–209.

Mouritsen, K. N., and R. Poulin. 2002. Parasitism, climate oscillations and the structure of natural communities *Oikos* 97:462–468.

Moyer, B. R., D. M. Drown, and D. H. Clayton. 2002. Low humidity reduces ectoparasite pressure: implications for host life history evolution. *Oikos* 97:223–228.

Muller, J. 1971. The effect of fox reduction on the occurrence of rabies. Observations from two outbreaks of rabies in Denmark. *Bulletin Office International Epizootie* 75:763–776.

Müller, G., P. Wohlsein, A. Beineke, L. Haas, I. Greiser-Wilke, U. Siebert, S. Fonfara, T. Harder, M. Stede, A. D. Gruber, and W. Baumgartner. 2004. Phocine distemper in German seals, 2002. *Emerging infectious Diseases* 10:723–725.

Müller, W. W. 1997. Where do we stand with oral vaccination of foxes against rabies in Europe. In *Viral Zoonoses and Food of Animal Origin,* edited by O.-R. Kaaden, C.-P. Czerny, and W. Ichorn, pp. 85–94. New York: SpringerWien.

Mulvey, M., and J. M. Aho. 1993. Parasitism and mate competition: liver flukes in white-tailed deer. *Oikos* 66:187–192.

Mundy, P. J., and J. A. Ledger. 1976. Griffon vultures, carnivores and bones. *South African Journal of Science* 72:106–110.

Munger, J. C., and W. H. Karasov. 1989. Sublethal parasites and host energy budgets: tapeworm infection in white-footed mice. *Ecology* 70:904–921.

————. 1991. Sublethal parasites in white-footed mice: impact on survival and reproduction. *Canadian Journal of Zoology* 69:398–404.

Munson, L. 2001. Feline morbillivirus infection. In *Infectious Diseases of Wild Mammals,* 3d ed., edited by E. S. Williams and I. K. Barker, pp. 59–64. Ames: Iowa State Press.

Murphy, F. A., and R. G. Webster. 1996. Orthomyxoviruses. In *Field Virology,* 3d ed., edited by B. N. Fields, D. M. Knipe, P. M. Howley, R. M. Chanock, J. L. Melnick, T. P. Monath, B. Roizman, and S. E. Straus, pp. 1397–1446. Philadelphia: Lippincott-Raven.

Murray, C. J. L., and A. D. Lopez. 1997. Mortality by cause for eight regions of the world: Global Burden of Disease Study. *Lancet* 349:1269–1276.

Murray, D. L., J. R. Cary, and L. B. Keith. 1997. Interactive effects of sublethal nematodes and nutritional status on snowshoe hare vulnerability to predation. *Journal of Animal Ecology* 66:250–264.

Mutze, G., B. Cooke, and P. Alexander. 1998. The initial impact of rabbit hemorrhagic disease on European rabbit populations in South Australia. *Journal of Wildlife Diseases* 34:221–227.

Nacci, D. E., D. Champlin, L. Coiro, R. McKinney, and S. Jayaraman. 2002. Predicting the occurrence of genetic adaptation to dioxinlike compounds in populations of estuarine fish *Fundulus heteroclitus*. *Environmental Toxicology and Chemistry* 21:1525–1532.

Naguib, M., K. Riebel, A. Marzhal, and D. Gil. 2004. Nestling immunocompetence and testosterone covary with brood size in a songbird. *Proceedings of the Royal Society, London B* 271:833–838.

Navarro, C., F. de lope, A. Marzal, and A. P. Møller. 2004. Predation risk, host immune response, and parasitism. *Behavioral Ecology* 15:629–635.

Neff, J. A. 1955. Outbreak of aspergillosis in mallards. *Journal of Wildlife Management* 19:415–416.

Neumann, G. B. 1997. Bovine tuberculosis—an increasingly rare event. *Australian Veterinary Journal* 77:445–446.

Newman, M. C. 2001. *Population Ecotoxicology.* Chichester: John Wiley & Sons, Ltd.

Newman, T. J., P. J. Baker, and S. Harris. 2002. Nutritional condition and survival of red foxes with sarcoptic mange. *Canadian Journal of Zoology* 80:154–161.

Newton, I. 1979. *Population Ecology of Raptors.* Berkhamsted: Poyser.

————. 1998. *Population Limitation in Birds.* San Diego: Academic Press.

Nichol, S. T., C. F. Spiropoulou, S. Morzunov, P. E. Rollin, T. G. Ksiazek, H. Feldmann, A. Sanchez, J. E. Childs, S. Zaki, and C. J. Peter. 1993. Genetic identification of a hantavirus associated with an outbreak of acute respiratory disease. *Science* 262:914–917.

Niklasson, B., B. Hörnfeldt, and B. Lundman. 1998. Could myocarditis, insulin-dependent diabetes mellitus, and Guillain-Barré syndrome be caused by one or more infectious agents carried by rodents? *Emerging Infectious Diseases* 4:1876–193.

Nilsen, E. B., J. C. Linnell, and R. Andersen. 2004. Individual access to preferred habitat affects fitness components in female roe deer *Capreolus capreolus*. *Journal of Animal Ecology* 73:44–50.

Nokes, D. J. 1992. Microparasites: viruses and bacteria. In *Natural Enemies. The Population Biology of Predators, Parasites and Diseases*, edited by M. J. Crawley, pp. 349–376. Oxford: Blackwell Scientific Publications.

Norrix, L. W., D. W. DeYoung, P. R. Krausman, R. C. Etchberger, and T. J. Glattke. 1995. Conductive hearing loss in bighorn sheep. *Journal of Wildlife Diseases* 31:223–227.

Nugent, G., J. Whitford, and N. Young. 2002. Use of released pigs as sentinels for *Mycobacterium bovis*. *Journal of Wildlife Diseases* 38:665–677.

Nygård, T., and J. O. Gjershaug. 2001. The effects of low levels of pollutants on the reproduction of golden eagles in western Norway. *Ecotoxicology* 10:285–290.

Oaks, J. L., M. Gilbert, M. Z. Virani, R. T. Watson, C. U. Meteyer, B. A. Rideout, H. L. Shivaprasad, S. Ahmed, M. J. I. Chaudry, M. Arshad, S. Mahmood, A. All, and A. A. Khan. 2004. Diclofenac residues as the cause of vulture population decline in Pakistan. *Nature* 427:630–633.

Oberheu, D. G., and C. B. Dabbert. 2001. Aflatoxin contamination in supplemental and wild foods of northern bobwhite. *Ecotoxicology* 10:125–129.

O'Brien, D. J., S. M. Schmitt, J. S. Fierke, S. A. Hogle, S. R. Winterstein, T. M. Cooley, W. E. Moritz, K. L. Diegel, S. D. Fitzgerald, D. E. Berry, and J. B. Kaneene. 2002. Epidemiology of *Mycobacterium bovis* in free-ranging white-tailed deer, Michigan, USA, 1995–2000. *Preventive Veterinary Medicine* 54:47–63.

Odum, E. P. 1993. *Ecology and Our Endangered Life-support Systems*. Sunderland: Sinauer Associates Incorporated.

Oh, P., R. Granich, J. Scott., B. Sun, M. Joseph, C. Strongfield, S. Thisdell, J. Stoley, D. Workman-Malcolm, L. Bornstein, E. Lehnkering, P. Ryan, J. Soukup, A. Nitta, and J. Flood. 2002. Human exposure following *Mycobacterium tuberculosis* infection of multiple animal species in a metropolitan zoo. *Emerging Infectious Diseases* 8:1290–1293.

Ohlendorf, H. L. 1996. Selenium. In *Noninfectious Diseases of Wildlife*, 2d ed., edited by A. Fairbrother, L. N. Locke, and G. L. Hoff, pp. 128–140. Ames: Iowa State University Press.

Olsen, N. J., and W. J. Kovacs. 1996. Gonadal steroids and immunity. *Endocrinological Reviews* 17:369–384.

Olsson, G. E., F. Dalerum, B. Hörnfeldt, F. Elgh, T.R. Palo, P. Juto, and C. Ahlm. 2003. Human hantavirus infections, Sweden. *Emerging Infectious Diseases* 9:1395–1401.

Orlando, E. F., and L. J. Guillette, Jr. 2001. A re-examination of variation associated with environmentally stressed organisms. *Human Reproduction Update* 7:265–272.

Ostfeld, R. S., E. M. Schauber, C. D. Canham, F. Keesing, C. G. Jones, and J. O. Wolff. 2001. Effects of acorn production and mouse abundance on abundance and Borrelia burgdorferi infection prevalence of nymphal *Ixodes scapularis* ticks. *Vector Borne Zoonotic Diseases* 1:55–63.

Ottinger, M. A., M. Abdelnabi, M. Quinn, N. Golden, J. Wu, and N. Thompson. 2002. Reproductive consequences of EDCs in birds. What do laboratory effects mean in field species? *Neurotoxicology and Teratology* 24:17–28.

Otto, G. F., and L. A. Jachowski. 1981. Mosquitos and canine heartworm disease. In *Proceedings Heartworm Symposium '80*, edited by G. F. Otto, pp. 17–32. Veterinary Medical Publishing Company.

Ould, P., and H. E. Welch. 1980. The effect of stress on the parasitism of mallard ducklings by *Echinuria uncinata* (Nematoda: Spirurida). *Canadian Journal of Zoology* 58:228–234.

Overstreet, R. M., and E. Rehak. 1981. Heatstroke in nesting least tern chicks from Gulfport, Mississippi, during June 1980. *Avian Diseases* 26:918–923.

Packer, C., R. D. Holt, K. D. Lafferty, and A. P. Dobson. 2003. Keeping the herds healthy and alert: implications of predator control for infectious disease. *Ecology Letters* 6:797–802.

Packer, C., S. Altizer, M. Appel, E. Brown, J. Martenson, S. J. O'Brien, M. Roelke-Parker, R. Hofman-Lehmann, and H. Lutz. 1999. Viruses of the Serengeti: patterns of infections and mortality in African lions. *Journal of Animal Ecology* 68:1161–1178.

Page, L. K., R. K. Swihart, and K. R. Kazacos. 1999. Implications of raccoon latrines in the epizootiology of baylisascariasis. *Journal of Wildlife Diseases* 35:474–480.

Palmer, M. V., D. L. Whipple, and S. C. Olsen. 1999. Development of a model of natural infection with *Mycobacterium bovis* in white-tailed deer. *Journal of Wildlife Diseases* 35:450–457.

Palmer, M. V., W. R. Waters, and D. L. Whipple. 2004. Shared feed as a means of deer-to-deer transmission of *Mycobacterium bovis*. *Journal of Wildlife Diseases* 40:87–91.

Palmer, S. R., Lord Soulsby, and D. I. H. Simpson. 1998. *Zoonoses: Biology, Clinical Practice, and Public Health Control*. Oxford: Oxford University Press.

Paré, J. A. 1997. *Vaccination of raccoons (Procyon lotor) against canine distemper: an experimental study*. Guelph, D.V.Sc. Thesis, University of Guelph, Ontario.

Parrish, J. M., and B. F. Hunter. 1969. Waterfowl botulism in the southern San Joaquin Valley, 1967–68. *California Fish and Game* 55:265–272.

Pavlovsky, E. N. 1966. *Natural Nidality of Transmissible Diseases, with Special Reference to the Landscape Epidemiology of the Zooanthroponoses.* Urbana: University of Illinois Press.

Pawelczyk, A., A. Bajer, J. M. Behnke, F. S. Gilbert, and E. Sinski. 2004. Factors affecting the component community structure of haemoparasites in common voles (*Microtus arvalis*) from the Mazury Lake district of Poland. *Parasitology Research* 92:270–284.

Pence, D. B., and E. Ueckermann. 2002. Sarcoptic mange in wildlife. *Revue Scientifique et Technique OIE* 21:385–398.

Pence, D. B., F. F. Knowlton, and L. A. Windberg. 1988. Transmission of *Ancylostoma caninum* and *Alaria marcianae* in coyotes (*Canis latrans*). *Journal of Wildlife Diseases* 26:560–563.

Peterson, C. A., S. L. Lee, and J. E. Elliot. 2000. Scavenging of waterfowl carcasses by birds in agricultural fields of British Columbia. *Canadian Field-Naturalist* 72:150–159.

Peterson, R. O. 1988. Increased osteoarthritis in moose from Isle Royale. *Journal of Wildlife Diseases* 24:461–466.

Petney, T. N., and R. H. Andrews. 1998. Multiparasite communities in animals and humans: frequency, structure and pathogenic significance. *International Journal of Parasitology* 28:377–393.

Petravy, A. F., F. Tenora, S. Deblock, and V. Sergent. 2000. *Echinococcus multilocularis* in domestic cats in France. A potential risk factor for alveolar hydatid disease contamination in humans. *Veterinary Parasitology* 87:151–156.

Pharo, H. 2002. New Zealand declares provisional freedom from hydatids. *Surveillance* 29:3–7.

Philibert, H., G. Wobeser, and R. G. Clark. 1993. Counting dead birds: examination of methods. *Journal of Wildlife Diseases* 29:284–289.

Phillips, B., and P. Harrison. 1999. Overview of the endocrine disruptor issue. In *Endocrine Disrupting Chemicals, Issues in Environmental Science and Technology 12,* edited by R. E. Hester and R. M. Harrisson, pp. 1–26. Cambridge: Royal Society of Chemistry.

Pienaar, U. de V. 1967. Epidemiology of anthrax in wild animals and the control of anthrax epizootics in the Kruger National Park, South Africa. *Federation Proceedings* 26:1496–1502.

Plagemann, P. G. W. 2003. Porcine reproductive and respiratory syndrome virus: origin hypothesis. *Emerging Infectious Diseases* 9:903–908.

Plaut, A. 1993. Microbial subversion of host defenses. In *Mechanisms of Microbial Disease,* edited by M. Schaechter, G. Medoff, and B. I. Einstein, pp. 154–161. Baltimore: Williams & Wilkins.

Plowright, W. 1982. The effects of rinderpest and rinderpest control on wildlife in Africa. *Symposium of the Zoological Society, London* 50:1–28.

Porter, W. P., R. Hinsdill, A. Fairbrother, L. J. Olson, J. Jaeger, T. Yuill, S. Bisgaard, W. G. Hunter, and K. Nolan. 1984. Toxicant-disease-environment interactions associated with suppression of immune system, growth, and reproduction. *Science* 224:1014–1017.

Potts, G. R. 1986. *The Partridge: Pesticides, Predation and Conservation.* London: Collins.

Poulin, R. 1996. Sexual inequalities in helminth infections: a cost of being male? *American Naturalist* 147:287–295.

Poulin, R., K. Hecker, and F. Thomas. 1998. Hosts manipulated by one parasite incur additional costs from infection by another parasite. *Journal of Parasitology* 84:1050–1052.

Pöysä, H., J. Elmberg, P. Nummi, and K. Sjöberg. 2004. Ecological basis of sustainable harvesting: is the prevailing paradigm of compensatory mortality still valid? *Oikos* 104:612–615.

Prusiner, S. B. 1998. Prions. *Proceedings of the National Academy of Science of the United States of America* 95:13363–13383

Pybus, M. J. 2001. Liver flukes. In *Parasitic Diseases of Wild Mammals.* 2d ed., edited by W. M. Samuel, M. J. Pybus, and A. A. Kocan, pp. 121–149. Ames: Iowa State University Press.

Quinn, J. L., and W. Cresswell. 2004. Predator hunting behaviour and prey vulnerability. *Journal of Animal Ecology* 73:143–154.

Qureshi, T., D. L. Drawe, D. S. Davis, and T. M. Craig. 1994. Use of bait containing triclabendazole to treat *Fascioloides magna* infection in free ranging white-tailed deer. *Journal of Wildlife Diseases* 30:346–350.

Ramsay, S. L., and D. C. Houston. 1999. Do acid rain and calcium supply limit eggshell formation for blue tits (*Parus caerulescens*) in the U.K.? *Journal of Zoology, London* 247:121–125.

Rand, P. W., C. Lubelczyk, G. R. Lavigne, S. Elias, M. S. Holman, E. H. Lacombe, and R. P. Smith, Jr. 2003. Deer density and the abundance of *Ixodes scapularis* (Acari: Ixodidae). *Journal of Medical Entomology* 40:179–184.

Randolph, S. E., C. Chemini, C. Furlanello, C. Genchi, R. S. Hails, P. J. Hudson, L. D. Jones, G. Medley, R. A. Norman, A. P. Rizzoli, G. Smith, and M. E. J. Woolhouse. 2001. The ecology of tick-borne infections in wildlife reservoirs. In *The Ecology of Wildlife Diseases,* edited by P. J. Hudson, A. Rizzoli, B. T. Grenfell, H. Heesterbeek, and A. P. Dobson, pp. 119–138. Oxford: Oxford University Press.

Rattner, B. A., and A. G. Heath. 1995. Environmental factors affecting contaminant toxicity in aquatic and terrestrial vertebrates. In *Handbook of Ecotoxicology,* edited by D. J. Hoffman, B. A. Rattner, G. A. Burton, Jr., J. Cairns, Jr., pp. 519–535. Boca Raton: Lewis Publishers.

Rattner, B. A., and J. R. Jehl, Jr. 1997. Dramatic fluctuations in liver mass and metal content of eared grebes (*Podiceps nigricollis*) during autumnal migration. *Bulletin of Environmental Contamation and Toxicology* 59:337–343.

Rau, M. E., and F. R. Caron. 1979. Parasite-induced susceptibility of moose to hunting. *Canadian Journal of Zoology* 57:2466–2468.

Read, A. F, and L. H. Taylor. 2001. The ecology of genetically diverse infections. *Science* 292:1099–1102.

Read, A. F., P. Aaby, R. Antia, D. Ebert, P. W. Ewald, S. Gupta, E. C. Holmes, A. Sasaki, D. C. Shields, F. Taddei, and E. R. Moxon. 1999. What can evolutionary biology contribute to understanding virulence? In *Evolution in Health and Disease,* edited by S. C. Stearns, pp. 205–215. Oxford: Oxford University Press.

Refsum, T., T. Vikøren, K. Handeland, G. Kapperud, and G. Holstad. 2003. Epidemiologic and pathologic aspects of *Salmonella typhimurium* infection in passerine birds of Norway. *Journal of Wildlife Diseases* 39:64–72.

Rehbein, S., M. Visser, R. Winter, B. Trommer, H.-F. Matthes, A. E. Maciel, and S. E. Marley. 2003. Productivity effects of bovine mange and control with ivermectin. *Veterinary Parasitology* 114:267–284.

Reichard, R. E. 2002. Area-wide biological control of disease vectors and agents affecting wildlife. *Revue Scientifique et Technique OIE* 21:179–185.

Reid, J. M., E. M. Bignal, S. Bignal, D. I. McCracken, and P. Monaghan. 2003. Age-specific reproductive performance in red-billed choughs *Pyrrhocorax pyrrhocorax*: patterns and processes in a natural population. *Journal of Animal Ecology* 72:765–776.

Relman, D. A. 1998. Detection and identification of previously unrecognized microbial pathogens. *Emerging Infectious Diseases* 4:382–389.

Relyea, R. A. 2003. Predator cues and pesticides: a double dose of danger for amphibians. *Ecological Applications* 13:1515–1521.

Reynolds, M. G., J. W. Krebs, J. A. Comer, J. W. Sumner, T. C. Rushton, C. E. Lopez, W. L. Nicholson, J. A. Rooney, S. E. Lace-Parker, J. H. McQuiston, C. D. Paddock, and J. E. Childs. 2003. Flying squirrel-associated typhus, United States. *Emerging Infectious Diseases* 9:1341–1344.

Rhyan, J. C. 2000. Brucellosis in terrestrial wildlife and marine mammals. In *Emerging Diseases of Animals,* edited by C. Brown and C. Bolin, pp. 161–184. Washington, D.C.: ASM Press.

Rhyan, J. C., T. Gidlewski, T. J. Roffe, K. Aune, L. M. Philo, D. R. Ewalt. 2000. Pathology of brucellosis in bison in Yellowstone National Park. *Journal of Wildlife Diseases* 37:101–109.

Rhyan, J. C., W. J. Quinn, L. S. Stackhouse, J. J. Henderson, D. R. Ewalt, J. B. Payeur, M. Johnson, and M. Meagher. 1994. Abortion caused by *Brucella abortus* biovar 1 in a free-ranging bison (*Bison bison*) from Yellowstone National Park. *Journal of Wildlife Diseases* 30:445–446.

Rigby, M. C., and Y. Moret. 2000. Life-history trade-offs with immune defenses. In *Evolutionary Biology of Host-parasite Relationships: Theory Meets Reality,* edited by R. Poulin, S. Morand, and A. Skoring, pp. 129–162. Amsterdam: Elsevier Science.

Robbins, C. T. 1993. *Wildlife Feeding and Nutrition.* San Diego: Academic Press.

Roberts, M. G., G. Smith, and B. T. Grenfell. 1995. Mathematical models for macroparasites of wildlife. In *Ecology of Infectious Diseases in Natural Populations,* edited by B. T. Grenfell and A. P. Dobson, pp. 177–208. Cambridge: Cambridge University Press.

Robinson, R. M., A. C. Ray, J. C. Reagor, and L. A. Holland. 1982. Waterfowl mortality caused by aflatoxicosis in Texas. *Journal of Wildlife Diseases* 18:311–313.

Robinson, R. M., L. P. Jones, T. J. Galvin, and G. M. Harwell. 1978. Elaeophorosis in Sika deer in Texas. *Journal of Wildlife Diseases* 14:137–141.

Rodenhouse, N. L., T. S. Sillett, P. J. Doran, and R. T. Holmes. 2003. Multiple density-dependence mechanisms regulate a migratory bird population during the breeding season. *Proceedings of the Royal Society, London B* 270:2105–2110.

Roelke-Parker, M. E., L. Munson, C. Packer, R. Kock, S. Cleaveland, M. Carpenter, S. J. O'Brien, A. Popischil, R. Hofmann-Lehmann, H. Lutz, G. L. M. Mwamengele, M. N. Mgasa, G. A. Machamge, B. A. Summers, and M. J. G. Appel. 1996. A canine distemper virus epidemic in Serengeti lions (*Panthera leo*). *Nature* 379:441–445.

Rogers, C. M., and J. M. Smith. 1993. Life-history theory in the nonbreeding period: trade-offs in avian fat reserves. *Ecology* 74:419–426.

Rolland, R. M. 2000. A review of chemically-induced alterations in thyroid and vitamin A status from field studies of wildlife and fish. *Journal of Wildlife Diseases* 36:615–635.

Root, J. J., C. H. Calisher, and B. J. Beaty. 1999. Relationships of deer mouse movement, vegetative structure and prevalence of infection with Sin Nombre virus. *Journal of Wildlife Diseases* 35:311–318.

Rosatte, R. C., D. Donovan, M. Allen, L.-A. Howes, A. Silver, K. Bennet, C. MacInness, C. Davies, A. Wandeler, and B. Radford. 2001. Emergency response to raccoon rabies introduction into Ontario. *Journal of Wildlife Diseases* 37:265–279.

Rosatte, R. C., M. J. Power, C. D. MacInness, and J. D. Campbell. 1992. Trap-vaccinate-release and oral vaccination for rabies control in urban skunks, raccoons and foxes. *Journal of Wildlife Diseases* 28:562–571.

Roscoe, D. E. 1993. Epizootiology of canine distemper in New Jersey raccoons. *Journal of Wildlife Diseases* 29:390–395.

Ross, J. 1982. Myxomatosis: the natural evolution of the disease. *Symposium of the Zoological Society, London* 50:77–95.

Ross, P. S., R. L. de Swart, P. J. H. Reijnders, H. Van Loveren, J. G. Vos, and A. D. M. E. Osterhaus. 1995.

Contaminant-related suppression of delayed-type hypersensitivity and antibody responses in harbour seals fed herring from the Baltic Sea. *Environmental Health Perspectives* 103:162–167.

Rothschild, B. M., L. D. Martin, G. Lav, H. Bercovier, G. K. Bar-Gal, C. Greenblatt, H. Donoghue, M. Spigelman, and D. Brittain. 2001. *Mycobacterium tuberculosis* complex DNA from an extinct bison dated 17,000 years before present. *Clinical Infectious Diseases* 33:305–311.

Rudolph, K. M., D. L. Hunter, W. J. Foreyt, E. F. Cassirer, R. B. Rimler, and A. C. Ward. 2003. Sharing of *Pasteurella* spp. between free-ranging bighorn sheep and feral goats. *Journal of Wildlife Diseases* 39:897–904.

Rupprecht, C. E., K. Stöhr, and C. Meredith. 2001. Rabies. In *Infectious Diseases of Wild Mammals,* 3d ed., edited by E. S. Williams and I. K. Barker, pp 3–36. Ames: Iowa State University Press.

Sacks, B. N., B. B. Chomel, and R. W. Kasten. 2004. Modeling the distribution and abundance of the nonnative parasite, canine heartworm, in California coyotes. *Oikos* 105:415–425.

Sagerup, K., E. O. Henriksen, A. Skorping, J. U. Skaares, and G. W. Gabrielsen. 2000. Intensity of parasitic nematodes increases with organochlorine levels in the glaucous gull. *Journal of Applied Ecology* 37:532–539.

Saino, N., L. Canova, M. Fasola, and R. Martinelli. 2000. Reproduction and population density affect humoral immunity in bank voles under field experimental conditions. *Oecologia* 124:358–366.

Saino, N., S. Calza, and A. P. Møller. 1997. Immunocompetence of nestling barn swallows in relation to brood size and parental effort. *Journal of Animal Ecology* 66:827–836.

Saito, K., N. Kurosawa, and R. Shimura. 2000. Lead poisoning in endangered sea-eagles in eastern Hokkaido through ingestion of shot Sika deer. In *Raptor Biomedicine III,* edited by J. D. Remple, P. T. Redig, M. Lierz, and J. E. Cooper, pp. 163–166. Lake Worth: Zoological Education Network.

Samuel, W. M., and D. A. Welch. 1991. Winter ticks on moose and other ungulates: factors influencing their population size. *Alces* 27:169–182.

Samuel, W. M., M. J. Pybus, and A. A. Kocan. 2001. *Parasitic Diseases of Wild Mammals,* 2d ed. Ames: Iowa State University Press.

Samuel, W. M., M. W. Barrett, and G. M. Lynch. 1976. Helminths in moose in Alberta. *Canadian Journal of Zoology* 54:307–312.

Sanderson, G. C. 2002. Effects of diet and soil on the toxicity of lead in mallards. *Ecotoxicology* 11:11–17.

Sanz, J. J., J. Moreno, E. Arrieroand, and S. Merino. 2002. Reproductive effort and blood parasites of breeding pied flycatchers: the need to control for interannual variation and initial health state. *Oikos* 96:299–306.

Sanz, J. J., J. Moreno, S. Merino, and G. Tomás. 2004. A trade-off between two resource-demanding functions:

post-nuptial moult and immunity during reproduction in male pied flycatchers. *Journal of Animal Ecology* 73:441–447.

Schaechter, M., G. Medoff, and B. I. Eisenstein. 1993. *Mechanisms of Microbial Disease,* 2d ed. Baltimore: Williams & Wilkins.

Schalk, G., and M. R. Forbes. 1997. Male biases in parasitism of mammals: effects of study type, host age, and parasite taxon. *Oikos* 78:67–74.

Schall, J. J. 2002. Parasite virulence. In *The Behavioural Ecology of Parasites,* edited by E.E. Lewis, J. F. Campbell, and M. V. K. Sukhdeo, pp. 283–313. New York: CAB International.

Schantz, P. M., J. Chai, P. S. Craig, J. Eckert, D. J. Jenkins, C. N. L. Macpherson, and A. Thakur. 1995. Epidemiology and control of hydatid disease. In *Echinococcus and Hydatid Disease,* edited by R.C.A. Thompson and A. J. L Lymbery, pp. 232–332. Wallingford: CAB International.

Schlaepfer, M. A., M. C. Runge, and P. W. Sherman. 2002. Ecological and evolutionary traps. *Trends in Ecology and Evolution* 17:471–480.

Schlessinger, D., and M. Schaechter. 1993. Bacterial toxins. In *Mechanisms of Microbial Disease.* 2d ed., edited by M. Schaechter, G. Medoff, and B. I. Eisenstein, pp.162–175. Baltimore: Williams & Wilkins.

Schmidt, R. L., C. P. Hibler, T. R. Spraker, and W. H. Rutherford. 1979. An evaluation of drug treatment for lungworm in bighorn sheep. *Journal of Wildlife Management* 43:461–467.

Schmidt-Posthaus, H., C. Breitenmoser-Würsten, H. Posthaus, L. Bacciarini, and U. Breitenmoser. 2002. Causes of mortality in reintroduced Eurasian lynx in Switzerland. *Journal of Wildlife Diseases* 38:84–92.

Schmitt, S. M., S. D. Fitzgerald, T. M. Cooley, C. S. Bruning-Fann, L. Sullivan, D. Berry, T. Carlson, R. B. Minnis, J. B. Payeur, and J. Sikarskie. 1997. Bovine tuberculosis in free-ranging white-tailed deer from Michigan. *Journal of Wildlife Diseases* 33:749–758.

Scholin, C. A., F. Gulland, G. J. Doucette, S. Benson, M. Busman, F. P. Chavez, J. Cordaro, R. Delong, A. De Vogelaere, J. Harvey, M. Haulena, K. Lefebvre, T. Lipscomb, S. Loscutoff, L. J. Lowenstine, R. Marin, III, P. E. Miller, W. A. Mclellan, P. D. R. Moeller, C. L. Powell, T. Rowells, P. Silvagni, M. Silver, T. Spraker, V. Trainer, and F. M. Van Dolah. 2000. Mortality of sea lions along the central California coast linked to a toxic diatom bloom. *Nature* 403:80–84.

Schultheiss, P. C., J. K. Collins, T. R. Spraker, and J. C. DeMartini. 2000. Epizootic malignant catarrhal fever in three bison herds: differences from cattle and association with ovine herpesvirus-2. *Journal of Veterinary Diagnostic Investigation* 12:497–502.

Scott, M. E. 1988. The impact of infection and disease on animal populations: implications for conservation biology. *Conservation Biology* 2:40–56.

Seip, D. R. 1992. Factors limiting woodland caribou populations and their interrelationships with wolves and moose in southeastern British Columbia. *Canadian Journal of Zoology* 70:1494–1503.

Sellers, R. F. 1980. Weather, host and vector—their interplay in the spread of insect-borne animal virus diseases. *Journal of Hygiene, Cambridge* 85:65–102.

Sellers, R. F., and D. E. Pedgley. 1985. Possible windborne spread to western Turkey of bluetongue virus in 1977 and akibane virus in 1979. *Journal of Hygiene, Cambridge* 95:149–158.

Shaman, J., J. F. Day, and M. Stieglitz. 2002a. Drought-induced amplification of Saint Louis encephalitis virus, Florida. *Emerging Infectious Diseases* 8:575–580.

———. 2002b. St. Louis encephalitis virus in wild birds during the 1990 south Florida epidemic: the importance of drought, wetting conditions, and the emergence of *Culex nigripalpus* (Diptera: Culicidae) to arboviral amplification and transmission. *Journal of Medical Entomology* 40:547–554.

Shaw, D. J., B. T. Grenfell, and A. P. Dobson. 1998. Patterns of macroparasite aggregation in wildlife host populations. *Parasitology* 117:597–610.

Shaw, G. G., and H. W. Reynolds. 1985. Selenium concentrations in forages of a northern herbivore. *Arctic* 38:61–64.

Shaw, J. L., and R. Moss. 1990. Effects of the caecal nematode *Trichostrongylus tenuis* on egg-laying by captive red grouse. *Research in Veterinary Science* 48:253.

Sheldon, B. C., and S. Verhuist. 1996. Ecological imuunity: costly parasite defenses and trade-offs in evolutionary ecology. *Trends in Ecology and Evolution* 11:317–321.

Shepard, T. H. 1998. *Catalog of Teratogenic Agents.* Baltimore: The Johns Hopkins University Press.

Shupe, J. L., A. E. Olson, H. B. Peterson, and J. B. Low. 1984. Fluoride toxicosis in wild ungulates. *Journal of the American Veterinary Medical Association* 185:1295–1300

Sibly, R. M., and P. Calow. 1989. A life-history theory of responses to stress. *Biology Journal of the Linnean Society* 37:101–106.

Sidor, I. F., M. A. Pokras, A. R. Major, R. H. Poppenga, K. M. Taylor, and R. M. Miconi. 2003. Mortality of common loons in New England, 1987–2000. *Journal of Wildlife Diseases* 39:306–315.

Sijtsma, S. R., J. H. W. M. Rombout, C. E. West, and A. J. vander Zijpp. 1990. Vitamin A deficiency impairs cytotoxic T lymphocyte activity in Newcastle disease virus-infected chickens. *Veterinary Immunology and Immunopathology* 26:191–204.

Sileo, L., and S. I. Fefer. 1987. Paint chip poisoning of Laysan albatross at Midway Atoll. *Journal of Wildlife Diseases* 23:432–437.

Sinclair, A. R. E. 1977. *The African Buffalo: A Study of the Resource Limitations of Populations.* Chicago: University of Chicago Press.

Skorping, A., and K. H. Jensen. 2004. Disease dynamics: all caused by males? *Trends in Ecology and Evolution* 19:219–220.

Slater, A. F. G., and A. E. Keymer. 1988. The influence of protein deficiency on immunity to *Heligmosoides polygyrus* (Nematoda) in mice. *Parasite Immunology* 10:507–522.

Slauson, D. O., and B. J. Cooper. 1990. *Mechanisms of Disease. A Textbook of Comparative General Pathology*, 2d ed. St. Louis: Mosby.

———. 2002. *Mechanisms of Disease. A Textbook of Comparative General Pathology.* 3d ed., St. Louis: Mosby.

Slomke, A. M., M. W. Lankester, and W. J. Peterson. 1995. Infrapopulation dynamics of *Parelaphostrongylus tenuis* in white-tailed deer. *Journal of Wildlife Diseases* 31:125–135.

Small, J. D., and B. Newman. 1972. Venereal spirochetosis of rabbits (rabbit syphilis) due to *Treponema cuniculi*: A clinical, serological, and histopathological study. *Laboratory Animal Science* 22:77–89.

Small, P. M., and U. M. Selcer. 2000. Tuberculosis. In *Hunter's Tropical Medicine and Emerging Infectious Diseases.* 8th ed., edited by G. T. Strickland, pp. 491–512. Philadelphia: W.B. Saunders Company.

Smit, T., A. Eger, J. Haagsma, and T. Bakhuizen. 1987. Avian tuberculosis in wild birds in the Netherlands. *Journal of Wildlife Diseases* 23:485–487.

Smith, G. C., and D. Wilkinson. 2003. Modeling control of rabies outbreaks in red fox populations to evaluate culling, vaccination, and vaccination combined with fertility control. *Journal of Wildlife Diseases* 39:278–283.

Smith, J. A., K. Wilson, J. G. Pilkington, and J. M. Pemberton. 1999. Heritable variation in resistance to gastro-intestinal nematodes in an unmanaged mammal population. *Philosophical Transactions of the Royal Society, London B* 339:493–497.

Soler, J. J., L. de Neve, T. Pérez-Contreras, M. Soler, and G. Sorci. 2002. Trade-off between immunocompetence and growth in magpies: an experimental study. *Proceedings of the Royal Society, London B* 270:241–248.

Solter, P. F., and V. R. Beasley. 2002. Phycotoxins. In *Handbook of Toxicologic Pathology*, 2d ed., Vol.1, edited by W. M. Haschek, C. G. Rousseaux and M. A. Wallig, pp. 631–643. San Diego: Academic Press.

Spalding, M. G., G. T. Bancroft, and D. J. Forrester. 1993. The epizootiology of eustrongylidosis in wading birds (Ciconiformes) in Florida. *Journal of Wildlife Diseases* 29:237–249.

Spieker, J. O., T. M. Yuill, and E. C. Burgess. 1996. Virulence of six strains of duck plague virus in eight waterfowl species. *Journal of Wildlife Diseases* 32:453–460.

Spitznagel, J. K. 1993. Constitutive defenses of the body. In *Mechanisms of Microbial Disease,* 2d ed., edited by M. Schaechter, G. Medoff, and B. I. Eisenstein, pp. 90–113. Baltimore: Williams and Wilkins.

Spratt, D. M. 1990. The role of helminths in the biological control of mammals. *International Journal of Parasitology* 20:543–550.

Spurlock, M. E., G. R. Frank, G. M. Willis, J. L. Kuske, and S. G. Cornelius. 1997. Effects of dietary energy source and immunological challenge on growth performance and immunological variables in growing pigs. *Journal of Animal Science* 75:720–726.

Spurrier, M. F., M. S. Boyce, and B. J. F. Manley. 1991. Effects of parasites on mate choice by captive sage grouse. In *Bird Parasite Interactions. Ecology, Evolution and Behaviour*, edited by J. E. Loye and M. Zuk, pp. 389–398. Oxford: Oxford University Press.

Sreevatsan, S., X. Pan, K. E. Stockauer, N. D. Connell, B. K. Kreiswirth, T. S. Whittam, and J. M. Musser. 1997. Restricted structural gene polymorphism in the *Mycobacterium tuberculosis* complex indicates evolutionarily recent global dissemination. *Proceedings of the National Academy of Science of the United States of America* 94:9869–9874.

Sréter, T., Z. Széll, Z. Egyed, and I. Varga. 2003. *Echinococcus multilocularis*: an emerging pathogen in Hungary and Central Eastern Europe? *Emerging Infectious Diseases* 9:384–386.

Stafford, K. C., III, A. J. Denicola, and H. J. Kilpatrick. 2003. Reduced abundance of *Ixodes scapularis* (Acarui: Ixodidae) and the tick parasitoid *Ixodiphagus hookeri* (Hymenoptera: Encyrtidae) with reduction of white-tailed deer. *Journal of Medical Entomology* 40:642–652.

Stallknecht, D. E., and E. Howerth. 2001. Pseudorabies (Aujeszky's Disease). In *Infectious Diseases of Wild Mammals*, 3d ed., edited by E. S. Williams and I. K. Barker, pp. 164–170. Ames: Iowa State University Press

Stallknecht, D. E., M. P. Luttrell, K. E. Smith, and V. F. Nettles. 1996. Hemorrhagic disease in white-tailed deer in Texas: A case for enzootic stability. *Journal of Wildlife Diseases* 32:695–700.

Stead, W. W., K. D. Eisenach, M. D. Cave, M. L. Beggs, G. L. Templeton, C. O. Thoen, and J. H. Bates. 1995. When did *Mycobacterium tuberculosis* infection first occur in the New World? *American Journal of Respiratory and Critical Care Medicine* 151:1267–1268.

Stear, M. J., K. Bairden, S. C. Bishop, G. Gettinby, Q. A. McKellar, M. Park, S. Strain, and D. S. Wallace. 1998. The processes influencing the distribution of parasitic nematodes among naturally infected lambs. *Parasitology* 117:165–171.

Stearns, S. C. 1992. *The Evolution of Life Histories*. Oxford: Oxford University Press.

Steck, F., A. Wandeler, P. Bichsel, S. Capt, U. Hafliger, and L. Schneider. 1982. Oral immunization of foxes against rabies, laboratory and field studies. *Comparative Immunology, Microbiology and Infectious Diseases* 5:165–171.

Stendall, R. C., R. J. Smith, K. P. Burnham, and R. E. Christensen. 1979. *Exposure of Waterfowl to Lead: a Nationwide Survey of Residues in Wingbones of Seven Species 1972–73.*, Washington, D.C.: US Fish and Wildlife Service, Special Scientific Report, Wildlife No. 223.

Stipkovits, L., Z. Varga, G. Czifra, and M. Dubos-Kovacs. 1986. Occurrence of mycoplasmas in geese associated with inflammation of the cloaca and phallus. *Avian Pathology* 15:289–299.

Stolley, D. S., J. A. Bissonette, J. A. Kadlec, and D. Coster. 1999. Effects of saline drinking water on early gosling development. *Journal of Wildlife Management* 63:990–996.

Stuen, S., P. Have, A. D. M. E. Osterhuis, J. M. Arnemo, and A. Moustard. 1994. Serological investigation of virus infection in harp seals (*Phoca groenlandica*) and hooded seals (*Chrystophora cristata*). *Veterinary Record* 134:502–504.

Stutzenbaker, C. D., K. Brown, and D. Lobpries. 1986. Special report: an assessment of the accuracy of documenting waterfowl die-offs in a Texas coastal marsh. In *Lead Poisoning in Wild Waterfowl*, edited by J.S. Feierabend and A.B. Russell, pp. 88–95. Washington, D.C.: National Wildlife Federation.

Suarez, D. L., and S. Schultz-Cherry. 2000. Immunology of avian influenza virus: a review. *Developmental and Comparative Immunology* 24:269–283.

Subak, S. 2002. Analysis of weather effects on variability in Lyme disease incidence in the northeastern United States. *Experimental and Applied Acarology* 28: 249–256.

Susser, M. 1973. *Causal Thinking in the Health Sciences: Concepts and Strategies of Epidemiology*. Oxford: Oxford University Press.

Sutherst, R. W., R. B. Floyd, A. S. Bourne, and M. J. Dallwitz. 1986. Cattle grazing behavior regulates tick populations. *Experientia* 42:194–196.

Swart, R. D., P. S. Ross, L. J. Vedder, H. H. Timmerman, S. Heisterkamp, H. Loveren, J. G. van Vos, P. J. H. Reijnders, A. D. M. E. Osterhaus, R. L. De Swart, and H. van Loveren. 1994. Impairment of immune function in harbor seals (*Phoca vitulina*) feeding on fish from polluted waters. *AMBIO* 23:155–159.

Swinton, J., D. MacDonald, D. J. Nokes, C.L. Cheeseman, and R. S. Clifton-Hadley. 1997. Comparison of fertility control and lethal control of bovine tuberculosis in badgers—the impact of perturbation induced transmission. *Philosophical Transactions of the Royal Society, London B* 352:619–631.

Swinton, J., M. E. J. Woolhouse, M. E. Begon, A. P. Dobson, E. Ferroglio, B. T. Grenfell, V. Guberti, R. S. Hails, J. A. P. Heesterbeek, A. Lavazza, M. C. Roberts, P. J. White, and K. Wilson. 2001. Microparasite transmission and persistence. In *The Ecology of Wildlife Diseases,* edited by P. J. Hudson, A. Rizzoli, B. T. Grenfell, H. Heesterbeek, and A. P. Dobson, pp. 83–101. Oxford: Oxford University Press.

Szaro, R. C. 1977. Effects of petroleum on birds. *Transactions of the North American Wildlife and Natural Resources Conference* 42:374–381.

Telfer, S., M. Bennett, K. Bown, R. Cavanagh, L. Crespin, S. Hazel, T. Jones, and M. Begon. 2002. The effects of cowpox virus on survival in natural rodent populations:

increases and decreases. *Journal of Animal Ecology* 71:558–568.

Temple, S. E. 1987. Do predators always capture substandard individuals disproportionately from prey populations? *Ecology* 68:669–674.

Tessaro, S. V., L. B. Forbes, and C. Turcotte. 1990. A survey of brucellosis and tuberculosis in bison in and around Wood Buffalo National Park, Canada. *Canadian Veterinary Journal* 31:174–180.

Thing, H., and B. Clausen. 1980. Summer mortality among caribou calves in Greenland. *Proceedings of the 2d International Reindeer/Caribou Symposium*, 434–437.

Thomas, F., and R. Poulin. 1998. Manipulation of a mollusc by a trophically transmitted parasite: convergent evolution or phylogenetic inheritance? *Parasitology* 116:431–436.

Thomas, N. J., C. U. Meteyer, and L. Sileo. 1998. Epizootic vacuolar myelinopathy of the central nervous system of bald eagles (*Haliaeetus leucocephalus*) and American coots (*Fulica americana*). *Veterinary Pathology* 35:479–485.

Thomas, R. E., A. M. Barnes, T. J. Quan, M. L. Beard, L. G. Carter, and C. E. Hopla. 1988. Susceptibility to *Yersinia pestis* in the northern grasshopper mouse (*Onchomys leucogaster*). *Journal of Wildlife Diseases* 24:327–333.

Thomson, G. R., R. G. Bengis, and C. C. Brown. 2001. Picornavirus infections. In *Infectious Diseases of Wild Mammals*, 3d ed., edited by E. S. Williams and I. K. Barker, pp. 119–130. Ames: Iowa State University Press.

Thompson, R. C. A., and J. Eckert. 1983. Observations on *Echinococcus multilocularis* in the definitive host. *Zeitschrift für Parasitenkunde* 69:335–345.

Thorne, E. T. 2001. Brucellosis. In *Infectious Diseases of Wild Mammals*, 3d ed., edited by E. S. Williams and I. K. Barker, pp. 372–395. Ames: Iowa State University Press.

Thorne, E. T., N. Kingston, W. R. Jolly, and R. C. Bergstrom. 1982. *Diseases of Wildlife in Wyoming*. 2d ed. Cheyenne: Wyoming Game and Fish Department.

Thrusfield, M. 1986. *Veterinary Epidemiology*. London: Butterworths.

Tilgar, V., R. Mänd, and A. Leivits. 1999. Effect of calcium availability and habitat quality on reproduction in pied flycatcher *Ficedula hypoleuca* and great tit *Parus major*. *Journal of Avian Biology* 30:383–391.

Tilgar, V., R. Mänd, and M. Mägi. 2002. Calcium shortage as a constraint on reproduction in great tits *Parus major*: a field experiment. *Journal of Avian Biology* 33:407–413.

Tizard, I. R. 2000. *Veterinary Immunology. An Introduction*. 6th ed. Philadelphia: W. B. Saunders Company.

Toma, B., B. Dufour, M. Eloit, F. Moutou, W. Marsh, J.J. Bénet, M. Sanaa, A. Louzã, and P. Michel. 1999a. *Dictionary of Veterinary Epidemiology*. Ames: Iowa State University Press.

Toma, B., B. Dufour, M. Sanaa, J. J. Bénet, F. Moutou, A. Louzã, and P. Ellis. 1999b. *Applied Veterinary Epidemiology and the Control of Disease in Populations*. Maisons-Alfort: AEEMA.

Tompkins, D. M., A. P. Dobson, P. Arneberg, M. E. Begon, I. M. Cattadori, J. V. Greenman, J. A. P. Heesterbeek, P. J. Hudson, , D. Newborn, A. Pugliese, A. P. Rizzoli, R. Rosà, F. Rosso, and K. Wilson. 2001a. Parasites and host population dynamics. In *The Ecology Of Wildlife Diseases*, edited by P. J. Hudson, A. P. Russoli, B. T. Grenfell, H. Heesterbeek, and A. P. Dobson, pp. 45–62. Oxford: Oxford University Press.

Tompkins, D. M., and M. Begon. 2000. Parasites can regulate wildlife populations. *Parasitology Today* 15:311–313.

Tompkins, D. M., D. M. B. Parrish, and P. J. Hudson. 2002. Parasite-mediated competition among red-legged partridges and other lowland gamebirds. *Journal of Wildlife Management* 66:445–450.

Tompkins, D. M., J. V. Greenman, P. A. Robertson, and P. J. Hudson. 2000. The role of shared parasites in the exclusion of wildlife hosts: *Heterakis gallinarum* in the ring-necked pheasant and the grey partridge. *Journal of Animal Ecology* 69:829–840.

Tompkins, D. M., J. V. Greenman, and P. J. Hudson. 2001b. Differential impact of a shared nematode parasite on two gamebird hosts: implications for apparent competition. *Parasitology* 122:187–193.

Torchin, M. E., K. D. Lafferty, and A. M. Kuris. 2002. Release from parasites as natural enemies: increased performance of globally introduced marine crab. *Biological Invasions* 3:333–345.

Torgerson, P.R., and C.M. Budke. 2003. Echinococcosis—an international public health challenge. *Research in Veterinary Science* 74:191–202.

Toth, T. E. 2000. Nonspecific cellular defense of the avian respiratory system: a review. *Developmental and Comparative Immunology* 24:121–139.

Tottin, S. C., R. R. Tinline, R. C. Rosatte, and L. L. Bigler. 2002. Contact rates of raccoons (*Procyon lotor*) at a communal feeding site in rural eastern Ontario. *Journal of Wildlife Diseases* 38:313–319.

Trudeau, K. M., H. B. Britten, and M. Restani. 2004. Sylvatic plague reduces genetic variability in black-tailed prairie dogs. *Journal of Wildlife Diseases* 40:205–211.

Tsai, T. F. 1987. Hemorrhagic fever with renal syndrome: mode of transmission to humans. *Laboratory Animal Science* 37:428–430.

Tschirren, B., P. S. Fitze, and H. Richner. 2003. Sexual dimorphism in susceptibility to parasites and cell-mediated immunity in great tit nestlings. *Journal of Animal Ecology* 72:839–845.

Turner, J. C., C. L. Douglas, C. R. Hallum, P. R. Krausman, and R. R. Ramey. 2004. Determination of critical habitat for the endangered Nelson's bighorn sheep in southern California. *Wildlife Society Bulletin* 32:427–448.

Twigg, L. E., T. J. Lowe, G. R. Martin, A. G. Wheeler, G. S. Gray, S. L. Griffin, C. M. O'Reilly, D. J. Robinson, and P. H. Hubach. 2000. Effects of surgically imposed sterility on free-ranging rabbit populations. *Journal of Animal Ecology* 37:16–39.

Urquhart, G. M., J. Armour, J. L. Duncan, A. M. Dunn, and F. W. Jennings. 1996. *Veterinary Parasitology.*, 2d ed. Oxford: Blackwell Science.

Van Campen, H., K. Frölich, and M. Hofmann. 2001. Pestivirus infections. In *Infectious Diseases of Wild Mammals*, 3d ed., edited by E. S. Williams and I. K. Barker, pp. 232–244. Ames: Iowa State University Press.

Van Pelt, R. W., and M. T. Caley. 1974. Nutritional secondary hyperparathyroidism in Alaskan red fox kits. *Journal of Wildlife Diseases* 10:47–52.

van Regenmortel, M. H. V., and B. W. J. Mahy. 2004. Emerging issues in virus taxonomy. *Emerging Infectious Diseases* 10:8–13.

van Riper, C., III, S. G. van Riper, M. L. Goff, and M. Laird. 1986. The epizootiology and ecological significance of malaria in Hawaiian landbirds. *Ecological Monographs* 56:327–344.

Villafuerte, R., C. Calvete, C. Gortzar, and S. Moreno. 1994. First epizootic of rabbit hemorrhagic disease in free living populations of *Oryctolagus cuniculus* at Doñana National Park, Spain. *Journal of Wildlife Diseases* 30:176–179.

Vŏrišek, P., J. Votýpka, K. Zvara, and M. Svobodová. 1998. Heteroxenous coccidia increase the predation risk for parasitized rodents. *Parasitology* 117:521–524

Wakelin, D. 1994. Host populations: genetics and immunity. In *Parasitic and Infectious Diseases*, edited by M. E. Scott and G. Smith, pp. 83–100. San Diego: Academic Press.

Walker, C. H. 2003. Neurotoxic pesticides and behavioural effects upon birds. *Ecotoxicology* 12:307–316.

Walter, H., F. Consolaro, P. Gramatica, M. Scholze, and R. Altenburger. 2002. Mixture toxicity of priority pollutants at no observed effect concentrations (NOECs). *Ecotoxicology* 11:299–310.

Wandeler, A., G. Wachendörfer, U. Förster, H. Krekel, U. Schale, J. Müller, and F. Steck. 1974. Rabies in wild carnivores in central Europe: I. Epidemiological studies. *Zentralblatt Veterinärmedizin Reihe B* 21:735–756.

Wanntorp., H., K. Borg, E. Hanko, and K. Erne. 1967. Mercury residues in wood pigeons (*Columbo p. palumbra* L.) in 1964 and 1966. *Nordsk Veterinaertidsskrift* 19:474– 477.

Warren, Y. 1994. *Protocalliphora braueri* (Diptera: Calliphoridae) induced pathogenesis in a brood of marsh wren (*Cistotothorus palustris*) young. *Journal of Wildlife Diseases* 30:107–109.

Webb, R. E., and F. Horsfall. 1967. Endrin resistance in the pine mouse. *Science* 156:1762.

Webster, J. P., C. F. A. Brunton, and D. W. MacDonald. 1994. Effect of *Toxoplasma gondii* upon neophobic behaviour in wild brown rats (*Rattus norvegicus*). *Parasitology* 109:37–43.

Webster, R. G., W. J. Bean, O. T. Gorman, T. M. Chambers, and Y. Kawaoka. 1992. Evolution and ecology of influenza A viruses. *Microbiology Reviews* 56:152–179.

Wegner, K. M., M. Kalbe, J. Kurtz, T. B. H. Reusch, and M. Milinski. 2003. Parasite selection for immunogentic optimality. *Science* 301:1343.

Wells, J. V., and M. E. Richmond. 1995. Populations, metapopulations, and species populations: what are they and who should care? *Wildlife Society Bulletin* 23:456–462.

Welshons, W. V., K. A. Thayer, B. M. Judy, J. A. Taylor, E. M. Curran, and F. S. vom Saal. 2003. Large effects from small exposures. I. Mechanisms for endocrine-disrupting chemicals with estrogenic activity. *Environmental Health Perspectives* 111:994–1006.

Wendelaar Bonga, S. E. 1997. The stress response in fish. *Physiologic Reviews* 77:591–625.

Westbury, H. A. 2000. Hendra virus disease in horses. *Revue Scientifique et Technique OIE* 19:151–159.

Whitaker, S., and J. Fair. 2002. The costs of immunological challenge to developing mountain chickadees, *Poecile gambeli*, in the wild. *Oikos* 99:161–165.

White, P. J., R. A. Norman, R. C. Trout, E. A. Gould, and P. J. Hudson. 2001. The emergence of rabbit haemorrhagic disease virus: will a non-pathogenic strain protect the UK? *Philosophical Transactions of the Royal Society, London B* 356:1087–1095.

Whittington, R. 2001. Chlamydiosis of koalas. In *Infectious Diseases of Wild Mammals*, 3d ed., edited by E. S. Williams and I. K. Barker, pp 423–434. Ames: Iowa State University Press.

WHO. 2001. *Nipah virus fact sheet.* WHO/OMS Fact Sheet No. 262, September 2001.

Wild, M. A., and M. W. Miller. 1991. Detecting non-hemolytic *Pasteurella haemolytica* infections in healthy Rocky Mountain bighorn sheep (*Ovis canadensis canadensis*): influences of sample site and handling. *Journal of Wildlife Diseases* 27:53–60.

Williams, E. S. 2001. Canine distemper. In *Infectious Diseases of Wild Mammals*, 3d ed., edited by E. S. Williams and I. K. Barker, pp. 50–58. Ames: Iowa State University Press.

Williams, E. S., and I. K. Barker. 2001. *Infectious Diseases of Wild Mammals*, 3d ed. Ames: Iowa State University Press.

Williams, E. S., E. T. Thorne, M. J. G. Appel, and D. W. Belitsky. 1988. Canine distemper in black-footed ferrets (*Mustela nigripes*) from Wyoming. *Journal of Wildlife Diseases* 24:385–398.

Williams, E. S., J. S. Kirkwood, and M. W. Miller. 2001. Transmissible spongiform encephalopathies. In *Infectious Diseases of Wild Mammals*. 3d ed., edited by E. S. Williams and I.K. Barker, pp. 292–301. Ames: Iowa State University Press.

Williams, T. M., J. McBain, R. K. Wilson, and R. W. Davis. 1990. Clinical evaluation and cleaning of sea otters affected by the T/V Exxon Valdez oil spill. In *Sea*

Otter Symposium: Proceedings of a Symposium to Evaluate the Response Effort on Behalf of Sea Otters after the T/V Exxon Valdez Oil Spill into Prince William Sound, Anchorage, Alaska, edited by K. Bayha and J. Kormendy. Washington, D.C.: United States Fish and Wildlife Service Biological Report 90(12).

Wilson, K., O. N. Bjørnstad, A. P. Dobson, S. Merler, G. Poglayen, S. E. Randolph, A. F. Read, and A. Skorping. 2001. Heterogeneities in macroparsite infections: patterns and process. In *The Ecology of Wildlife Diseases*, edited by P. J. Hudson, A. Rizzoli, B. T. Grenfell, H. Heesterbeek, and A. P. Dobson, pp. 6–44. Oxford: Oxford University Press.

Windingstad, R. M., F. X. Kartch, R. K. Stroud, and M. R. Smith. 1987. Salt toxicosis in waterfowl in North Dakota. *Journal of Wildlife Diseases* 23:443–446.

Windingstad, R. M., R. J. Cole, P. E. Nelson, T. J. Roffe, R. R. George, and J. W. Dorner. 1989. Fusarium mycotoxins from peanuts suspected as a cause of sandhill crane mortality. *Journal of Wildlife Diseases* 25:38–46.

Wingfield, J. C., and L. M. Romero. 2001. Adrenocortical responses to stress and their modulation in free-living vertebrates. In *Handbook of Physiology. Section 7: The endocrine System. Volume IV: Coping with the Environment: Neural and Endocrine Mechanisms*, edited by B. S. McEwen and H. M. Goodman, pp. 211–234. New York: Oxford University Press.

Wingfield, J. C., K. Hunt, C. Breuner, K. Dunlap, G. S. Fowler, L. Freed, and J. Lepson. 1997. Environmental stress, field technology, and conservation biology. In *Behavioral Approaches to Conservation in the Wild*, edited by J. R. Clemmons and R. Buchholz, pp. 95–131. Cambridge: Cambridge University Press.

Wingfield, J. C., K. M. O'Reilly, and L. B. Astheimer. 1995. Modulation of the adrenocortical responses to acute stress in arctic birds: A possible ecological basis. *American Zoologist* 35:285–294.

Winn, D. S. 1973. *Effects of Sublethal Levels of Dieldrin on Mallard Breeding Behaviour and Reproduction*. M.Sc. Thesis, Utah State University, Logan.

Wobeser, G. 1992. Avian cholera and waterfowl biology. *Journal of Wildlife Diseases* 28:674–682.

———. 2001. Tyzzer's disease. In *Infectious Diseases of Wild Mammals*, 3d ed., edited by E. S. Williams and I. K. Barker, pp.510–513. Ames: Iowa State University Press.

———. 2002. Disease management strategies for wildlife. *Revue Scientifique et Technique OIE* 21:159–178.

Wobeser, G., and A. G. Wobeser. 1992. Carcass disappearance and estimation of mortality in a simulated die-off of small birds. *Journal of Wildlife Diseases* 28:548–564.

Wobeser, G., and C. J. Brand. 1982. Chlamydiosis in 2 biologist investigating disease occurrences in wild waterfowl. *Wildlife Society Bulletin* 10:170–172.

Wobeser, G., and D. J. Rainnie. 1987. Epizootic necrotizing enteritis in wild geese. *Journal of Wildlife Diseases* 23:376–385.

Wobeser, G., and E. A. Galmut. 1984. Internal temperature of decomposing duck carcasses in relation to botulism. *Journal of Wildlife Diseases* 20:267–271.

Wobeser, G., and J. Howard. 1987. Mortality of waterfowl on a hypersaline wetland as a result of salt encrustation. *Journal of Wildlife Diseases* 23:127–134.

Wobeser, G., and M. Swift. 1976. Mercury poisoning in a wild mink. *Journal of Wildlife Diseases* 12:335–340.

Wobeser, G., and W. Kost. 1992. Starvation, staphylococcosis, and vitamin A deficiency among mallards overwintering in Saskatchewan. *Journal of Wildlife Diseases* 28:215–222.

Wobeser, G., and W. Runge. 1975. Rumen overload and rumenitis in white-tailed deer. *Journal of Wildlife Management* 39:596–600.

Wobeser, G., D. B. Hunter, and P.-Y. Daoust. 1978. Tyzzer's disease in muskrats: occurrence in free-living animals. *Journal of Wildlife Diseases* 14: 325–328.

Wobeser, G., H. J. Barnes, and K. Pierce. 1979. Tyzzer's disease in muskrats: re-examination of specimens of hemorrhagic disease collected by Paul Errington. *Journal of Wildlife Diseases* 15:525–527.

Wobeser, G., R. J. Cawthorn, and A. A. Gajadhar. 1983. Pathology of *Sarcocystis campestris* infection in Richardson's ground squirrels (*Spermophilus richardsoni*). *Canadian Journal of Comparative Medicine* 47:198–202.

Wobeser, G., T. Bollinger, F. A. Leighton, B. Blakley, and P. Mineau. 2004. Secondary poisoning of eagles following intentional poisoning of coyotes with anticholinesterase pesticides in western Canada. *Journal of Wildlife Diseases* 40:163–172.

Wobeser, G. A. 1981. *Diseases of Wild Waterfowl*. New York: Plenum Press.

———. 1994. *Investigation and Management of Disease in Wild Animals*. New York: Plenum Press.

———. 1997. *Diseases of Wild Waterfowl*, 2d ed. New York: Plenum Press.

Wobeser, G. A., and M. C. Finlayson. 1969. *Salmonella typhimurium* infection in house sparrows. *Archives of Environmental Health* 19:882–884.

Wolfe L. L., M. W. Miller, and E. S. Williams. 2004. Feasibility of "test-and-cull" for managing chronic wasting disease in urban mule deer. *Wildlife Society Bulletin* 32:500–505.

Woods, R. E., and A. A. Hoffmann. 2000. Evolution in toxic environments: quantitative versus major gene approaches. In *Demography in Ecotoxicology*, edited by J. Kammenga and R. Laskowski, pp. 129–145. Chichester: John Wiley & Sons Ltd.

Woolf, A., D. R. Shoemaker, and M. Cooper. 1993. Evidence of tularemia regulating a semi-isolated cottontail rabbit population. *Journal of Wildlife Management* 57:144–157.

Worley, D. E., C. K. Anderson, and K. R. Greer. 1972. Elaeophorosis in moose from Montana. *Journal of Wildlife Diseases* 8:242–244.

Worley, M. 2001. Retrovirus infections. In *Infectious Diseases of Wild Mammals,* 3d ed., edited by E. S. Williams and I. K. Barker, pp. 213–222. Ames: Iowa State University Press.

Yaremych, S. A., R. E. Warner, P. C. Mankin, J. D. Brawn, A. Raim, and R. Novak. 2004. West Nile virus and high death rate in American crows. *Emerging Infectious Diseases* 10:709–711.

Yekutiel, P. 1980. *Eradication of Infectious Diseases: A Critical Study, Contributions to Epidemiology and Biostatistics.*, Vol. 2. Basel: S. Karger.

Young, S., and R. F. Slocombe. 2003. Prion-associated spongiform encephalopathy in an imported Asian golden cat (*Catopuma temmincki*). *Australian Veterinary Journal* 81:295–296.

Ytrehus, B., H. Skagemo, G. Syuve, T. Sivertsen, K. Handeland, and T. Vikøren. 1999. Osteoporosis, bone mineralization, and status of selected trace elements in two populations of moose calves in Norway. *Journal of Wildlife Diseases* 35:204–211.

Yuill, T. M. 1987. Diseases as components of mammalian ecosystems: mayhem and subtlety. *Canadian Journal of Zoology* 65:1061–1066.

Yuill, T. M., and C. Seymour. 2001. Arboviral infections. In *Infectious Diseases of Wild Mammals*. 3d ed., edited by E. S. Williams and I. K. Barker, pp. 98–118. Ames: Iowa State University Press.

Ziegler, H. K. 1993. Induced defenses of the body. In *Mechanisms of Microbial Disease*, 2d ed., edited by M. Schaechter, G. Medoff, and B. I. Eisenstein, pp. 114–153. Baltimore: Williams and Wilkins.

Zinkl, J. G., J. M. Hyland, and J. J. Hurt. 1977a. Aspergiloosis in common crows in Nebraska, 1974. *Journal of Wildlife Diseases* 13:191–193.

Zinkl, J. G., J. M. Hyland, J. J. Hurt, and K. I. Heddleston. 1977b. An epornitic of avian cholera in waterfowl and common crows in Phelps County, Nebraska, in the spring 1975. *Journal of Wildlife Diseases* 13:194–198.

Zuk, M., and A. M. Stoehr. 2002. Immune defense and host life history. *American Naturalist* 160:S9–S22.

Zúñiga, M. C. 2002. A pox on thee! Manipulation of the host immune system by myxoma virus and implications for viral-host co-adaptation. *Virus Research* 88:17–33.

Index